Work, Worklessness, and the Political Economy of Health

Work, Worklessness, and the Political Economy of Health

Clare Bambra

Professor of Public Health Policy,
Department of Geography, Wolfson Research Institute,
Durham University, UK

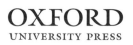

OXFORD
UNIVERSITY PRESS

OXFORD

UNIVERSITY PRESS

Great Clarendon Street, Oxford ox2 6DP

Oxford University Press is a department of the University of Oxford.
It furthers the University's objective of excellence in research, scholarship,
and education by publishing worldwide in

Oxford New York

Auckland Cape Town Dar es Salaam Hong Kong Karachi
Kuala Lumpur Madrid Melbourne Mexico City Nairobi
New Delhi Shanghai Taipei Toronto

With offices in

Argentina Austria Brazil Chile Czech Republic France Greece
Guatemala Hungary Italy Japan Poland Portugal Singapore
South Korea Switzerland Thailand Turkey Ukraine Vietnam

Oxford is a registered trade mark of Oxford University Press
in the UK and in certain other countries

Published in the United States
by Oxford University Press Inc., New York

British Library Cataloguing in Publication Data
Data available

Library of Congress Cataloging in Publication Data
Data available

Typeset in Minion by Cenveo, Bangalore, India
Printed and bound by
CPI Group (UK) Ltd, Croydon, CR0 4YY

ISBN 978–0–19–958829–9

10 9 8 7 6 5 4 3 2 1

Whilst every effort has been made to ensure that the contents of this book are as complete,
accurate and up-to-date as possible at the date of writing, Oxford University Press is not able
to give any guarantee or assurance that such is the case. Readers are urged to take appropriately
qualified medical advice in all cases. The information in this book is intended to be useful to
the general reader, but should not be used as a means of self-diagnosis or for the prescription
of medication.

For Frances

Foreword

A characteristic of our times, in both developed and developing countries, has been the growth of social inequalities, including health inequalities. These inequalities have been even more accentuated in the current economic and financial crises. As a consequence, we have seen a spectacular increase in the scientific literature of studies analyzing the growth of health inequalities and the reasons for that growth.

For the most part, these studies have analyzed inequalities in populations according to status, income, gender, race, education, place of residence, and other attributes considered important to an understanding of inequalities. These studies have been very useful and informative, and their contribution to revealing the extent of such inequalities has been substantial.

Within this extensive bibliography, the focus on the causes of the existence and growth of health inequalities varies, but a dimension that has taken up considerable space in this literature is the analysis of collective and individual behaviours. And most preventive and public health measures have focused on interventions to change these behaviours. Here again, the studies have been useful and relevant, but remarkably insufficient, as has the larger bibliography on status and the other attributes mentioned above.

The reason for the limitations and insufficiencies of these studies is their use of a conceptual frame that focuses on status and categories related to consumption (behavioural patterns such as smoking, diet, physical exercise) rather than on production and work to explain health and quality of life. The limited (at least until recently) scholarship focusing on work and relations of production, which are the most important variables in explaining the health and quality of life of populations, is quite remarkable.

This limited interest within academia contrasts with the full awareness among the population in every country that work is of enormous importance in determining their lives. When, on the street level, one person meets another, the most frequently asked question in getting to know one another is 'What do you do?'—meaning, what type of work do you do?—because when we know someone's occupation, we immediately know the likely income that individual has, the type of housing and neighborhood he or she lives in, his or her cultural tastes, and a long list of other important facts (including health). In other words, in our societies, for the majority of the population, what you have (income, status, housing, etc.) depends on what you do, not the other way around.

In spite of this reality, work and work conditions, as a cause of health and inequalities, have been remarkably underdeveloped in the medical literature. An indicator of this is that even today, few practitioners of medicine include, in taking their patients' medical histories, questions related to work life, even though we know that the type of work people have done throughout their lives is the most important variable in explaining longevity among people ready to retire. Work and type of work are indeed the most important variables in explaining the health and quality of life of our populations.

It is a most important indictment of our societies that work, for most people, is a mere instrument to get the resources they need to realize themselves through the world of consumption. It is consumption and status that are supposed to be important. A decent and humane society, however, is one in which work helps develop the enormous potential for creativity and enjoyment that every human being has. There is an urgent need to change the focus of public health research from status and consumption to work and production. And this volume, *Work, Worklessness and the Political Economy of Health*, by Clare Bambra, is an important step in that direction.

But work is also important because it is the link between the individual and the society in which he or she lives. His or her place in society is primarily determined by the place he or she occupies in the production and distribution of goods and services. The relations of production are the critical relations for understanding our societies and how power is exercised within their institutions, including their political institutions. The type, nature, and purpose of work depend very much on the power relations derived from the articulation of individuals within the relations of production—that is, the class structure. It is this class structure and the individual's position within it that determine his or her health. In the US, a steel worker makes much more money than a teacher, yet the teacher has a longer life expectancy than the steel worker. It is not income but class that determines health. In Glasgow, Scotland, an unskilled working class person has a life expectancy 28 years shorter than that of a businessman. And in east Baltimore in the US, an unemployed young worker has a life expectancy 32 years shorter than that of a corporate lawyer. These mortality differentials depend on the power relation derived primarily from the class structure and class relations. Mortality differentials are larger in societies where the owners of capital have more power than labourers than in societies where labourers have more power. The poor health indicators of the US are based on the enormous power of the dominant class (known popularly as the corporate class). One area where class power appears is at the level of the state. As many researchers have shown, the type of welfare state (including the health services) depends on the power relations in our societies, particularly class power relations, those derived from the relations of production. The literature on welfare state regimes proves this to be so, and Clare Bambra's work here is a significant expansion of this topic.

Needless to say, other characteristics besides class, such as race and gender, also play an important role in determining health. But for too long, the importance of class has been dismissed. This volume is a welcome reminder that class and work continue to be of paramount importance. I strongly recommend this volume as a way of stimulating a change of direction in the literature on the determinants of health and health inequalities, recognizing the value of work and the relations of power within and outside work in configuring the health of our populations.

Vicente Navarro
Professor of Health and Public Policy
The Johns Hopkins University & Professor of Public Policy
Pompeu Fabra University

Preface

'. . . and at least I know this, that if a man is overworked in
any degree he cannot enjoy the sort of health I am speaking of;
nor can he if he is continually chained to one dull round of
mechanical work, with no hope at the other end of it; nor if he
lives in continual sordid anxiety for his livelihood'.

William Morris (1884)

Work is the most important determinant of population health and health inequalities in advanced market democracies. Work, and the socio-economic class
polarities it creates, are the key organisational features of modern societies.
Work is the main source of income, via wages and salaries, for most of the
population and it thus mediates other life chances and exposures to the wider
social determinants of health. Work, both paid and unpaid, dominates adult
life, and even much of modern childhood is spent as preparation for it. Work is
a salient part of self-definition. It is often the basis of citizenship and social
rights. At both the micro (e.g. work environment, unemployment) and macro
levels (e.g. welfare state regulation and labour market structures), therefore, it
plays a fundamental role in determining the prevalence and distribution of
morbidity and mortality. This can be directly, via industrial accidents, or indirectly, as in the increased risk of death from coronary heart disease as a result of
psychosocial work related stress. Exposures to physical hazards and psychosocial risks in the workplace, as well as the distribution of shift work and irregular
working arrangements are all socially distributed with a higher prevalence
amongst the least educated. This is also the case with respect to exclusion from
the labour market and the absence of paid work—worklessness—which is also
negatively associated with health and contributes to health inequalities.
In this book, I examine the relationships between work, worklessness and
health within the broader welfare state context in which they are situated: a
political economy of work, worklessness and health is set out.

The book has two central themes: that paid work, or lack of it, is the most
important determinant of population health and health inequalities in
advanced market democracies; and that this is a result of the role that work
plays within the wider political economy of health. These two themes are
examined in various ways across the following eight chapters:

- ◆ *Chapter 1—Introduction* This introductory chapter examines the key concepts of work and worklessness within the broader framework of social and

political organisation. It also provides an empirical and theoretical over-view of health inequalities and it outlines the social determinants of health.

- *Chapter 2—Welfare state capitalism and health* This chapter examines the wider welfare state and labour market contexts in which the relation-ships between work, worklessness and health are experienced. It outlines the different types of welfare state, and the development of welfare states especially in relation to economic and employment changes. It also examines international differences in health and health inequalities.

- *Chapter 3—Health hazards in the physical work environment* In this chapter, the health effects of three material dimensions of the physical work environment are examined: chemical hazards; environmental factors; and ergonomic hazards. The continuing importance of the physical work envi-ronment with regard to health inequalities is also examined and differences by welfare state are explored.

- *Chapter 4—The psychosocial work environment and risks to health* This chapter outlines the key theories and debates in the field of psychosocial health in relation to the work environment. Evidence on the health effects of the demand-control-support model, the effort-reward imbalance model and the organisational justice approach are summarised. The contribution of the psychosocial work environment to socio-economic health inequali-ties is also examined. Differences by welfare state are examined.

- *Chapter 5—Recession, unemployment, and health* This chapter initially examines the health effects of economic recessions before exploring the longstanding negative relationship between unemployment and health, specifically examining issues of causality and the importance of the wider welfare state context. The contribution of unemployment to health inequalities is also examined.

- *Chapter 6—Health related worklessness* This chapter explores the compli-cated relationship between ill health, sickness absence and unemployment. Social policy debates as well as the politics of health and worklessness are examined. The chapter also examines variation by welfare state regime as well as inequalities in ill health related worklessness.

- *Chapter 7—Work, health, and welfare interventions* This chapter presents evidence on the effectiveness of interventions which are intended to change the experience of work and worklessness. It provides examples of how to create healthier work environments, healthier experiences of worklessness, and a healthy return to work, within the constraints of unequal societies.

◆ *Chapter 8—Conclusion* This concluding chapter summarises the previous chapters, and then presents a model of the political economy of health inequalities. This is used to show how different types of public policy interventions can mitigate health inequalities. The model is applied to the case of work and worklessness. The chapter concludes by arguing that politics matter in the aetiology of health inequalities.

These chapters each examine a different aspect of the role of work and worklessness in the political economy of health and health inequalities. However, they all explore variations by time, by place and by socio-economic class and how these relate to international variations in the role of the welfare state in the regulation of work and the labour market.

My book is aimed primarily at advanced level undergraduate and postgraduate students and researchers in health policy, medical geography, public health, epidemiology and occupational health. It will also be of interest to those studying medical sociology, health management, and social policy as well as medical and health practitioners with an interest in the wider determinants of health.

Acknowledgements

This book originated in lecture courses given over a number of years at Durham University, UK. Special thanks are owed to Kerry Joyce who contributed material to Chapters 3 and 4 and without whose input the book would not have been completed in a timely manner. Thanks also to Kayleigh Garthwaite and Jon Warren who contributed material to Chapter 6. I would also like to thank Sharon Gollan for creating the front cover. I am also grateful to the following: Danielle Moore and Susan Easton who conducted literature searches and provided research notes for Chapter 5; Jack Briggs for formatting the references and helping with data entry; Jennifer Cook for general administrative assistance; and Chris Orton for helping to format the figures and tables. I would like to thank the following for permission to reproduce copyrighted material: *British Medical Journal, Critical Public Health, European Journal of Public Health, Health and Place, Health Policy, Health Promotion International, Humanity and Society, International Journal of Health Services, Journal of Epidemiology and Community Health, Population, Space and Place.* I am also indebted to Dr Alex Scott-Samuel and members of the UK Politics of Health group who encouraged me to apply a political economy perspective to the study of population health. Finally, thanks are also due to my friends and family who supported me through the shingles I suffered whilst writing the book.

Contents

List of figures

List of tables

List of boxes

Chapter 1

Introduction

In this introductory chapter, I show how work and worklessness are not the discrete activities of individuals but essential parts of the way in which the totality of society is organised politically, socially and economically. Work based hierarchies are reflected to greater or lesser extents in wider societal hierarchies, and socio-economic class is determined largely by occupation and work related income. Work and worklessness and their relationships with health and health inequalities therefore exist within the broader political and economic structures of society. The chapter is divided into three main sections: the first examines the key concepts of work and worklessness, focusing on their relationship with the state in advanced market democracies; the second section provides an overview of the social determinants of health and health inequalities; the final part of the chapter reflects on matters of structure and agency in explaining the relationship between work, worklessness and health.

1.1 **Work, worklessness, and the state**

The state is active in constituting work and working conditions, as well as influencing the level of worklessness and the extent to which a certain standard of living can be maintained regardless of labour market performance (decommodification). Definitions of the state vary, although perhaps the most widely used is the pluralist theory of the state as simply the institutions of central and local government, the police, the army, and the civil service. In this view, the state is considered to be neutral and independent above party political disputes or the conflicts of economic interests. Political power is thus dispersed amongst a wide variety of social groups which compete with one another for dominance and control of independent state institutions. On the other hand, political economists broaden the parameters of the state to include many aspects of civil society including schools, the health care system, the professions (such as medicine) and the media (Althusser, 1971). Certainly, the emergence of the welfare state enlarged the size and responsibilities of the state. In this way, the state is seen as being primarily concerned with the maintenance of capitalism and capitalist social relations with the economic interests of capital dominating those of labour. Alongside capital, work (in the form of wage labour) is a vital element of the capitalist economy. The state is therefore important as it shapes the circumstances in which work and worklessness occur with the intention of rewarding work (both ideologically and politically) and disincentivising worklessness (economically and politically). These issues are explored further below.

1.1.1 **Work**

Work literally means to labour, or to produce, *'to engage in activity designed to achieve a particular purpose and requiring an expenditure of considerable effort'* (Longman's Dictionary, 1976). More narrowly, it means *'to be employed or to have a job'* (Webster's Dictionary, 2002). At both an individual and a collective level, work, both paid and unpaid, is one of the most fundamental and defining activities of humankind. Work is the process whereby the essential prerequisites of survival—food, shelter, security—are obtained. It is the means of human production. Debate about what exactly constitutes work is longstanding and ongoing (for example see Grint, 2005). What is most commonly referred to as work in European societies is 'wage labour'. All other forms of work, such as domestic labour or voluntary work are not given the same social status as wage labour. Barbrook (2006) argues that the term 'wage labour' has several meanings, denoting an employment status, a method of hiring labour, a method of payment and also an indicator of civil or legal status within a society. Labour relations where work is exchanged for wages, are indicative of societies that are not based on slavery or feudalism. These economic rights can in turn be argued as being a step towards political emancipation and are the root of the linkage between work and citizenship.

The organisation of work thus clearly differs by time, place and culture. In pre-capitalist Europe, for example, work in feudal societies was often organised around the home and the family, was focused on the land and there was little demarcation between work and non-work time, between the workplace and the home. The emergence of industrial capitalism from the eighteenth century onwards resulted in the more systematic organisation of work, with clear spatial and social divisions between the productive sphere of the industrial workplace (e.g. factories, offices or mines) and the domestic or reproductive sphere of the home and the family. Work was thus clearly constituted as waged work, differentiated from leisure and consumption (non-work time) or unpaid household reproduction (unpaid work). Capitalism thus organised the everyday world, providing a *'closed circuit of production-consumption-production'* (Lefebvre, 1984: 59). The emergence of capitalism also massified waged work, whereby people (largely men until the late twentieth century) sold their labour power via the market in return for wages: what is referred to as the commodification of labour. Labour thus became separated (alienated) from work as wages enabled the extraction of surplus value (profit) by the owners of production (capitalists) (Marx, [1844] 1970). This led to the emergence of clear divisions into broad socio-economic classes: the working classes (alienated wage labour) and the middle and upper classes (initially the property-owning capitalists, but later also encompassing the salaried professions). Each of these classes had a different relationship with the means of production as a result of their different work. How socio-economic class is now constituted has changed considerably since the eighteenth and nineteenth centuries, not least due to the changed nature of economic production and the shift from industrial and manufacturing to a more service based economy. Property ownership (at least in terms of homes if not capital) has also been more dispersed, and changing patterns of consumption have also impacted upon the character of classes. The traditional Marxian definition of class—as a singular economic position— therefore needs to be broadened to mean *'positionality in relation to capital circulation and accumulation'*: being a labourer can involve multiple positions as *'a worker, consumer, saver, lover, and bearer of culture, and can even be an occasional employer and landed proprietor'* (Harvey, 2000: 102). Social or occupational class is still the most fundamental social determinant of health and of life chances. Following the materialist viewpoint, in which the production and exchange of commodities is the basis of all social structure (Engels, [1877] 1969), work is therefore the source of the most fundamental division in society: socio-economic class. Workplace hierarchies thus reflect, and are reflected in, societal ones.

Whilst the economic growth associated with capitalism (and industrialisation) eventually facilitated improvements in the overall health of the population (e.g. improved infant mortality rates and life expectancy), there are clear contradictions between health and profit (Doyal and Pennell, 1979). Doyal and Pennell (1979: 25), identify three ways in which capitalist production and the ensuing organisation of work and the labour market impact negatively on health. Firstly, production is driven by the needs of capital accumulation rather than the health of workers. Shift work, overtime, low wages, the use of dangerous materials all result from the need to increase profit (Doyal and Pennell, 1979: 25). Similarly, stressful and health-damaging competition between workers is encouraged. Secondly, commodity production has impacts beyond the workplace, in terms of the role of work related (class based) social hierarchies, and the physical effects of the production process on the environment and on pollution levels. Thirdly, capitalist production is concerned with generating profit and so concerns about the effects on health of a product will usually arise only in the context of saleability: *'many health-damaging products will continue to be made simply because they are profitable'* (e.g. cigarettes) (Doyal and Pennell, 1979: 25). Drawing on Wilkinson and Pickett, a fourth link between capitalist production and ill health could be added, that of inequality. Social and economic inequality are an inevitable outcome of capitalist production and this results not just in socio-economic health inequalities, but also in varying levels of overall population health: more equal societies are more healthy (Wilkinson and Pickett, 2009).

The economic role of work is clearly not limited to the macro level organisation of production within society; it is also present at the individual and household level: for most people, work is the main source of income whereby they are able to feed, clothe and shelter themselves and their families, as well as take part in other forms of consumption. Work is thus a vital determinant of individual material wellbeing, but it is also the means whereby labour is produced and reproduced. It is a key part of the everyday way in which capitalist societies exist and re-exist (Lefebvre, 1984). Work provides the income whereby individual families can reproduce, so that a certain standard of labour power is provided on a consistent basis to fuel the capitalist economy on both a day-to-day basis, and on an inter-generational one: *'if the owner of labour power works today, tomorrow he must be able to repeat the same process in the same conditions'* (Marx, 1976). Healthy, productive, motivated and conciliatory workers (and consumers) are required on an ongoing basis. Particularly aggressive forms of capitalism risk instability and collapse in the long run if they suppress wages or working conditions too much in the pursuit of profit, and labour is thus unable to reproduce (Peck, 1996). Of course, the unpaid labour carried out in the home largely by women, is also a vital element in the system of social reproduction both physically and ideologically (e.g. instilling the work ethic, legitimising the system, role preparation) (Doyal and Pennell, 1979: 42). The separation between the productive (public) and the reproductive (private) spheres has also resulted in the gendered division of work.

Paid work is vital on several fronts to the maintenance of a successful capitalist economy and work itself is also an everyday way of reinforcing capitalist relations. It is therefore given high status within public and political discourses, lack of paid work is stigmatised and the social rights of citizenship are often entwined with work history. Although the emergence of welfare states across advanced market democracies since 1945 has meant that it is possible for labour to be reproduced even without the presence of paid work (via social benefits such as unemployment benefit), the premium given to work both financially and socially is still very high. Work is promoted ideologically as a fundamentally *good thing.* Work thereby constitutes an important element of the self-identity of many people, especially men (Bambra, 2010a). It is often how people define themselves and how in turn they are defined by others. Not to work (that is not to be in paid work), is seen as lesser than to be working. It is from this ideological construction of work that stigma is attached to those who do not, or cannot, work. The loss of work can in turn lead to a loss of identity and social role; the relationship between work and health is psychosocial as well as material.

Work and its value can be considered on three levels: work as an economic relationship, work as self-identity, and work as a social contract. At an economic level, *'working is the exchange of labour for cash, and the only sure test of the value of work to the individual and to society is financial profit'* (Marsden and Duff, 1975: 35). Motivation to work is considered to be purely financial and labour is required to be flexible in terms of location, hours and pay, and unattached to particular jobs or skills. In contrast, understandings of work as a sense of self move beyond rational economic arguments and treat workers as creative human beings with attachments to particular jobs, skills and locations: workers obtain rewards from work that are not just economic—control, responsibility, achievement, pride, and social support. Alienation ensues when these aspects of work are ignored and Marxist political economy analysis constructs work as oppression and wage slavery: *'Labourers are necessarily alienated because their creative capacities are appropriated as the commodity labour power by capitalists'* (Harvey, 2000: 102). Work understood as a social contract between society and the worker takes this one step further and sees work not as the actions of individuals but as service to society and a means of social integration: work forms a vital part of the fabric of social cohesion and social responsibility (Marsden and Duff, 1975: 37).

These are not just different meanings of work, but effectively, different political understandings of the role of work within societies. Different public policy implications flow from each of these positions. The purely economic, liberal view of work as a cash commodity limits the role of the state and public policy to the removal of restrictions on free trade and the free movement of labour. Employment policy is thus largely the concern of employers, not the state. The view of work as a form of self-identity implies that there should be interventions within the labour market and work environment to ensure that work is both available (even if it is unpaid) and of a quality sufficient enough to provide meaning and identity to people. The final view of work as a social contract between the state and society implicitly dominated public policy in Western Europe until the mid-1970s and requires the state actively to pursue a policy of full employment with *'high unemployment figures, the failure to ensure work security and poor quality in working relationships [considered to be] a failure of policy'* (Marsden and Duff, 1975: 38). State intervention is therefore vital, with regional and industrial subsidies if necessary. These competing political views of the value and meaning of work also have implications for how worklessness is constructed as a social problem.

1.1.2 **Worklessness**

In simple terms, worklessness is the absence of paid work. Worklessness in its broadest sense would therefore encompass a variety of states of non-employment including unemployment, ill health and incapacity for work, homemaking and lone parenthood, retirement, education and training. However, in the UK and other developed welfare states, the term is most often used to refer to people out of work and who are in receipt of welfare benefits for one of three reasons: unemployment (e.g. Jobseekers Allowance recipients in the UK or Arbeitslosenhilfe in Germany), lone parenthood or ill health (e.g. incapacity related benefits in the UK, disability pensions in other countries). For example, the UK government defines the workless as those who are unemployed (people who are without a job, want a job, have actively sought work in the last four weeks and are available to start work in the next two weeks, or are out of work, have found a job and are waiting to start it in the next two weeks) and the economically inactive (those who are of working age and not in work; not in full-time education or training; and those who are not actively seeking work) (Office for National Statistics, 2009). Sometimes within academic discourse, worklessness is also referred to as joblessness, acknowledging the fact that being without paid work does not necessarily mean that you are not 'working' (e.g. unpaid domestic labour in the home or voluntary work).

Worklessness is a comparatively new concept; or rather a new reconceptualisation of unemployment in the light of changes to the nature of work and labour markets. Worklessness first emerged as a term in the UK during the economic crisis and high unemployment of the 1970s (see for example Marsden and Duff, 1975). Previously, for example in the 1930s, unemployment was the most common phrase to define people (men) who were out of work. In the 1970s and 1980s, worklessness was used fairly synonymously with unemployment (see for example, Showler and Sinfield, 1981). However, in the twenty-first century, the term is used to capture far more than the traditional understanding of 'the unemployed' (defined as those out of work but looking for work), it also encompasses those who have never worked and those who are deemed unable to work (for example, due to ill health or lone parenthood). The evolution of the term and its more frequent use within policy discourses, particularly in the UK, since the late 1990s reflects the changing nature of advanced economies and specifically the demise of full employment. From the late 1940s until the mid-1970s, the advanced economies of the West experienced full (male) employment (broadly understood either as registered unemployment rates of less than 3% or employment rates of over 80%). To a large extent this ended with the economic crisis of the 1970s, the industrial restructuring and the end of the informal social contract around employment that followed it (Showler and Sinfield, 1981). Since then, structural worklessness has been a feature to a greater or lesser extent of all advanced economies.

Structural worklessness is the term used to describe the emergence of large numbers of people who are out of paid work and in receipt of social assistance for long periods of time. It is not related to the economic cycle (non-cyclical) as it exists even during periods of economic growth. Across advanced market democracies, it has gradually emerged as a major public policy issue since the 1990s, with the rates of people claiming workless benefits increasing rapidly (Blondal and Pearson, 1995; McCormick, 2000). This is particularly the case with health related worklessness (Chapter 6) where, for example in the UK, rates of incapacity benefit receipt have increased from 0.5 million in 1975 to 2.7 million in 2009. Internationally, 5.8% of the working age population in the Organisation for Cooperation and Development (OECD) countries is in receipt of health related benefits (Organisation for Economic Cooperation and Development, 2009). Whilst there is a debate as to the exact causes of this—the hidden unemployment versus ill health debate (Beatty and Fothergill [2002] versus Bambra and Norman [2006])—it is clear that it is related to the restructuring of market economies and the shift to post-industrialism. This has led to large geographical variations in worklessness with some post-industrial regions (e.g. North East England, Northern France, North Eastern Canada) having major long-term concentrations of worklessness across all ages and both genders (although concentrated amongst the semi-skilled and unskilled) with up to a fifth of the adult population in receipt of health related benefits. This is in the context of overall improvements in morbidity and mortality. This conundrum has led to media and policy talk of 'cultures of worklessness', in which whole families grow up in a community in which work is no longer the norm and lack of paid work is no longer stigmatised (Fletcher, 2007).

This structural worklessness represents the breakdown of work as part of the social contract between state and society. During the 1980s the social contract was 'renegotiated', leading to an expansion in those obliged to work, at the same time as a contraction in the role of the state in guaranteeing full employment. Groups of people previously outside the social contract (such as women, lone parents and those with a disability or chronic ill health) were brought in, and paid work became the expected norm for a wider range of people. However, whilst almost all those of working age are now expected to work (or at least be economically active e.g. participate in training), the state no longer pursues full employment. In all welfare states then, structural worklessness represents a form of macro-level state restructuring (in the sense of the renegotiation of the role of full employment within the social contract), whilst also acting as a catalyst for micro level welfare reforms. Policy responses have varied by welfare state context, with 'workfare' (compulsory 'work-for-benefit' programmes) being pursued in the USA, whilst in Europe the focus has largely been on active labour market policies (work experience, job search, skills, training etc.) (Burghes, 1987; Robinson, 1998). The UK's main strategy has been 'welfare to work', a hybrid of both workfare and active labour market policies. Countries have also reformed their benefit systems, reducing the prevalence of *passive* out of work benefits which are received as entitlements (such as Incapacity Benefit in the UK) and replacing them with more *active* benefits which require participation in active labour market policies (such as Employment and Support Allowance).

1.2 **Health and health inequalities**

Work and worklessness are widely recognised as important determinants of health and health inequalities. Definitions of health have changed over time: its etymological roots lie in the Old English for 'whole' implying that a person who is healthy is 'whole'. The World Health Organisation (WHO) attempted to encompass this in its 1948 definition of health as '*a state of complete physical, mental and social well-being, and not merely the absence of disease or infirmity*'. In contemporary Western societies, several competing theories of health co-exist (Seedhouse, 1986): Health as an ideal state; health as a personal strength or ability; health as physical and mental fitness to do socialised tasks; health as a commodity; and health as the foundation for achievement of potentials. More radically, following Marx, Harvey has noted that within capitalist economic systems, the productiveness and value of a person is reduced to their ability to produce surplus value and that sickness and ill health thereby signify a lack of productivity, an inability to produce profit: sickness is defined as the inability to work and, by association, health is the ability to work (Harvey, 2000: 106). Naidoo and Wills (2000) suggest that in the West a gradual shift in the meaning of health occurred during the eighteenth century as the increasing dominance of medicine encouraged a mechanistic view of the body. In this mechanical/medical conceptualisation, health is simply the absence of disease, and ill health is the presence of disease. The causation of disease presence or non-presence, and hence of a state of ill health or health, is thus atomised and examined at the level of the individual. However, population health arises from the complex interactions of individual, environmental, material and social relations (Dahlgren and Whitehead, 1991). In short, the level of health experienced or attainable by an individual, community or population is a direct result of the interaction and quality of the relationships between the various genetic, environmental, economic, social and political determinants of health (Bambra *et al.*, 2005a; Bambra, 2007a). The social determinants of health and health inequalities are examined in this section.

1.2.1 Social determinants of health

The social determinants of health are the conditions in which people work and live—what have been referred to as the 'causes of the causes' (Marmot, 2006). In addition to working conditions and worklessness, the main social determinants of health are widely considered to be: access to essential goods and services (specifically water, sanitation and food); housing and the living environment; access to health care; and transport (Dahlgren and Whitehead, 1991; Marmot and Wilkinson, 2006).

Working conditions

The work environment has long been acknowledged as an important determinant of health and health inequalities. Historically, physical working conditions (e.g. exposure to dangerous substances such as lead, asbestos, mercury etc., as well as physical load or ergonomic problems) were a major cause of ill health in the working age population and, because of the steep social gradient in physical working conditions, still remain an important factor behind social inequalities in health (Chapter 3). Stressful psychosocial work environments, however, have become more prominent as determinants of health, and exposure exhibits a strong social gradient which influences inequalities in health amongst employees (Chapter 4).

Worklessness

Unemployment is associated with an increased likelihood of morbidity and mortality (Chapter 5). The negative health experiences of unemployment are not limited to the unemployed only but also extend to families and the wider community. Links between unemployment and poorer health have conventionally been explained through two inter-related concepts: the material consequences of unemployment (e.g. wage loss and resulting changes in access to essential goods and services), and the psychosocial effects of unemployment (e.g. stigma, isolation and loss of self-worth). Lower socio-economic classes are disproportionately at risk of unemployment and it is a key determinant of the social gradient in health. Health related worklessness is also concentrated in more deprived areas and amongst less skilled workers (Chapter 6).

Access to essential goods and services

Access to clean water and hygienic sanitation systems are the most basic pre-requisites for good public health. In the advanced capitalist democracies, access to water and sanitation were amongst the first major public health reforms of nineteenth century Europe, although it was often only with the slum clear-ances and the advent of the post-war welfare state that access became univer-sal. Agricultural policies affect the quality, quantity, price, and availability of food, all of which are important for public health (Dahlgren *et al.*, 1996). While overall increases in life expectancy may be partly attributed to better nutrition, increases in the prevalence of obesity in many countries point to the contribu-tion food policies also make to over-nutrition. Obesity is associated with an increased risk of disease (e.g. diabetes, heart disease) and premature mor-tality (Bambra *et al.*, 2009a). Rates of obesity are higher amongst lower socio-economic classes. Access to healthy food is often restricted by what have been termed 'obesogenic environments': geographic areas (usually low income areas) with little access to fresh fruit and vegetables, high access to fast foods combined with low access to green space or sports facilities in terms of exercise (Lake and Townshend, 2006).

Housing and the living environment

Housing has long been recognised as an important material determinant of health, and health concerns underpinned the slum clearances that accompa-nied the advent of the post-war welfare state. Damp housing can lead to breath-ing diseases such as asthma; infested housing leads to the rapid spread of infectious diseases; overcrowding can result in higher infection rates and is associated with an increased prevalence of household accidents. Expensive housing (e.g. as a result of high rents) can also have a negative effect on health as expenditure in other areas (such as diet) is reduced (Stafford and McCarthy, 2006). The wider living environment is also an important determinant of population health. In the past, environmental issues tended to focus on pollu-tion from factories. However, more recently psychosocial concerns such as crime levels leading to stress and fear (as well as preventing people from exer-cising or walking) or the negative reputation of deprived areas resulting in the poor self-esteem of the inhabitants, have also been recognised as potentially important influences on health.

Access to health care

Access to health care is a fundamental determinant of health, particularly in terms of the treatment of pre-existing conditions. In most advanced capitalist countries, access to health care is universal. However, there are variations in terms of how health care is funded (e.g. social insurance, private insurance or general taxation), the role and level of co-payments for treatment, and the extent of provision—what has been collectively termed 'health care decommodification' (Bambra, 2005). Provision can vary within countries. For example, in the nationalised UK health system, it has long been the case that an 'inverse care law' operates whereby there are fewer doctors in areas of higher need (Tudor-Hart, 1971). People in lower socio-economic classes are also less likely to access health care services than those in higher socio-economic classes with the same health need (*ibid.*).

Transport

Transport works as a social determinant of health in three ways: as a source of pollution, as a cause of accidents, and as a form of exercise. Traffic pollution from exhaust fumes is associated with increased rates of asthma (particularly amongst children). Road traffic accidents are a leading cause of premature mortality amongst the young and road traffic statistics show that most children killed are from lower social class backgrounds (Bambra *et al.*, 2009a). The increased use of automated transport over the latter part of the twentieth century is also considered to be a factor in terms of the increased levels of obesity in advanced capitalist countries. From a more positive perspective, walking and cycling are healthier forms of transport which act as a form of exercise as well as transportation (McCarthy, 2006). Lower socio-economic classes tend to live in areas with higher traffic density.

This book argues that work and worklessness are not only determinants in themselves but they are also the main determinants of exposure to the social determinants: the 'causes of the causes of the causes'. Firstly, this is because work is to a large extent the underlying measure of inequality in any definition of socio-economic health inequalities (see Section 1.2.3). This is directly the case for occupational class, or indirectly for income. Even educational achievement is highly correlated with parental occupation, and the type and quality of work engaged in are usually related to prior education and skills. Secondly, as already mentioned, work is the basis of the major division within capitalist societies, creating social hierarchies and income inequalities which exist beyond the workplace. Thirdly, worklessness is far more likely to be experienced by lower socio-economic classes (Popham and Bambra, 2010) as are the lower quality, more insecure and more dangerous jobs (Marmot *et al.*, 2006). Finally, work and the workplace are central aspects of many of the theories of health inequalities (see Section 1.2.4). For example, the psychosocial theory of health inequalities to a large degree focuses on the psychosocial work environment (see Chapter 4). Similarly, materialist theories focus on physical working conditions (Chapter 3) and on how income determines access to services and the main source of income for the majority of the population derives from work. Even the cultural-behavioural model acknowledges the role of work-place stress or lack of income in contributing to unhealthy lifestyles.

1.2.2 Health inequality

The term 'health inequality' is usually used to refer to the systematic differences in health which exist between socio-economic classes (although there are other inequalities for example by gender or race). Health inequality can be defined in a purely descriptive way. For example, Kawachi and colleagues refer to health inequality as '*a term used to designate differences, variations, and disparities in the health achievements of individuals and groups*' (Kawachi *et al.*, 2002). More commonly though (and in this book), the moral and ethical dimensions of the term are emphasised: inequalities in health are thereby '*systematic differences in health between different socio-economic groups within a society. As they are socially produced, they are potentially avoidable and widely considered unacceptable in a civilised society*' (Whitehead, 2007). Inequalities in health between socio-economic classes are not restricted to differences between the most privileged groups and the most disadvantaged; health inequalities exist across the entire social gradient (Marmot, 2006). The social gradient in health is not confined to the poorest in society, it runs from the top to the bottom of society and '*even comfortably off people somewhere in the middle tend to have poorer health than those above them*' (Marmot, 2006): '*the higher the social position, the better the health*' (Lundberg and Lahelma, 2001). Health inequalities are thus not '*natural*' or '*inevitable*'; they are socially distributed and socially and politically determined.

Data presented in the Marmot Review of Health Inequalities in England (Marmot, 2010) show that infant mortality rates were 16% higher in children of routine and manual workers as compared to professional and managerial workers; deaths from cardiovascular diseases were 2.7 times higher in the 20% most deprived areas compared to the 20% least deprived; smoking rates were 28% and 24% respectively amongst men and women routine and manual workers as compared to 16% and 14% amongst men and women professional and managerial workers; alcohol related hospital admissions were 2.6 times higher amongst men and 2.4 times higher amongst women in the 20% most deprived areas compared to the 20% least deprived areas; and obesity rates were 27% and 34% amongst men and women routine and manual workers as compared to 21% and 14% amongst men and women professional and managerial workers. Socio-economic inequalities in health are universal within capitalist countries. Table 1.1 presents comparative data from the 2002 and 2004 waves of the

Table 1.1 Age-adjusted absolute and relative differences in rates of limiting longstanding illness for the highest compared to the lowest income tertile for men and women in 23 European countries

Country	Men		Women	
	Absolute difference in prevalence rates	Relative difference (odds ratio, 95% CI)	Absolute difference in prevalence rates	Relative difference (odds ratio, 95% CI)
Austria	10.8	1.80 (1.20–2.71)	4.2	1.47 (1.02–2.11)
Belgium	7.4	1.43 (0.99–2.07)	8.3	1.92 (1.33–2.78)
Czech Rep	4.0	1.13 (0.80–1.58)	7.7	1.19 (0.83–1.70)
Denmark	15.1	1.94 (1.38–2.73)	20.0	2.07 (1.46–2.93)
Estonia	22.8	3.20 (1.85–5.52)	12.4	2.60 (1.64–4.11)
Finland	14.8	1.97 (1.49–2.61)	15.4	1.97 (1.47–2.65)
France	11.7	1.91 (1.34–2.74)	10.5	2.01 (1.42–2.83)
Germany	11.5	2.23 (1.71–2.91)	12.1	2.04 (1.58–2.63)
Greece	8.9	2.15 (1.40–3.29)	12.0	2.22 (1.58–3.12)
Hungary	23.5	1.64 (1.16–2.33)	13.4	2.17 (1.59–2.94)
Ireland	8.0	2.24 (1.50–3.29)	10.8	1.88 (1.31–2.69)
Italy	13.9	2.80 (1.06–7.40)	−0.2	1.07 (0.40–2.87)
Luxembourg	11.9	1.78 (1.16–2.71)	8.0	1.42 (0.87–2.31)
Netherlands	12.9	1.92 (1.43–2.58)	6.0	1.22 (0.95–1.57)
Norway	10.9	1.75 (1.33–2.31)	13.9	2.15 (1.61–2.88)
Poland	17.0	2.49 (1.80–3.46)	10.6	1.83 (1.33–2.51)
Portugal	14.6	2.75 (1.54–4.92)	7.1	1.37 (0.89–2.13)
Slovakia	16.2	2.38 (1.22–4.64)	9.6	2.53 (1.43–4.50)
Slovenia	18.8	2.16 (1.52–3.07)	19.1	2.19 (1.55–3.10)
Spain	13.3	1.93 (1.16–3.22)	6.8	1.53 (0.95–2.48)
Sweden	11.6	1.67 (1.28–2.19)	13.1	1.52 (1.16–2.00)
Switzerland	9.5	1.83 (1.24–2.71)	6.1	1.40 (0.99–1.96)
UK	20.8	3.05 (2.17–4.30)	17.5	2.63 (1.92–3.60)

Source: Adapted from Eikemo *et al.* (2008a) with the permission of Oxford University Press.

representative European Social Survey, and shows absolute and relative income inequalities in limiting longstanding illness for men and women in 23 European countries (highest income tertile compared to the lowest income tertile) (Eikemo *et al.*, 2008a).

1.2.3 **Measuring inequality**

How health inequalities are measured is also an important issue. There are two major measurement issues in health inequalities: measuring social class, and measuring health. Measures for the former will determine the 'inequality' part of the concept, whilst measures for the latter will define the 'health' aspect.

Social class can be measured in a number of different ways, most commonly in terms of occupational class, income or education. Of course, class, income and education are inter-related and so the term 'socio-economic' class can be used to refer to these collectively. The public health literature often utilises a more neutral and less political term—socio-economic status—which reflects the Weberian rather than the Marxist tradition and can be interpreted as a way of depoliticising class inequality (Johnson, 2009). In the Marxist tradition of political economy, social class is a multi-faceted concept which incorporates ownership (property owner versus worker), skills and credentials (level of education and qualifications) as well as organisational assets (manager versus subordinate) (Wright, 1985). It reflects the economic and political relationships between those who own the means of production and those who are employed by this class (Johnson, 2009). Prior to 2001, social class was measured in official UK government statistics using occupation as measured by the 1911 Registrar General's Social Class. Individuals with similar levels of occupational skill were grouped into six categories (Figure 1.1).

Since 2001, a new eight point classification—the Socio-economic Classification NS-SEC—has been used (Figure 1.2).

I	Professional occupations
II	Managerial and technical occupations
IIIN	Skilled non-manual occupations
IIIM	Skilled manual occupations
IV	Semi-skilled occupations
V	Unskilled occupations

Fig. 1.1 Registrar General's Social Class (1911).

1	Higher managerial and professional occupations
	1.1 Large employers and higher managerial occupations
	1.2 Higher professional occupations
2	Lower managerial and professional occupations
3	Intermediate occupations
4	Small employers and own account workers
5	Lower supervisory and technical occupations
6	Semi-routine occupations
7	Routine occupations
8	Never worked and long-term unemployed

Fig. 1.2 Socio-economic Classification NS-SEC (2001).

This again largely divides the population up on the basis of occupation, but employment status and size of establishment, as well as managerial responsibilities, are also taken into account. The physical nature of work is given less prominence in the new typology, reflecting the more service based nature of the contemporary UK economy. Importantly, the last stratum of 'never worked' highlights the naturalisation of structural worklessness. Both of the scales are however hierarchical, reflecting the importance of work to societal organisation.

Income is usually measured using a proportional measure such as quartiles or quintiles so groups are formed based on how close to the top or bottom of the income scale they are. Education can be measured in terms of a specific cut-off such as no qualifications versus a higher degree, or it can be used as a scale variable measuring the number of years in education. Clearly each of these measures captures a different aspect of social inequality and the magnitude of health inequalities can vary depending on which measure is used. Socio-economic status is the term most frequently used within current public health research as it encapsulates the most easily measurable aspects of class: income and education. It is of course, a far less political term than social class. So, in this book the cross-over term 'socio-economic class' will be used.

In terms of measuring health, studies look at either mortality (such as infant mortality rates, adult mortality, all-cause mortality or cause specific mortality) or morbidity (illness, disease prevalence etc). Mortality data is considered to be more objectively measured (although there can be problems with how deaths are recorded in some countries e.g. for suicides). Morbidity can also be objectively measured (e.g. through medical examination) but more usually it is self-reported. Self-reported health is a more subjective measure of health and there is some debate over its validity especially in terms of cross-national comparisons. Some commentators have questioned whether we can compare self-reported measures of illness between countries and cultures, especially over time (Mitchell, 2005). In contrast, others have shown that self-reported health is strongly associated with later mortality across all socio-economic classes (Burstrom and Fredlund, 2001).

One further issue in measuring health inequalities is whether absolute or relative measures are used. Absolute measures of health inequality refer to the difference in the actual numbers of people who get ill or who die. In contrast, relative health inequality compares the percentage difference in ill health or mortality between groups (Bartley, 2004). So, for example, if the life expectancy of population A is 80 years and the life expectancy of population B is 70, the absolute inequality in health between groups A and B is 10 years. However, the relative difference is 80:70; population A lives 1.14 times—14%—longer than population B. There is debate about the use of relative and absolute measures: best practice in cross-national comparisons is to present both measures of health inequality. The relative index of inequality (RII) is an example of a well used regression based measure of relative inequality. It is the ratio between the estimated mortality or morbidity prevalence among the lowest socio-economic class (rank 1) and the highest (rank 0) (Mackenbach *et al.*, 2008). A high score on the RII represents large health inequalities. Table 1.1 presents European data using income as the measure of health inequality.

1.2.4 Explaining health inequalities

The influential Black report published in 1980 in the UK was the first government-commissioned report anywhere that systematically collated data on social inequalities in health (Black *et al.*, 1980). It also outlined several explanatory theories for why health inequalities existed between socio-economic classes in countries with advanced welfare states. In the years since Black, these theories have been elaborated and expanded. There are now five commonly used theories of health inequalities: cultural-behavioural, materialist, psychosocial, life course and political economy (Bartley, 2004; Mackenbach *et al.*, 2002). These theories are not mutually exclusive as, for example, material and psychosocial conditions (such as the work environment) impact on cultures and behaviours.

Cultural-behavioural

The cultural-behavioural approach asserts that the link between socio-economic class and health is a result of differences between socio-economic class in terms of their health related behaviour: smoking rates, alcohol and drug consumption, dietary intake, physical activity levels, risky sexual behaviour, and health service usage. Such differences in health behaviour, it is argued, are themselves a consequence of disadvantage, and unhealthy behaviours may be more culturally acceptable amongst lower socio-economic class. The 'hard' version of the cultural-behavioural approach asserts that the differences in health between socio-economic classes are wholly accounted for by differences in these unhealthy behaviours. The 'softer' version posits that behaviour is a contributory factor to the social gradient but not the entire explanation (MacIntyre, 1997). Risky health behaviours are more concentrated amongst poorer socio-economic classes due to the concentration of individuals with less self-control, lower responsibility, poorer coping abilities, lower health knowledge, and a more short-term outlook on life: an agency-focused explanation which can be summed up as the 'feckless poor' argument. A more recent version of the behavioural model (the cultural-behavioural approach) takes into consideration the more structural role of culture and how different cultural norms can pattern the distribution of unhealthy behaviours. Unhealthy behaviours are more common in lower socio-economic classes where these behaviours represent the cultural norm and are more acceptable (possibly as a result of longstanding industrial work cultures). The cultural-behavioural explanation does not take into account possible wider reasons for why unhealthy behaviours are more prevalent and/or more acceptable in lower socio-economic classes, namely the social determinants of health and other more structural factors such as the experience of deprivation and feelings of powerlessness. Simplistic behavioural explanations therefore merely lend authority to policies which stigmatise already disadvantaged individuals and communities (Joyce and Bambra, 2010).

Materialist

The materialist explanation focuses on income, and the neo-materialist approach on what income enables, in the relationship between socio-economic class and health. Important dimensions of what income enables include access to goods and services and the limitation of exposures to physical and psychosocial risk factors. By way of illustration, a decent income enables access to health care, transport, an adequate diet, quality housing and opportunities for social participation; all of which are health promoting. Material wealth also enables people to limit their exposures to known risk factors for disease such as physical hazards at work or adverse environmental exposures. Materialist approaches give primacy to structure in their explanation of health and health inequalities, looking beyond individual level factors (agency) in favour of the role of public policy and services such as schools, transport and welfare in the social patterning of inequality (Bartley, 2004; Skalická *et al.*, 2009). Cross-national comparisons demonstrate the importance of material factors on health and health inequalities (Bartley, 2004). In general, countries with narrower income differences between rich and poor have better health and wellbeing e.g. obesity, drug misuse, teenage conceptions, stress, mental ill health (Wilkinson and Pickett, 2009). These countries also have better welfare services and so access to education, social housing, transport, health care provision and green spaces tend to be better and more fairly distributed across the population. This may partly account for how lower income inequality translates into better health outcomes (Bartley, 2004). This evidence augments Wilkinson and Pickett's (2009) theory that everyone does better in conditions where income equality is higher.

Psychosocial

Psychosocial explanations focus on how social inequality makes people feel and the effects of the biological consequences of these feelings on health. Bartley describes how feelings of subordination or inferiority stimulate stress responses which can have long term consequences for physical and mental health especially when they are prolonged (chronic) (Bartley, 2004). The socio-economic class gradient is therefore explained by the unequal social and economic distribution of psychosocial risk factors. Psychosocial risk factors associated with the workplace include low levels of control over how work is undertaken, limited autonomy over work tasks, monotonous work and time pressures, low levels of support from co-workers and supervisors, an imbalance between efforts exerted and rewards received and organisational injustice (Marmot *et al.*, 2006). Bartley underscores how it is the way stress makes people feel that is important in relation to health outcomes rather than straightforward exposures to stressors. In this way the model combines both structure and agency. For example, it may not simply be income level or an adequate working environment alone that leads to good health, but rather how good income and good quality work can make people feel, especially in relation to others (Bartley, 2004). Here perceptions of social status and in particular perceptions of status in comparison to other people in society are significant constructs: what matters is how individuals value themselves. If these value judgements are negative, feelings of inferiority or subordination can invoke harmful stress responses.

Life course

The life course approach combines aspects of the other explanations, thereby allowing different causal mechanisms and processes, as well as structure and agency, to explain the social gradient in different diseases. Health inequality between socio-economic classes is therefore a result of inequalities in the accumulation of social, psychological, and biological advantages and disadvantages over time: *'the social is literally embodied; and the body records the past'* (Blane, 2006: 54). The notion of critical social transitions is also used to explain how certain important changes in social status (e.g. entry into the labour market or movement between jobs) can have long term consequences for health and future life chances (Blane, 2006). Longitudinal cohort studies have shown that disadvantage tends to cluster in the present and accumulate over time (Blane, 2006). In this way, individuals who are exposed to adverse conditions in one respect, for example work, are also more likely to encounter disadvantage in others, such as poor and damp housing, exposure to environmental pollution, inadequate nutrition, limited social participation, and lack of access to green spaces. Moreover, any disadvantage encountered in the past, such as unemployment, is likely to increase the chances of accumulating further disadvantage in the future. The life-course explanation captures some of the complexity of the interrelationships between social class, society, political economy and health by combining aspects of the neo-materialist, psychosocial and behavioural-cultural approaches.

Political economy

The political economy approach combines aspects of the materialist and psychosocial explanations with the recognition that the meso-level social determinants of health are shaped by macro level structural determinants: politics, the economy, the state, the organisation of work, and the labour market. This is referred to collectively in this book as the *political economy of health* (Doyal and Pennell, 1979). Notable aspects of the political economy approach include the epidemiology of Navarro and colleagues (e.g. Navarro *et al.*, 2006 and Borrell *et al.*, 2007) and Krieger (e.g. Beckfield and Krieger, 2009), the classic text by Doyal and Pennell (1979), and Bambra *et al.* (2005a) on the politics of health as well as Wilkinson and Pickett's (2009) influential work on economic inequality. Harvey's work on the body and the definition of sickness as the inability to work can also be viewed as part of the political economy analysis of health (Harvey, 2000). In this explanation, politics is understood in its broadest terms as *'the process through which the production, distribution and use of scarce resources is determined in all areas of social existence'* (Bambra *et al.*, 2005a), not simply the actions of governments or political parties. Public health and health inequalities are thus considered as politically determined (Beckfield and Krieger, 2009). In democratic societies, politics is the process whereby the levels of acceptable inequality are set (Bambra *et al.*, 2007a).

A wide range of research has demonstrated that even within the constraints of unequal societies, the social determinants of health are themselves amenable to public policy interventions (for examples see Marmot, 2010). Not all advanced welfare state economies have the same levels of inequality, and political choices are responsible for these differences with, for example, long term rule by Social Democratic parties resulting in better health outcomes than that of more neo-liberal governments (Navarro *et al.*, 2006; Chung and Muntaneer, 2006). Politics and the balance of power between key political groups—labour and capital—determine whether there are collective interventions by the state to reduce inequality (via the welfare state—see Chapter 2), and whether these interventions are individually, environmentally or structurally focused. In this way, health inequalities are politically as well as economically determined. A *political economy* explanation of health and health inequalities is developed within this book.

1.3 **Structure and agency**

The economic crisis of 2007 and 2008 has led to resurgence in structural political economy accounts of social change (e.g. Gamble, 2009). Structuralism *'privileges structure within the structure-agency debate, seeking to account for observable social and political events, processes and outcomes in terms of the operation of unobservable social and political structures of which actors are merely bearers'* (Hay, 1995: 193). Structuralism became unfashionable in the social sciences in the mid-1980s with the dominance of postmodernist and poststructuralist perspectives which focused on individuals and agency (intentionalism) to the exclusion of the social and the collective (structuralism). Intentionalist accounts seek to provide political and social explanation through the actions of individual agents: *'intentionalism is an 'insider' account that focuses on social practices, human agency and the rich texture of social and political interaction'* (Hay, 1995: 194). In mainstream sociology and geography for example, intentionalism resulted in a focus on consumption rather than production, and as a consequence the study of work and worklessness has been marginalised. Similarly, research on the social determinants of health has tended to ignore or marginalise the political and economic aspects of health and health inequalities (Bambra *et al.*, 2005a).

Political economy perspectives have tended to privilege structure over agency in their explanations of social and political phenomena. However, both structuralist and intentionalist accounts have been discredited in recent years because of their simplistic understanding of the complicated relationship that exists between structure and agency: Structuralist accounts fail to acknowledge the roles of intentional actors in the process of social and political change; and agency-centred accounts regard structures as merely the products of intentional action (Hay, 1995). This has led to attempts within political economy perspectives to 'reconcile' structure and agency in more sophisticated accounts which attempt to overcome the artificial dualism of structure and agency by moving towards a truly dialectical understanding of their inter-relationship (Hay, 1996). One example is Jessop's strategic-relational approach. Jessop asserts that social and political relationships exist through the inter-action of both structures and agents, but that the role of agency is constrained by the existing structural terrain. He argues that *'systems, and the structures that comprise them, are strategically selective'* (Hay, 1995: 199) and that the state and its institutions, systems and structures, *'are more open to some forms of political strategy than others'* (Jessop, 1990: 260). The strategic-relational approach suggests that *'systems . . . are not level playing fields—their complex, sloping contours favour certain strategies and actors over others'* (Hay, 1995: 199). The contradictory processes of capitalism and the multiple interactions between work and worklessness as determinants of health and health inequalities, all point to the complexity of public health and the need to reconcile structure (economy) and agency (politics) in explaining the influences of social, political and economic systems upon it.

1.4 **Conclusion**

In this book, I present a broad political economy analysis of the influence of work and worklessness on health and health inequalities. However, my aim is not to take an exclusively structural or deterministic approach, as a balance must be struck between the constraining and conditioning roles of economic, social and political structures of capitalism, and the intervening effects of agency (be it individual or collective e.g. state action). This account acknowledges the complexity of the political and social worlds and how these vary temporally and spatially. Too many contemporary accounts of health and health inequalities focus exclusively on the social determinants of health without recognising that these meso-level social determinants are themselves shaped by macro-level structural determinants: politics, the economy, the (welfare) state, the organisation of work, and the labour market—the political economy of health. This book aims to update more structurally-orientated political economy accounts, particularly of the labour market and the welfare state, and apply their insights to the complex relationships between work, worklessness and health.

1.5 **Further reading**

Bartley, M. (2004). *Health Inequality: An Introduction to Theories, Concepts and Methods.* Cambridge, Polity Press.

Doyal, L. and Pennell, I. (1979). *The Political Economy of Health.* London, Pluto Press.

Marmot, M. and Wilkinson, R.G. (2006) (eds.). *Social Determinants of Health.* Oxford, Oxford University Press.

Chapter 2

Welfare state capitalism and health

The welfare state developed as a particular polity across advanced market democracies in the early post-war period as a way of regulating capitalism and structuring the labour market. It therefore sets the parameters of the broader macro political and economic context within which work, worklessness and the associated social and health inequalities are experienced. It is also the key mediator in terms of governing the exposure of populations and sub-population groups to the social determinants of health and health inequalities. It is impossible to understand the relationships between work, worklessness and health without placing them within their broader political and economic context, which in the post-war period in advanced market democracies has been characterised by the emergence and restructuring of welfare state capitalism.

In very broad terms (as the timings of these periods of welfare state development vary by country and by welfare state regime), the development of welfare capitalism can be divided into four distinctive periods: pre-welfare state, the golden age of the welfare state, crisis and restructuring, and the emergence of post-Fordist workfare states (Bambra *et al.*, 2010a). For most of the nineteenth century, there was minimal state welfare beyond very basic 'poor relief'—the provision of basic food rations and shelter (e.g. the English Poor Laws and workhouse system). Beyond these provisions, welfare came via family members or charity. This began to change in the late nineteenth and early twentieth centuries with the introduction of rudimentary and highly selective state organised welfare systems which provided basic pensions, unemployment, and sickness benefits funded via social insurance payments (e.g. the 1911 National Insurance Act in the UK or the Bismarckian welfare reforms of 1880s Germany). It was not until after the experiences of the Great Depression of the 1930s and the Second World War (1939–1945) that what is here referred to as the Fordist welfare state was established. To a greater or lesser extent, the Fordist welfare state was characterised by centralism, universalism, and Keynesian demand-management, full (male) employment and high public expenditure, and the promotion of mass consumption via a redistributive welfare system and the social wage. There was also a mainstream political consensus in favour of the welfare state: it was acceptable to Social Democrats on the grounds of equality and poverty alleviation, and to the right (Christian Democrats, Liberals, and Conservatives) on the grounds of economic efficiency. Welfare state expansion effectively ended with the economic crisis of the 1970s. The welfare state was subject to ongoing reforms characterised by a reduction in the size of the welfare state, cuts to social benefits, the privatisation and marketisation of welfare services; a shift away from business taxation; and an increased emphasis on an active rather than a passive welfare system. This restructuring of the welfare state can be viewed as part of the shift from Fordist welfare to post-Fordist workfare. Post-Fordist workfare states are characterised by welfare pluralism, labour market flexibility, supply-side economics, and a desire to minimise social expenditure. Like Fordist welfare states, there are variants on the post-Fordist model reflecting welfare state regimes and their path dependent responses to common challenges (Jessop, 1991).

In this chapter, I examine the development of the welfare state from a political economy perspective. Initially, the emergence of post-war welfare state capitalism is examined (particularly through reference to the classic works of Piven and Cloward (1971/1993), O'Connor (1973), Gough (1979), Korpi (1983), Offe (1984), Esping-Andersen (1985) and Jessop (1991, 1994a, 1994b)) and subsequently international variations—Fordist welfare state regimes—are outlined and compared (Esping-Andersen, 1990). The crisis and reform of developed welfare states as forms of labour market regulation and capital accumulation are then examined and contextualised within the wider economic and political structural shifts from Fordism to post-Fordism (Jessop, 1991, 1994a, 1994b). The emergence of new forms of welfare—post-Fordist workfare state regimes—is also described. In the final section, the role of the welfare state as mediator in the social determinants of health is outlined and differences in population health and health inequalities by welfare state regime are examined.

2.1 **Welfare state capitalism**

The 'welfare state' is a contested term within social and political analysis (Eikemo and Bambra, 2008). Conventionally, the phrase has been used in a narrow sense, as a means of referring to the various post-war state measures for the provision of key welfare services or those state policies that permit, encourage or discourage the decommodification of labour. The welfare state is thus understood as the state's role in education, health, housing, poor relief, social insurance and other social services in developed capitalist countries during the post-war period (Ginsburg, 1979: 3). Welfare state responsibility and structures include not only the direct provision of cash benefits (such as unemployment benefit) and welfare services (such as health care), but also the regulation and subsidy of private forms of welfare (Ginsburg, 1992:1). The welfare state is thus a term which is often used as shorthand for the post-war social systems which developed in the West and comprise a mixed economy, a liberal polity and a social welfare sector (Mishra, 1984: xi). In contrast, the welfare state can be considered more broadly as a particular form of state, or a specific type of society which emerged in advanced market democracies in the post-war period (Pierson, 1998: 7). In political economy terms, the welfare state is understood as a particular form of the capitalist state (Hay, 1996: 9), the fundamental concern of which is the maintenance and reproduction of capitalist social relations and the use of state power to modify the reproduction of labour power and to maintain (and discipline) the non-working population (Ginsburg, 1979: 2; Gough, 1979: 44–5). The welfare state is thereby understood as more than a set of transfers and services, it consists of systems and processes which themselves shape society and structure socio-economic and demographic stratifications.

Political economy explanations for the emergence of post-war welfare state capitalism are three-fold (Bambra, 2009): (1) that it developed as a result of working class pressure (the 'power resources model'), (2) that it emerged as a result of the need to ensure the accumulation, legitimation and reproduction of capitalism (the 'requirements of capital' thesis), or (3) that it is a result of the congruence of interests of both labour and capital (the post-Fordist position). These are examined in more detail below.

2.1.1 Power resources model

The 'power resources model' (associated with Korpi (1983) and Esping-Andersen (1985)) has one central assertion: that the welfare state is a product of working class power and the organisation of labour and political rule by parties that represent their interests (social democratic/labour parties). Thus, as Korpi argues, the class struggle produces the welfare state and the level of class struggle shapes the institutions and ongoing development of the welfare state: the welfare state expands and retracts in accordance with the industrial, economic and political position of the working class (Korpi, 1983: 312). In this view, the more successful the forces of the organised working class, the more extensive, entrenched and institutionalised the welfare state will be (Pierson, 1991: 29). This model is a very useful way of explaining cross-national differences in welfare states (welfare state regimes) as it is the comparative power of organised labour and its' representatives that determines both the nature of the initial post-war welfare state which emerges in each country, and its subsequent development and response to internal and external pressures. This explanation therefore favours agency over structure.

2.1.2 Requirements of capital

In contrast, the 'requirements of capital' thesis prioritises a structural explanation of the emergence and development of welfare states. It asserts that the welfare state is a response to problems or needs generated by capitalism (Piven and Cloward, 1971 [1993]: 413), and specifically, the growth of Fordist capitalism (O'Connor, 1973:159) and the subsequent need to expand consumption within domestic markets (O'Connor, 1973: 150–1). Capitalism is unable to self-reproduce because of the competition of individual capitals. Its continuation is therefore dependent on interventions made in the collective interest of all capitals. The only institution/body relatively autonomous from any one type of capital (manufacturing, finance, agriculture etc.) is the state. Similarly, as Offe (1984: 51) asserts, capitalism consists of three interacting subsystems; economic, administrative and normative. These systems cannot operate efficiently independently, and the welfare state emerged as a means of managing their interaction. The welfare state exists as a form of crisis management which is designed to oversee the three systems. The state is thereby regarded as the ideal collective capitalist as, in the form of the welfare state, it intervenes in the economy in order to enable the continued accumulation, reproduction and legitimation of capitalism.

In terms of accumulation, Fordist capitalism produces the paradox of surplus goods (created by overproduction) and an impoverished surplus population (as a result of the unemployment caused by technological change and the subsequent decline in demand for unskilled manual labour), and the welfare state is the means by which the paradox is resolved as it gives (albeit limited) purchasing power to the surplus population whereby the surplus goods are consumed (O'Connor, 1973: 151). Furthermore, the problem of the surplus population is partially resolved by the employment created by the public sector welfare state agencies which are established to control what remains of the surplus population (O'Connor, 1973: 151). Therefore, the Fordist welfare state is a means of absorbing surplus goods and stimulating demand within the domestic market (leading to mass production and mass consumption), thus enhancing capital accumulation. This was a successful approach to capital accumulation in the immediate post-war period resulting in an inflationary boom until the mid-1970s (Gamble, 2009).

The welfare state also fulfils a legitimation function whereby it must maintain the conditions for profitable capital accumulation whilst also providing social harmony and the political-ideological legitimacy of capitalism (O'Connor, 1973; Habermas, 1976; Offe, 1984). Coercion is no longer a tool which could be used regularly to ensure accumulation (as had occurred in the nineteenth century when the use of the army to break up strikes and force workers back to work was common), as in the changed political dynamics of the Cold War, this would decrease the popular legitimacy of the liberal democratic state. The state therefore takes a more conciliatory and ideological approach whereby the social inequalities that are a fundamental and essential element of the capitalist economy are justified and legitimised by the presence of the social wage (social security benefits and welfare state services such as health care) and, in the early post-war period, by the incorporation of organised labour into the regulatory functions of the state via corporatist economic management (Offe, 1984). The welfare state therefore operates as a factor of social cohesion within the capitalist system which ensures unity and cohesion by concentrating and sanctioning class domination (Poulantzas, 1975: 24–5).

The welfare state is also a means of subsidising the cost to capital of the production and reproduction of labour power and therefore the cost of the production and (generational) reproduction of the capitalist system itself (Gough, 1979: 55). The production/reproduction of labour is a complex and costly task requiring food, shelter, health and increasingly in advanced capitalist economies, education. The welfare state places the financial burden for this upon the taxation system which is funded disproportionately through the taxation of the working population as opposed to businesses (O'Connor, 1973: 161). Previously these costs were borne in the wages paid out; the welfare state thus enables the capitalist class to avoid the total cost of the reproduction of labour by redistributing resources within the working population. This serves to expand productivity, and accelerate accumulation and profits (O'Connor, 1973: 162).

2.1.3 Post-Fordist perspective

Combining elements of both the agency orientated 'power resources model' and the structural 'requirements of capital' thesis is the post-Fordist position (most notably associated with Schumpeter (1942 [2010]) and Jessop (1991, 1994a, 1994b, 1995)). Fordism is commonly defined as the means of intensive capitalist accumulation via mass production techniques that occurred in the immediate post-war era (1945 to early 1970s). The Fordist labour process was distinctive as it was characterised by assembly line mass production which used the labour of a semi-skilled workforce. Although not all production was organised on a mass production basis and not all workplaces and workers were engaged directly in this labour process, mass production dominated the economy and was the dynamic behind economic growth (Jessop, 1991: 136). In terms of accumulation, Fordism provided a stable form of economic growth through the combination of mass production, rising productivity, productivity related income rises, increased profit; and increased mass demand due to wage rises and the social wage. Regulation in Fordism was provided through the Keynesian welfare state which enabled monopoly pricing, wage rises, collective bargaining, demand management and the social wage. Fordism involved the mass consumption of standardised, mass produced commodities in traditional nuclear family households and the provision of standardised welfare services (Jessop, 1991: 136–7).

The welfare state was a crucial element of the post-war Fordist regulation system (1950s–1980s) as politically it reconciled the interests of capital and labour, and economically because it regulated the economy as well as becoming a large consumer of national output. The post-war Fordist welfare state provided full employment in relatively closed national economies and did so through the use of Keynesian demand-side economic management. At the regulatory level, the welfare state aided accumulation by restricting collective bargaining over wage levels to within the rate of growth provided by the full employment economy; and it generalized mass consumption to all workers. The provision of a social wage, via a redistributive welfare system, spread the benefits of productivity and economic growth even to the economically inactive (Torfing, 1999a). This process not only helped to stimulate domestic demand for Fordist mass produced consumer goods, but it also provided conditions of full employment and social welfare in which it was possible for the state to reconcile the interests of organised capital and organised labour (Jessop, 1994a: 255). Thus the welfare state under Fordism was shaped by both the accumulation needs of capital and the defensive strength of the organised working class (Pierson C., 1994: 97). The Keynesian welfare state was the ideal type Fordist state. However, there were national variations on this general picture—welfare state regimes. The development of these different types of welfare state capitalism reflects historical differences in the comparative power and resources of the working class and their political representatives (power resources model), and the differing needs of capital (requirements of capital thesis).

2.2 Worlds of welfare state capitalism

In *The Three Worlds of Welfare State Capitalism*, Esping-Andersen (1990) presented a typology of Fordist welfare states based largely upon measuring decommodification. Decommodification is the extent to which individuals and families can maintain a normal and socially acceptable standard of living without being reliant on wages gained from the labour market (Esping-Andersen, 1987: 86). Commodification on the other hand refers to the extent to which workers and their families are reliant upon the market sale of their labour (Eikemo and Bambra, 2008). Labour became extensively commodified during the industrial revolution as workers became entirely dependent upon the market for their survival (Esping-Andersen, 1990: 21). In the early twentieth century, the introduction of some rights to social welfare brought about a 'loosening' of the pure commodity status of labour. The post-war Fordist welfare state, to a greater or lesser extent, fully decommodified labour because certain services and a certain standard of living became a right of citizenship (although the basis or extent of citizenship was often related to previous engagement with the labour market, work history and prior earnings), and reliance on the market (i.e. earnings from work) for survival decreased (Esping-Andersen, 1990: 22). Decommodification is most often used to refer to cash benefits, but it can also be used in relation to access to welfare services such as health care (Bambra, 2005). Social stratification (the role of welfare states in maintaining or breaking down market created socio-economic and demographic stratification) and the private-public mix in welfare (the relative roles of the state, the family and the market in welfare provision) were also examined. This analysis led to a division of Fordist welfare states into three ideal regime types: Liberal, Conservative and Social Democratic (Table 2.1).

2.2.1 **Liberal regime**

In the welfare states of the Liberal regime, state provision of welfare is minimal and benefits have strict entitlement criteria. Recipients are usually means-tested and benefit receipt is stigmatised (Esping-Andersen, 1990: 26). In this model, the dominance of the market is encouraged by guaranteeing only a minimum and by subsidising private welfare schemes. In areas such as health and pensions a stark division exists between those, largely the poor, who rely on state aid and those who are able to afford private provision. The Liberal welfare state regime therefore minimises the decommodification effects of state welfare and restricts social rights. There is a basic equality amongst state welfare recipients within this Beveridgian system but it is an equality of poverty. Many benefits are universal but of such little value that there is a clear division both politically and economically between those who can and those who cannot source additional welfare support by virtue of their position in the labour market (Esping-Andersen, 1990: 27). The welfare mix in Liberal regimes is stratified into three layers: the bottom layer of those who are reliant on public relief, the middle layer who are predominantly served by social insurance schemes and the 'privileged' top group whose welfare needs are satisfied almost

Table 2.1 Main welfare state typologies

Author	Welfare state regimes				
Esping-Andersen (1990)	**Liberal**	**Conservative**	**Social Democratic**		
	Australia	Finland	Austria		
	Canada	France	Belgium		
	Ireland	Germany	Netherlands		
	New Zealand	Japan	Denmark		
	UK	Italy	Norway		
	US	Switzerland	Sweden		
Leibfreid (1992)	**Anglo-Saxon**	**Bismarck**	**Scandinavian**	**Latin Rim**	
	Australia	Austria	Denmark	France	
	New Zealand	Germany	Finland	Greece	
	UK		Norway	Italy	
	US		Sweden	Portugal	
				Spain	
Castles and Mitchell (1993)	**Liberal**	**Conservative**	**Non-Right Hegemony**		**Radical**
	Ireland	Germany	Belgium		Australia
	Japan	Italy	Denmark		New Zealand
	Switzerland	Netherlands	Norway		UK
	US		Sweden		
Ferrera (1996)	**Anglo-Saxon**	**Bismarck**	**Scandinavian**	**Southern**	
	Ireland	Austria	Denmark	Greece	
	UK	Belgium	Finland	Italy	
		France	Norway	Portugal	
		Germany	Sweden	Spain	
		Luxembourg			
		Netherlands			
		Switzerland			
Bonoli (1997)	**British**	**Continental**	**Nordic**	**Southern**	
	Ireland	Belgium	Denmark	Greece	
	UK	France	Finland	Italy	
		Germany	Norway	Portugal	
		Luxembourg	Sweden	Spain	
		Netherlands		Switzerland	

Table 2.1 (*continued*) Main welfare state typologies

Author	Welfare state regimes			
Korpi and Palme (1998)	**Basic Security**	**Corporatist**	**Encompassing**	**Targeted**
	Canada	Austria	Finland	Australia
	Denmark	Belgium	Norway	
	Ireland	France	Sweden	
	Netherlands	Germany		
	New Zealand	Italy		
	Switzerland	Japan		
	UK			
	US			
Navarro and Shi (2001)	**Liberal-Anglo-Saxon**	**Christian Democrat**	**Social Democratic**	**Ex-Fascist**
	Canada	Belgium	Sweden	Spain
	Ireland	Netherlands	Norway	Greece
	UK	Germany	Denmark	Portugal
	US	France	Finland	
		Italy	Austria	
		Switzerland		

Source: Reproduced from Bambra (2007a) with permission from BMJ Publishing Group Ltd.

exclusively by the market (Esping-Andersen, 1990: 65). Private provision is therefore comparatively high and this leads to the description of the countries of the Liberal regime as residualist because the market prevails (Esping-Andersen, 1990: 86). In terms of gender stratification, this regime is to varying degrees associated with a paternalistic male breadwinner model of the family (Lewis, 1992; Esping-Andersen, 1999). The UK is often (but not exclusively) considered to be a key example of the Liberal regime type.

2.2.2 Conservative regime

In contrast, the Conservative welfare regime is concerned with the preservation of status divisions, and social rights are therefore attached to class and occupational status (Esping-Andersen, 1990: 27). This welfare state regime is distinguished by its status differentiating welfare programmes in which benefits are often earnings related and geared towards maintaining existing social patterns. This regime is characterised by the principle of social insurance and so the redistributive impact of this type of welfare state is minimal as benefits usually reflect previous earnings. In terms of gender stratification, this regime actively promotes a male breadwinner model of the family (Lewis, 1992; Esping-Andersen, 1999). However, as the role of the market is marginalised, in terms of decommodification, it lies between the low decommodifying Liberal regime and the highly decommodifying Social Democratic regime. The private-public mix is strongly weighted towards the latter although this is largely provided by voluntary (charities, especially churches) rather than statutory agencies. In terms of stratification, the Conservative regime is highly stratified with numerous different state-run and status-differentiated social insurance schemes. Status distinction, hierarchy and privilege characterise welfare provision in these countries (Esping-Andersen, 1990: 61). In terms of demand-management, these states operate highly corporatist systems of governance but with the intention of preserving existing inter- and intra-occupational class differences. Germany is considered to be the clearest example of a Conservative welfare state.

2.2.3 Social Democratic regime

The third 'world of welfare', the Social Democratic, is the smallest regime cluster in which the principles of universalism and the decommodification of social rights are not limited to the very poorest but extended across the working and middle classes (Esping-Andersen, 1990: 27). Its provision is therefore characterised by universal and comparatively generous benefits, a commitment to full employment and income protection and a strongly interventionist state. The state is used to promote social equality in two main ways: firstly via pre-taxation wage compression organised via strong collective bargaining and the incorporation of the trade union movement within the state; and secondly by using the taxation system to redistribute via the welfare state social security system. Unlike the other welfare state regimes, the Social Democratic regime type therefore promotes an equality of the highest standards, not an equality of minimal needs (Esping-Andersen, 1990: 27) and income inequalities are the smallest in these countries, particularly the Scandinavian countries (Ritakallio and Fritzell, 2004). The Social Democratic regime is also the least socially stratified of the three regimes as it is firmly based around principles of collectivism, solidarity and universalism. The state provides the majority of benefits which are set at relatively generous levels and thus incorporate both the working class and the middle classes (Esping-Andersen, 1990: 69). Similarly, these universalistic state-dominated systems minimise the role of the market. Social benefits are set at a level that is attractive to a broad population base and the need for market provision to supplement state benefits is therefore minimal. Widespread entitlement eradicates both status privilege and market provision (Esping-Andersen, 1990: 87). In terms of gender stratification, this regime uses publicly funded child care and parental leave to promote a dual earner family model in which both and men and women are expected to work (Lewis, 1992; Esping-Andersen, 1999). Sweden is widely considered to be the ideal-type Social Democratic welfare state.

2.2.4 Beyond the Three Worlds

The *Three Worlds of Welfare Capitalism* typology sparked a volatile debate (for overviews see Abrahamson (1999); Bambra (2007a))about which principles should be used to classify welfare states; in which regimes particular countries belong; the number of countries and the different regime types; the methodology of regime construction (for an overview see Bambra (2006b, 2007a)); and the nature of gender stratification within different types of welfare state (for an overview see Bambra (2004)). The entire concept of welfare state regimes has also been challenged on the basis that it incorporates two flawed assumptions: that most of the key social policy areas within a welfare regime will reflect a similar, across the board approach to welfare provision; and secondly, that each regime type itself reflects a set of principles that establishes a coherence in each country's welfare package (Kasza, 2002). A comprehensive discussion of these criticisms and how they link into public health research is presented by Bambra (2007a). It should be noted that welfare state regimes are ideal, not real, types: no single country adheres to all aspects and there is internal policy variation within individual welfare states and between the countries of each welfare state regime (most notably in terms of health care provision in the Liberal countries, see Bambra (2005)). Some countries are more consistently placed in each regime than others and most notably the Scandinavian countries are most consistently placed together in one regime and in most typologies they are considered to be the only Social Democratic countries (see Table 2.1). However, the concept is still very useful in analysing the complexity of welfare state formations and social provision across different countries and different times. Subsequently, the main outcome of the *Three Worlds* debate has been the development of alternative typologies (the most prominent ones in public health research are presented in Table 2.1) and of most significance here, is the suggestion that there are more than three types of welfare state capitalism.

Commentators such as Bonoli (1997), Ferrera (1996), and Leibfreid (1992) have asserted that when the Latin rim countries of the European Union (Spain, Portugal, Greece) are added into the analysis, a fourth 'Southern' world of welfare emerges into which Italy can also be placed (see Table 2.1). The Southern welfare states are described as 'rudimentary' because they are characterised by their fragmented system of welfare provision which consists of diverse income maintenance schemes that range from the meagre to the generous and a health care system that provides only limited and partial coverage (Bonoli, 1997; Ferrera, 1996; Leibfreid, 1992). Reliance on the family and voluntary sector is also a prominent feature. Similarly, Navarro and colleagues have argued strongly for the existence of a 'late democracy' regime consisting of Greece, Portugal and Spain (Navarro and Shi, 2001; Navarro et al., 2003, 2006). These countries were not democratic until the mid-1970s, and had until then the most regressive fiscal policies in Europe and underdeveloped welfare services, the legacy of which is still evident today. The Ferrera typology in particular has been used extensively in public health research as it has been shown to be the most empirically accurate of the various typologies in terms of within-regime homogeneity and between-regime heterogeneity (Bambra, 2007b).

In addition, Castles and Mitchell (1993) suggested that the UK, Australia and New Zealand constitute a 'Radical', targeted form of welfare state, in which poverty and income inequality are tackled through redistributive instruments rather than by high expenditure levels (see Table 2.1). In the same vein, Korpi and Palme describe the existence of a 'targeted' welfare state regime (Korpi and Palme, 1998). More recently, research into East Asian welfare states (South Korea, Taiwan, Hong Kong, Singapore) has suggested that these countries, sometimes including Japan, form a further 'Confucian' welfare state regime (Asphalter, 2006; Croissant, 2004; Walker and Wong, 2005). The Confucian welfare state is characterised by low levels of government intervention and investment in social welfare, underdeveloped public service provision, and the fundamental importance of the family and voluntary sector in providing social safety nets. This minimalist approach is combined with Confucian social ethics (obligation for immediate family members, thrift, diligence, and a strong education and work ethic). The formerly Communist countries of Eastern Europe (Czech Republic, Estonia, Hungary, Poland, Slovakia, and Slovenia) have also increasingly begun to be analysed as a separate welfare state regime (Cerami and Vanhuysse, 2009). However, they have experienced extensive economic upheaval and have been radically reformed so that the universalism of the Communist welfare state has been replaced by a more liberal welfare system (Eikemo and Bambra, 2008).

2.3 **Crisis and reform**

There have been two clear crises in the development of advanced capitalism: the first was the deflationary Great Depression of the 1930s and the second was the stagflation crisis of the 1970s. As discussed later in this chapter, it is possible that the financial collapse of 2008 will develop into the third major crisis (Gamble, 2009). Experiences of the Great Depression and the laissez-faire non-interventionist approach of governments (particularly Hoover's administration in the US) which was widely blamed in retrospect for the deflationary spiral, in part led to the more interventionist Keynesian state approach to the management of capitalism in the post-war period (as described above). Initially, Keynesian demand-management seemed to be successful in preventing major slumps as it resulted in the long inflationary boom of the 1950s and 1960s. However, by the 1970s growth was faltering and with the oil crisis of 1973, the boom ended and a period of severe economic recession ensued. The recession of the 1970s (and before that the 1930s) is widely considered to be a 'crisis of capitalism' because unlike the usual cyclical recessions considered to be an inevitable aspect of capitalist growth, this was both economic (stagflation, the slowdown in economic growth, the end of full employment, and the fiscal crisis of the state) and political (loss of confidence in the Fordist welfare state's ability to provide economic growth and political legitimacy) in nature. Previous orthodoxies were challenged, new political discourses took over and new policy regimes emerged: the crisis of the 1970s and 1980s was therefore constructed as a crisis of the interventionist welfare state, the solution to which was its reform and restructuring. This led to the emergence of a new 'post-Fordist' economy and new forms of state—'workfare' states. Thus, the crisis did not signify the end of capitalism but rather its fundamental restructuring (Gamble, 2009).

2.3.1 Workfare state capitalism

The crisis of Fordism and its corresponding state form prompted a process of economic, social and political restructuring in the quest to establish a new basis for capitalist accumulation. In global terms, this restructuring has taken the form of the deregulation of international markets, the abandonment of fixed exchange rates and the development of new financial institutions designed to increase capital mobility (collectively such processes are often referred to as globalisation). In industry, a number of structural changes have occurred such as the displacement of mass production and assembly line techniques by the batch production of diversified products, niche marketing and the use of new technologies. In accumulation terms, post-Fordism can be identified through its flexibility and permanent innovation (Jessop, 1994b: 19). Economic growth is based upon increased productivity from economies of scope/innovation, increased demand for differentiated goods and services, access to international markets, and rising incomes for skilled labour and the service class (Jessop, 1994b: 19). The workforce has become individualised (de-massified) and there has been a significant decrease in the role of the trade union movement and a shift in the balance of class power towards capital. There has been a growth in different employment patterns such as non-unionised work, insecure and temporary work, casual work, shift work, sub-contracting, part-time employment and other forms of flexible working (Jessop, 1991, 1994a, 1994b). However, unlike the Fordist regime, post-Fordism does not need to generalise the income rises of core workers to other sections of labour to stimulate demand. This limits the spread of prosperity and subsequently, new occupational structures have emerged as whilst Fordism was characterised by the key role of the affluent mass worker (or semi-skilled worker), post-Fordism has seen growing divisions between a full-time skilled and affluent core workforce, a semi- and unskilled peripheral workforce who are precariously employed (the 'precariat'), and a third group who are largely surplus to the requirements of the new system of capital accumulation (structural worklessness) (Jessop, 1991:88). Political dualisms and rising social and spatial inequalities have resulted.

2.3.2 **Workfare state**

The shift from a Fordist to a post-Fordist accumulation regime and the crisis of welfare state capitalism led to a need for a new type of regulatory state: the workfare state. In response to the changed political and economic environment (caused by the shift to post-Fordism, the globalisation of national economies, and the rise of new technologies), the state has experienced significant structural alterations over the last two decades and the emerging new post-Fordist workfare state differs significantly from the previous state form. The post-Fordist workfare state aids capital accumulation through the promotion of flexibility and innovation in production, processes, organisation, and market innovation. It has 'opened up' and deregulated national economies (Jessop, 1994b: 24) and its interventions are largely supply-side and concerned with increasing the international competitiveness of domestic export-orientated industries. Domestic full employment is therefore de-prioritised, redistribution is restricted, taxation on income and profit decreased and social rights undermined. This re-orientation of the state has made it more suited to the accumulation needs of the emerging post-Fordist economy. It has also resolved the crisis of the Fordist welfare state as low economic growth and stagflation have been tackled with supply-side interventions to promote innovation and structural competitiveness, and the fiscal crisis resulting from high social expenditure has been addressed through retrenchment and the restructuring of social welfare.

In terms of social regulation, the post-Fordist state is described as a workfare state because it subordinates social policy to the demands of greater labour market flexibility and lower social expenditure (Torfing, 1999a). Fordist welfare provision was provided through a redistributive state-dominated centralised system and it was characterised by the passive and unconditional nature of the benefits it provided. These benefits were passive, as they provided a 'safety net' of cash benefits, and they were also unconditional, as entitlement usually came through citizenship. In contrast, the post-Fordist workfare state is decentralised and pluralist, or in Jessop's words 'hollowed-out', as power has shifted on the one hand to supra-national and regional forms of governance; and on the other hand to private agencies and multi-national corporations (Jessop, 1994b; Torfing, 1999b). Welfare services are sourced by a number of different agencies including central and local public authorities, the market, social enterprises, private charities and the family. The state thereby becomes more a regulator or a financer than a direct provider, facilitating competition and 'choice' between welfare service providers (Moran, 2007). Post-Fordist welfare is also active in nature, providing a 'trampoline' effect whereby through training and work experience, welfare recipients are expected to return quickly to the market and regain their self-sufficiency (Torfing, 1999b: 8). Welfare rights under the workfare state are, to varying degrees, conditional upon fulfilling certain obligations—workfare. Workfare is not just compulsory 'work-for-benefits' but also includes training, education, job search and work experience schemes that form part of an active labour market policy (Torfing,1999a). This interconnection of social entitlements and market obligations under post-Fordist workfare capitalism has meant that welfare is no longer a right of citizenship and that therefore, labour has experienced a process of recommodification.

2.3.3 Workfare state regimes

Welfare state restructuring operates within pre-existing institutional, political and policy paradigms and so change is incremental rather than revolutionary: it is path-dependent (Pierson P., 1994: 180). Therefore, just as it was argued that there were different types of welfare state under Fordism, there are also variants of the post-Fordist workfare state: neo-liberal, neo-corporatist, and neo-statist (Esping-Andersen, 1999; Jessop, 1991).

The neo-liberal post-Fordist workfare state emphasises the recommodification of labour power, the privatisation of state enterprise and welfare services and the deregulation of the private sector (Jessop, 1991: 95). This has resulted in a number of changes to the state structure, intended to shift the balance of power in the labour market towards capital. For example, corporatist institutions have been dismantled, trade unions' capacity for strike action has been reduced, expectations about rising wage levels have been curbed, and the disciplinary force of social security has been heightened (Jessop, 1991). The neo-corporatist workfare state is characterised by its reliance on corporatist structures to introduce the flexibility required to complement the post-Fordist accumulation regime. However, economic policy is increasingly geared to the micro-economic level. Similarly, the state steps back as key welfare services, such as health or pensions, become increasingly self-regulated and welfare becomes more pluralistic and privatised (Jessop, 1991: 97). The neo-statist response relies on a state guided approach to reorganisation. Flexibility is provided through an active labour market policy, which emphasises training, skills and mobility (Torfing, 1999b) whilst retaining a strongly decommodifying out of work benefit system. A strong example of the neo-statist approach is the Danish 'flexicurity' system. Denmark has one of the most flexible and least regulated labour markets in Europe and it is very easy for employers to hire and fire. However, this is supported by a generous benefits system which provides a high standard of living for those out of work. It also invests heavily in training and education schemes to ensure that the work force is highly skilled and adapted to changes in the demand for different types of labour (Viebrock and Clasen, 2009). Welfare provision is also more mixed but the new providers are more likely to be from the charitable and voluntary sectors than private capital.

2.3.4 Post-Fordist crisis?

The deregulation and flexibility which typified the Post-Fordist approach to capital accumulation were particularly apparent in the relation to the financial capital sector. Lack of regulation of financial capital was considered to be one of the major factors in the first crisis of capitalism—the Great Depression of the 1930s. As a result, there was comparatively strong state regulation of the financial markets in the post-war period with faith placed on the efficiency of governments to mediate the irregularities and cyclical nature of capitalist growth. However, as the 'withering' away of state intervention and an increased faith in the efficiency of markets were widely argued to be the solution to the second crisis of capitalism in the 1970s, the financial sector was given considerable freedom in the 1980s. This was particularly the case in the neo-liberal welfare states of the UK and the US. This deregulation alongside the other facets of Post-Fordist capitalism (especially labour market flexibility and the availability of low cost consumer goods from places such as China and India as a result of globalisation) led to a second long boom in the global economy. This post-Fordist boom (1992–2007) was characterised by increased reliance on individual and public debt (in 2008, household, banking and corporate debt amounted to 350% and 300% of US and UK GDP respectively), especially mortgage credit (Gamble, 2009).

The period of post-Fordist growth ended in 2007 with financial collapse across the advanced market economies in 2008 and subsequent recession from

2009 (Gamble, 2009). The catalyst for the slump was a downturn in the US housing market which led to a massive collapse in financial markets across the world. Banks increasingly required state bailouts (e.g. in the UK the retail bank Northern Rock was nationalised, whilst in the US, Lehmann Brothers investment bank filed for bankruptcy and the mortgage companies Freddie Mac and Fannie Mae were given major government bailouts). Stock markets posted massive falls which continued as the effects in the 'real' economy began to be felt with rising unemployment rates of around 10% in the US and the Eurozone. Further bank bailouts were announced during 2009, with the IMF announcing that the global economy was experiencing its worst period for 60 years (Gamble, 2009). The recession continued throughout 2009 and whilst governments attempted to inject liquidity, this was accompanied by predictions of widespread tax increases and public expenditure cuts from 2010 onwards. This is by necessity a very simplistic summary of the emergence of the 'crisis', for a more detailed and eloquent account see Gamble (2009).

Many parallels have been drawn between the Great Depression of the 1930s, the crisis of the welfare state in the 1970s and this more recent financial crisis. The majority of commentators have initially regarded this recession as the third crisis of capitalism, and therefore structural rather than cyclical (Gamble (2009) is a notable proponent of this thesis). Certainly, in terms of depth it has much in common with the previous crises and to date it has operated across both the economic and the political domains. Certainly in the initial stages, the legitimacy of the post-Fordist economy and the workfare state appeared to be fundamentally challenged and the initial policy responses were certainly neo-Keynesian (most notably bank and company nationalisations and bailouts such as Northern Rock Bank in the UK, or Chrysler, Ford and General Motors in the US). However, unlike the 1970s and 1980s with the New Right politics of Thatcherism and Reaganism, there was no pre-existing alternative vision with enough currency in the mainstream to fill the political vacuum created by the economic crisis and provide a narrative to shape and 'solve' it (Hall and Jacques, 1983). Further, the initial neo-Keynesian state responses were only short-term measures (which were also accompanied by Monetarist mechanisms such as increasing the money supply using quantitative easing) and in the medium to longer term, this crisis management period was followed by a return to, and indeed extension of, 'normal post-Fordist business', that is, further welfare state retrenchment and a decrease in public expenditure and further reductions in the role of the welfare state as provider and employer (particularly in the UK). It is too early to determine whether this downturn is on the same scale as the upheavals of the 1930s and 1970s and therefore whether it will lead to a radical restructuring of capitalism and be retrospectively constructed as the third crisis of capitalism: the crisis of post-Fordism. It seems likely that it is merely the crisis of one form of post-Fordism, that of neo-liberal finance led growth, and that another form of post-Fordist capitalist growth will emerge, that of the knowledge economy with a corresponding resurgence of productive capital (Jessop, 2010).

2.4 Welfare states, health, and health inequalities

In its narrow definition as the state's role in education, health, housing, poor relief, social insurance and other social services, the welfare state clearly plays a key role as mediator in the influence of the material and social determinants of health and health inequalities. This is most obvious in terms of the strong relationship between universal health care systems, higher levels of health care decommodification (Bambra, 2005), better population health and lower health inequalities (for an overview see Beckfield and Krieger (2009)). However, as has been shown already in this chapter, the *welfare state* cannot be reduced to a set of specific social benefits and welfare services: it is a complex system of stratification, and the economic, political and social relationships enshrined within welfare state, or more recently workfare state, capitalism are therefore the most important macro-level determinants of individual and population health. In its broadest definition, welfare (workfare) state capitalism sets the parameters in which the social determinants of health (including the work environment, unemployment and so forth) take place. Further, the way in which the *welfare state* distributes financial resources and welfare services has consequences for social and economic hierarchies. As outlined above, there are different types of Fordist and post-Fordist welfare states offering varying levels of welfare provision and labour market decommodification. These have mediated the impact of the social determinants of health and also of socio-economic class on health to varying degrees. International research on the social determinants of health has therefore increasingly started to examine how population health and health inequalities vary by welfare state regime type.

2.4.1 Welfare state regimes and population health

Given the characteristics of the different types of welfare/workfare states and their varying influence on the social determinants of health, it would be expected that population health would be better in the more decommodifying Social Democratic welfare states of the Scandinavian countries, particularly in comparison to the Liberal welfare states of the Anglo-Saxon countries. This is certainly the general pattern found by those epidemiological studies that have used welfare state regime typologies to analyse cross-national differences in population health—specifically in terms of infant mortality rates (IMR), low birth weight (LBW), life expectancy (LE) and self-reported health (Chung and Muntaner, 2007; Coburn, 2004; Navarro *et al.*, 2003, 2006; Eikemo *et al.*, 2008b). Studies have consistently shown that IMR vary significantly by welfare regime type, with rates lowest in the Social Democratic Scandinavian countries and highest in the Liberal and Southern regimes. For example, Chung and Muntaneer's (2007) multilevel longitudinal analysis of welfare state regimes found that around 20% of the difference in IMR between countries, and 10% for LBW, could be explained by the type of welfare state. Social Democratic countries had significantly lower IMR and LBW rates, compared to all other welfare state regimes. Similarly, a study by Karim *et al.* (2010), found that LE ($R^2=0.58$, adjusted $R^2=0.47$, $p<0.05$) differed significantly by welfare state regime with 47% of the variation explained by welfare state regime type. By way of example, Table 2.2 presents data on infant mortality rates and life expectancy by welfare state regime.

Explanations for the better performance of the Social Democratic Scandinavian welfare state regime have varied. For example, Coburn (2004) has suggested that the key characteristics of the Scandinavian welfare state package (universalism, generous replacement rates, extensive and high quality welfare services) result in narrower income inequalities and higher levels of decommodification, both of which are associated with better population health. Coburn (2004), along with Navarro *et al.* (2003, 2006), has highlighted the importance of the accumulative positive effect on income inequalities of governance by pro-redistribution political parties in the Scandinavian countries. Other commentators (e.g. Stanistreet *et al.*, 2005) have suggested that increased gender equality within the Scandinavian welfare states may be another incremental factor behind their better health outcomes. Perhaps most influentially, Wilkinson and Pickett have highlighted the beneficial population health effects of higher levels of social equality (Wilkinson and Pickett, 2009). Furthermore, proponents of the social capital approach have highlighted the high levels of social cohesion and integration within Scandinavian societies (e.g. Putnam, 2000), something that has also been associated with better population health (e.g. Kawachi *et al.*, 1997). However, each of these explanations tries to pinpoint one or other aspect of the regime as the cause of the relatively better health in these societies. It is unlikely that it is one particular facet of the Scandinavian welfare model that leads to better health outcomes—rather it is the entire approach to accumulation, legitimation and reproduction taken by this particular type of welfare state/workfare capitalism. The relative reduction in material and social inequality in this form of capitalism is a result of the interaction and combination of a variety of policies (e.g. universal access

Table 2.2 Infant mortality rates and life expectancy at birth for 30 countries and 6 welfare state regimes in 2003

Welfare state regime and country	Infant mortality rate (deaths per 1,000 live births)	Life expectancy at birth (in years)
Scandinavian	3.98	78.52
Denmark	4.90	77.10
Finland	3.73	77.92
Norway	3.87	79.09
Sweden	3.42	79.97
Liberal	5.53	78.49
Australia	4.83	80.13
Canada	4.88	79.83
Ireland	5.34	77.35
New Zealand	6.07	78.32
United Kingdom	5.28	78.16
United States	6.75	77.14
Conservative	4.40	78.65
Austria	4.33	78.17
Belgium	4.57	78.29
France	4.37	79.28
Germany	4.23	78.42
Luxembourg	4.65	77.66
Netherlands	4.26	78.74
Switzerland	4.36	79.99
Southern	5.65	78.47
Greece	6.12	78.89
Italy	6.19	79.40
Portugal	5.73	76.35
Spain	4.54	79.23
Eastern	6.83	74.19
Hungary	8.58	72.17
Czech Republic	5.37	75.18
Poland	8.95	73.91
Slovenia	4.42	75.51
East Asian	5.29	78.70
Japan	3.30	80.93

Table 2.2 (*continued*) Infant mortality rates and life expectancy at birth for 30 countries and 6 welfare state regimes in 2003

Welfare state regime and country	Infant mortality rate (deaths per 1,000 live births)	Life expectancy at birth (in years)
Korea	7.31	75.36
Hong Kong	5.63	79.93
Singapore	3.57	80.42
Taiwan	6.65	76.87

Source: Reproduced from Karim *et al.* (2010) with permission from Elsevier.

to welfare services, higher replacement rates) resulting in higher levels of decommodification and lower inequality sustained over a long period of time (Chung and Muntaner, 2007; Navarro *et al.*, 2006).

2.4.2 Welfare state regimes and health inequalities

Until the late 1990s, the few comparative studies that had been conducted into socio-economic inequalities in health had concluded that the Social Democratic Scandinavian welfare states (particularly Norway and Sweden) had the smallest socio-economic health inequalities (Black *et al.*, 1980). For example, a study by Valkonen that examined educational inequalities in mortality in six European countries in the 1970s, found that relative inequalities were smallest in Denmark, Norway and Sweden (Valkonen, 1989). This result was in keeping with the fact that the Social Democratic countries performed better in terms of overall health, and also that from a theoretical perspective, it would be expected that labour market generated socio-economic class inequalities in health would be smaller in the more highly decommodifying and egalitarian Social Democratic Scandinavian countries. However, studies of health inequalities in this period were criticised as they only covered a few countries, they often compared differing time periods, and used different methods of analysis (Lundberg and Lahelma, 2001). As a result, in the 1990s, a large scale European Union funded comparative study of health inequalities was set up (Mackenbach *et al.*, 1997).

This study was designed to compare as many Western European countries (n=11) as possible over similar time periods, using representative national data and comparable measures of health (mortality and morbidity) and inequality. The study found that in the 1980s, relative educational, income and occupational class inequalities in morbidity (self-reported health) were present in all the European countries studied (Mackenbach *et al.*, 1997). The Scandinavian countries did not have smaller relative educational inequalities in self-reported health than the other European countries, but they did have smaller relative income inequalities in self-reported health for men (but not women). Mortality was lower for non-manual occupations in all the countries studied but there were little differences in the sizes of relative inequalities by country (Mackenbach *et al.*, 1997). However, the Social Democratic Scandinavian countries did exhibit smaller absolute differences in mortality by occupational class. These findings were confirmed by a follow-up European-wide study of relative health inequalities conducted in the 2000s (Mackenbach *et al.*, 2008).

This unexpected finding resulted in a surge of comparative studies examining cross-national differences in the magnitude of socio-economic health inequalities by welfare state regime. Overall, they have all found that socio-economic inequalities in health are present in all types of welfare state. However, the comparative performance of different types of welfare state varies by the measure of inequality used. For example, the Social Democratic welfare states have the smallest income-based relative inequalities in health (Eikemo *et al.*, 2008a), but in terms of education-based relative health inequalities, the various studies have found that there is little evidence of '*systematically smaller relative inequalities in heath across the whole population in the Nordic countries*' (Mackenbach *et al.*, 2008). Beyond relative measures of health inequality though, there is clear evidence which shows that amongst the most vulnerable social groups— the old (Avendano *et al.*, 2009), the sick (van der Wel *et al.*, 2010), and children (Zambon *et al.*, 2006; Lundberg *et al.*, 2007)—there are much smaller socio-economic inequalities in the Social Democratic Scandinavian welfare states— particularly Norway and Sweden. Further, in absolute terms everyone does better in the Social Democratic countries. There is evidence that while relative mortality inequities are not smaller in welfare states with more generous, universal, social protection systems, absolute mortality levels among disadvantaged groups do appear to be lower (Lundberg *et al.*, 2007). Taking the case of mortality amongst middle-aged men in Sweden, Lundberg and Lahelma (2001) comment that:

> 'On the basis of relative risk it would be possible to draw the conclusion that more than half a century of egalitarian policies have failed, since inequalities in mortality among middle-aged men are as large in Sweden as elsewhere in Europe. This sort of simplistic conclusion would ignore the fact that Swedish working class men have extremely good survival rates compared to similar men in other European countries, which in turn may very well result from the wide range of welfare state policies implemented since the 1930s.'

> Lundberg and Lahelma (2001: 64)

The life expectancy of all socio-economic classes is comparatively higher than the equivalent groups in other developed countries, and premature mortality risks are also lower (especially in Norway and Sweden) (Lundberg and Lahelma, 2001; Fritzell and Lundberg, 2005). The focus of comparative epidemiological research on relative, as opposed to absolute, measures of health and inequality has meant that the Scandinavian countries are effectively 'victims of their own success', as whilst they have substantially improved the health of all, the high level of health of the middle classes has meant that relative social inequalities remain. This is the real issue in terms of why the Scandinavian countries perform comparatively poorly in terms of relative health inequalities, and, as Lundberg *et al.* (2008) have pointed out, this is an achievement, not something to be criticised. The use of absolute or relative measures of health inequality also raises important normative and political issues about whether the role of the welfare state is to improve the status of those at the very bottom of society or whether it is about promoting general equality. Implicitly, relative measures of inequality are based on the latter view, and absolute ones on the former. Absolute measures are also more amenable to public policy interventions as was noted by the renowned epidemiologist Geoffrey Rose:

'Relative risk is not what decision taking requires . . . relative risk is only for research ers; decisions call for absolute measures'.

Rose (1992: 19)

2.5 **Conclusion**

In this chapter, I have argued that the welfare state sets the broader political, social and economic parameters within which work and worklessness and their health effects are experienced. I have briefly overviewed the origins and functions of welfare state capitalism and described the various forms of welfare state regime. I have discussed the nature of welfare state reform and the role of economic crisis in shaping labour market and social policies. The chapter has also shown how these different types of welfare state have impacted on health and health inequalities. The chapter has shown that different models of capitalism have different health effects, with better population health in the more equal Social Democratic welfare states, particularly in comparison to the more unequal Liberal welfare states. This shows that political (state) action, such as income redistribution, higher investment in welfare services, and universal benefits, can make a substantial difference to health and absolute inequalities in health, even within the constraints of unequal capitalist societies. In subsequent chapters, I will show the importance of the macroeconomic context to the interactions between work, worklessness and population health and health inequalities by examining differences by welfare state regime.

2.6 **Further reading**

Bambra, C. (2011b). 'Social inequalities in health: Interrogating the Nordic welfare state puzzle'. In: J. Kvist, J. Fritzell, B. Hvinden and O. Kangas (eds.) *Changing Equality: The Nordic Welfare Model in the 21st Century*. Bristol, Policy Press.

Esping-Andersen, G. (1990). *The Three Worlds of Welfare Capitalism*. London, Polity.

Gamble, A. (2009). *The Spectre at the Feast: Capitalist Crisis and the Politics of Recession*. Basingstoke, Palgrave.

Chapter 3

Health hazards in the physical work environment

Physical working conditions first became a public health concern with indus
trialisation, urbanisation and the emergence of capitalism in the eighteenth
and nineteenth centuries. Industrial work in this period was severely unhealthy
with men, women and children mentally and physically exhausted from regularly working sixteen hour days. Repetitive, intensive, heavy, unskilled work
was the norm, usually conducted in damp and unsanitary conditions with few,
if any, rest breaks. Employers had little concern for the health of workers who
were cheap, unskilled, and easily replaceable. Mechanisation merely served to
intensify production. Fatal and severely disabling non-fatal industrial injuries
were rife as a result of exhaustion, the high pace of work, and the failure of
employers to undertake any safety precautions. Work related diseases were
widespread and often occupation-specific with, for example, chest diseases
commonplace amongst miners and mill workers, eye diseases and blindness
amongst weavers, lead and arsenic poisoning amongst potters, and consumption amongst dressmakers (Doyal and Pennell, 1979). The physical work environment was clearly an important social (material) determinant of health.

Technological improvements, shifts in economic demand for more skilled
labour (with the associated costs to employers of higher wage and reproduction costs), reforms to the length of the working day and week (the eight hour
day and the forty hour week) (Dobson and Schnall, 2009), as well as the introduction of workplace health and safety legislation, and the emergence of sickness benefits as part of the post-war welfare state settlements, gradually saw
improvements in occupational health and the physical work environment over
the twentieth century. The physical work environment continued to be a major
focus of public health discourse in advanced market democracies, and for
example, research in the 1960s into physical hazards, such as asbestos exposure, led to legal restrictions on its use in most countries (e.g. the 1969 UK
legislation). However, there is a noticeable lack of contemporary discussion of
the physical work environment as a social determinant of health or as a contributory factor behind socio-economic inequalities in health. For example,

recent policy reports (e.g. the 2010 Marmot Review of Health Inequalities in England) as well as prominent academic books on the social determinants of health (e.g. Marmot and Wilkinson, 2006), have marginalised or completely ignored the contribution of physical work hazards in favour of psychosocial ones. This may be because there has been an increased focus on psychosocial, as opposed to material, explanations of health (Lynch *et al.*, 2000) or it is perhaps a result of the decline in the advanced capitalist economies of those manufacturing and traditional heavy industries, such as mining or steel, which have conventionally been most associated with physical hazards. For example, in Britain in 1983 there were approximately 200,000 miners working in 200 pits, in 2010 there were only 4,000 or so miners working in fewer than ten mines (Pattison and Peace, 2010). However, European Union survey data (Box 3.1) on the physical work environment show that around one in six workers are still exposed to hazardous chemicals at work, a fifth are exposed to vibrations, and a third are exposed to noise, heavy loads, or repetitive work. Further, over 15% of the European workforce is involved in shift work. The physical work environment therefore remains an important issue for a sizeable number of workers

Box 3.1 The European Working Conditions Survey

The European Working Conditions Survey is carried out every five years by the European Foundation for the Improvement of Living and Working Condition, an autonomous European Union agency. The 2010 survey interviewed almost 45,000 European workers across 34 countries: all 27 European Union member states (Austria, Belgium, Bulgaria, Cyprus, the Czech Republic, Denmark, Estonia, Finland, France, Germany, Greece, Hungary, Ireland, Italy, Latvia, Lithuania, Luxembourg, Malta, the Netherlands, Poland, Portugal, Romania, Slovak Republic, Slovenia, Spain, Sweden and the United Kingdom) plus Albania, Croatia, Macedonia, Montenegro and Kosovo, Norway, Turkey and Switzerland. The survey included more than 100 questions on a wide range of issues regarding employment and working conditions. It is a unique source of comparative information. The survey sample is representative of employed people (employees and self-employed) in each of the countries covered. In each country, sampling followed a multi-stage, stratified and clustered design with a 'random walk' procedure for the selection of the respondents at the last stage. All interviews were conducted face-to-face in the respondents' homes. The overall response rate was 48%. More details on the survey method can be obtained at: http://www.eurofound.europa.eu/ewco/surveys/index.htm.

in advanced market economies, as well as to the majority of workers in the newly industrialising economies such as China, India, and Brazil.

In this chapter I examine the health effects of three traditional dimensions of the physical work environment: chemical hazards including exposure to toxic substances used in industrial processes (asbestos, silica, coal dust, and lead); environmental factors such as noise, vibration, and workplace injuries; as well as ergonomic hazards such as repetitive movements, heavy lifting and including shift work. I also highlight the continuing importance of the physical work environment with regard to health inequalities. Differences by welfare state in the physical work environment and health are also considered.

3.1 **Chemical hazards and health**

There is a plethora of different chemical hazards in the workplace that can have adverse effects on health including aluminium, cadmium, lead, mercury, benzene, as well as toxic gases such as carbon monoxide and hydrogen cyanide (Harrington *et al.*, 1998). Table 3.1) shows that 15.3% of workers in the European Union currently handle dangerous chemicals for at least 25% of their working time, with men (17.0%) having a slightly higher exposure than women (13.2%). Exposure also potentially goes beyond the workplace, with evidence to suggest that workers can bring toxic substances home from work such as lead in their clothes or in their hair (Doyal and Pennell, 1979). The health effects of such chemical hazards can thus extend beyond the worker to the family and community. Industrial pollution from factories, refineries and power plants can also have potentially damaging health effects on communities. In areas that have experienced de-industrialisation (such as the North East of England, South Wales, Northern France, or Michigan in the US), there is also chemical contamination of hundreds of thousands of hectares of previously industrialised land (so called Brownfield land) which requires extensive remediation and is unlikely ever to be suitable for return to agricultural use. This section focuses on what have historically been the most health damaging chemical hazards: asbestos, silica, coal dust and lead.

3.1.1 **Asbestos**

The term asbestos refers to a group of naturally occurring mineral fibres known as silicates. There are two categories of asbestos fibre—serpentine and ambiphole—both of which are carcinogenic (World Health Organisation, 2006). Asbestos was commonly used in building and construction (in fibre cement, roofing and shingles as well as in insulation materials); in shipbuilding (for the insulation of boilers, steam and hot water pipes) and in the automotive industry (in brake linings, clutches, gaskets and pads) (National Cancer

Table 3.1 Exposure to common physical work environment health hazards amongst the European Union workforce (2010)

Physical hazard		Percentage of workforce (16–64) regularly exposed[a]			High risk work settings	Known adverse health consequences
		EU-27[b] All	EU-27[b] Men	EU-27[b] Women	EU-15[c]		
Chemical	Handling chemical substances[d]	15.3	17.0	13.2	15.7	Construction and maintenance, auto repair, painting, and construction, mining, and agriculture.	Respiratory diseases, cancers, hypertension.
Environment	Noise	29.0	37.4	18.8	28.0	Call/contact centres, construction, demolition work, road repair, engineering, manufacturing.	Acoustic shock injuries, tinnitus, hypertension, stress, fatigue.
	Vibrations	22.5	33.2	9.6	21.6	Construction, road repair, mining, machinery operators, drivers.	Vibration syndrome and vibration induced white finger, musculoskeletal disease (particularly hand and arm, lower back)

Ergonomic					
Heavy loads	33.5	41.7	23.5	32.8	Health care, air transportation, food processing, mining, goods manufacturing.	Musculoskeletal disease (particularly lower back)
Repetitive work	30.5	30.7	30.5	31.3	Assembly line packaging, machinery operators, clerical work, call/contact centres.	Musculoskeletal disease (particularly repetitive strain injuries), stress and anxiety.
Shift Work	17.0	16.9	17.4	15.9	Assembly line health care, mining, manufacturing, retail.	Gastrointestinal problems, cardiovascular disease, fatigue, sleep problems, injuries.

[a] 25% of working time or more.

[b] EU-27: The 15 pre-2004 European Union member states (Austria, Belgium, Denmark, Finland, France, Germany, Greece, Ireland, Italy, Luxembourg, the Netherlands, Portugal, Spain, Sweden and the United Kingdom) plus 10 who joined in 2004 (Malta, Cyprus, Slovenia, Estonia, Latvia, Lithuania, Poland, the Czech Republic, Slovak Republic, and Hungary) and 2 who joined in 2007 (Romania and Bulgaria).

[c] EU-15: The 15 pre-2004 European Union member states.

[d] This exposure data includes all workplace chemical hazards not just asbestos, silica, coal dust or lead.

Source: Based on data from the European Working Conditions Observatory (2010) and the European Agency for Safety and Health at Work (2006).

Institute, 2009; World Health Organisation, 2000a). Given its widespread use in lagging, asbestos was also common in any industrial location in which there were pipes (e.g. institutional heating systems). The most common route of asbestos exposure is occupational, with workers in the construction and ship-building industries being at an increased risk of exposure. Exposure to asbestos in contemporary workplaces in developed countries usually occurs during the demolition or renovation of asbestos containing materials.

Asbestos has been implicated in the aetiology of a number of diseases including asbestosis (a slow developing non-malignant pulmonary fibrosis), lung cancer, mesothelioma (malignant tumours of the pleura and peritoneum) and other pleural disorders (World Health Organisation, 1989, 2000a; National Cancer Institute, 2009). Mesothelioma is almost exclusively associated with asbestos exposure (Concha-Barrientos et al., 2004). The association between lung cancer and asbestos exposure was first noted in the US by Lynch and Smith in 1935, and confirmed by studies in the 1950s by Doll (1955) (UK) and Breslow (1955) (US). Several studies have demonstrated consistent results for a dose-response relationship between asbestos and lung cancer and prospective cohort studies have strongly suggested a causal relationship (Concha-Barrientos et al., 2004). For example, in a systematic review of the association between asbestos and lung cancer, the relative risk (RR) of lung cancer for a worker exposed to asbestos was twice that of a non-exposed worker (RR = 2.0, 95% confidence interval [CI] 1.90 to 2.11) (Steenland et al., 1996). In terms of carcinoma of the lung, asbestos also has a synergistic effect with cigarette smoking (Harrington et al., 1998). There is also emerging evidence that asbestos exposure is a risk factor for other forms of cancer including laryngeal, gastrointestinal and colorectal carcinomas (National Cancer Institute, 2009; World Health Organization, 2006).

Despite legal restrictions on the use of abestos in the majority of advanced market democracies in the later part of the twentieth century (e.g. in the UK in 1969 or Sweden in 1975), cases of asbestos related lung cancer and mesothelioma are increasing due to the long latency period of the disease (which can be up to 35 years). It is estimated that the incidence of asbestos related deaths will peak in Europe between 2010 and 2020 (Hogstedt and Lundberg, 2002). For example, in the UK in 2008, there were 429 asbestosis related deaths and 2249 from mesothelioma (up from 153 in 1968) (Health and Safety Executive, 2009). It is estimated that a similar number of lung cancer deaths are asebestos related (Health and Safety Executive, 2009).

3.1.2 Silica

Silicosis, which is caused by exposure to dust containing free crystalline silica (SiO_2), is known to be one of the oldest occupational diseases (World Health

Organisation, 2000b). Silicosis is defined as '*a fibrotic nodular disease of the lung parenchyma*' (Rees and Murray, 2007: 474) but exposure to silica dust is also causally linked to tuberculosis, lung cancer, chronic obstructive pulmonary disease, autoimmune and renal diseases (National Institute for Occupational Safety and Health, 2002; Rees and Murray, 2007). Silica is one of the most common minerals in the earth's crust and is found in sand, granite, sandstone, flint, slate and some types of coal. Exposure usually occurs when silica is liberalised into the air though processes such as crushing or blasting (World Health Organisation, 2000b). Thus, occupations associated with an increased risk of exposure to silica dust include coal mining, quarrying, foundry working, rock cutters, stone masons, granite workers, pottery workers, construction workers and manufacturers of glass and ceramics (Concha-Barrientos, *et al.*, 2004; World Health Organisation, 2000b). Cases of silicosis have become rare in developed nations due to the decline in the sort of work which has a higher exposure. For example, there were 10 silicosis deaths and 80 Industrial Injuries and Disablement Benefits Scheme recognised new cases of the disease in the UK in 2008 (Health and Safety Executive, 2009). However in low and middle income countries (including India, China, Vietnam, Brazil and South Africa), silicosis is a much more common disease (World Health Organisation, 2000c; Rees and Murray, 2007). New exposure pathways are also being reported such as denim sandblasting, a process used in clothing manufacture to create a distressed denim using silica as an abrasive (Ozmen *et al.*, 2010).

Although preventable, once exposure has occurred, pulmonary damage is not reversible (Ozmen *et al.*, 2010). The route of transmission is airborne and due to the light weight nature of the particles, silica can travel quite a distance from the source of exposure (World Health Organisation, 2000b). A clear dose response relationship between silica exposure and silicosis has been consistently reported in cohort studies which have compared silica-exposed and non-exposed workers (Concha-Barrientos *et al.*, 2004). For example, a prospective cohort study which followed 3,260 workers (half of whom were exposed to industrial particulates, and half not) over a fifty year period, found that exposure to particulates reduced the average life expectancy by 1.6 years (Moshammer and Neuberger, 2004). Individuals with silicosis are also at an increased risk of lung cancer. For example, a meta-analysis of cohort studies found that the risk of lung cancer was 69% greater in subjects with diagnosed silicosis (RR = 1.69, 95% CI 1.32 to 2.16) (Pelucchi *et al.*, 2006).

3.1.3 Coal dust

Coal miners working in enclosed and poorly ventilated spaces are at high risk of adverse health effects from the inhalation of coal dust. Cumulative exposure to coal dust is causally linked to a number of lung diseases including coal worker's pneumoconiosis, progressive massive fibrosis, chronic bronchitis and emphysema (Schins and Borm, 1999). Coal worker's pneumoconiosis, or 'black lung', is a condition which develops over a long period, with symptoms sometimes only appearing after retirement (Carta et al., 1996). It was initially a struggle for coal miners and their unions to get black lung recognized as an occupational illness (for an account of this in the US see Smith (1983)). Wagner (1996: 14) describes coal workers pneumoconiosis as '*a chronic and irreversible disease of insidious onset, usually requiring ten or more years of dust exposure before becoming apparent on routine chest radiographs*'. Although there is a trend towards decreasing numbers of workers being employed in the mining industry in Europe, it remains a significant employer in countries such as China, Poland, India, Africa, Australia and South America (Ross and Murray, 2004). The increased mechanisation of mining processes has only served to increase coal dust exposures (Smith, 1983; Ross and Murray, 2004). This might be an explanatory factor in the findings of a recent US study, which found that the prevalence of pneumoconiosis amongst working coal miners has increased over the last 40 years (Laney and Attfield, 2010). Given the industrial heritage of the UK and other parts of Western Europe and the long latency period of the disease, cases of pneumoconiosis and other lung disorders are likely to continue over the next decade (Health and Safety Executive, 2010a). In 2008 for example, 255 new cases of coal worker's pneumoconiosis were recognized by the UK's Industrial Injuries and Disablement Benefits Scheme.

Pneumoconiosis occurs in two forms: simple and complicated, the latter is characterized by larger macular and nodular lesions in the lung and can give rise to more serious and disabling diseases including pulmonary tuberculosis, *cor pulmonale* (failure of the right side of the heart), congestive heart failure and bronchopneumonia (Duguid and Lambert, 1964; Wagner, 1996). Progression of the disease after exposure ends is less common in coal worker's pneumoconiosis when compared with silicosis or asbestosis (two other types of pneumoconiosis). Risk factors for the development and progression of coal worker's pneumoconiosis include age, immunological status, the presence of tuberculosis, length of dust exposure and the total dust burden in the lungs. Another important determinant is the carbon content and grade of the coal. Higher grade coal dust, usually containing a higher carbon content (for example anthracite), is more pathogenic due to its greater surface area, higher surface free radicals and greater silica content (Ross and Murray, 2004). For example, a prospective cohort study of 909 new mine workers in Italy (with a follow-up period of approximately seven years) found that even moderate exposures to mixed coal dust were associated with a decline in lung function and an increased prevalence in respiratory symptoms such as breathlessness, wheeze and chronic bronchitis: moderate exposure to mixed coal dust resulted in a doubling of the relative risk of developing respiratory symptoms amongst coal miners compared to non-exposed office staff (RR of 3.74 mg/m^2 per year exposure = 2.26, 95% CI 1.72 to 2.96) (Carta et al., 1996). A recent US study also found a significantly higher prevalence of pneumoconiosis in workers of small mines (<50 workers) compared to those employed by large mines (p<0.0001) (Laney and Attfield, 2010).

3.1.4 Lead

The heavy metal lead (Pb) is omnipresent in the environment due to its involvement in a number of industrial processes including mining, smelting, battery plants, and the ceramics, plastic and rubber industries (Paoliello and Capitani, 2007). It is a bluish-white metallic element, which forms the alloys pewter and solder and has a half-life in soil of several hundred years (Thornton et al., 2001). In the environment, lead can spread from source to receptor by inhalation, but also by ingestion, and is thought to exhibit a spectrum of physiological effects depending on the level of exposure (Prasad and Nazareth, 2000). Lead can accumulate in organs, particularly the brain, heart, kidneys, nervous, and reproductive systems (National Academy of Sciences, 1993). The effects of long-term lead exposure include anaemia, anorexia, fatigue, depression, vomiting, hypertension, gastrointestinal conditions and, in some cases, renal failure (Batuman et al., 1983; Prasad and Nazareth, 2000; Lin et al., 2003). Maternal lead exposure has been associated with elevated risks of miscarriage, foetal development problems, and preterm births (Gardella, 2001). Lead is an accumulative toxin, which tends to be deposited in the skeletal system where it can persist for decades (Millstone, 1997). Lead exposure at work is an important health issue in industrialising countries. However, exposure is comparatively low in developed countries and has decreased over the last 30 years, largely as a result of declining industrial employment levels as well as better regulation and monitoring. For example, during 2008 and 2009, around 6,800 people in the UK were under medical surveillance for occupational lead exposure, as opposed to 26,700 in 1990 to 1991 (Health and Safety Executive, 2009). Regulation 10 of the UK's Control of Lead at Work Regulations (Health and Safety Executive, 2002), specifies that medical surveillance is required for 'significant exposure levels' defined as blood lead levels (PbB level) of 35µgdL^{-1} (or 20µgdL^{-1} for women workers of reproductive age). However, evidence is emerging to suggest that the effects of long-term lead exposure can be observed at levels as low as 10µgdL^{-1} (Canfield et al., 2003).

Lead has also been classified as a possible human carcinogen by the International Agency for Research on Cancer since 1980. The first international meta-analysis by Fu and Bofetta (1995) of the epidemiological evidence (cohort and case-control studies) on the carcinogenicity of occupational exposure to inorganic lead found *'slight to moderate but significant excess risks for all the cancer sites of interest'* with exposed workers 11% more likely to develop any cancer as compared to non-exposed workers (pooled RR 1.11, 95% CI 1.05 to 1.17). Bladder cancer had the highest pooled relative risk (RR 1.41, 95% CI 1.16 to 1.71), followed by stomach (1.33, 95% CI 1.18 to 1.49) and lung cancers (1.29, 95% CI 1.10 to 1.50). There was an increased risk of kidney cancer, although this did not reach statistical significance (RR 1.19, 95% CI 0.96 to 1.48). The likelihood of stomach (pooled RR 1.50, 95% CI 1.23 to 1.83) and lung (RR 1.44, 95% CI 1.29 to 1.62) cancers increased amongst those workers with higher exposure levels (e.g. workers in the battery or smelter industries).

3.2 **Environmental factors**

In this section, the health effects of exposure to noise and vibration are examined, as well as workplace injury rates. Table 3.1 shows that around 30% of workers in the Europe Union are exposed to noise and 20% to vibrations, for at least 25% of their working time and, as Table 3.2 shows, the incidence of injury rates across the Europe Union is 2.5 per 100,000. Men have a much higher exposure to both occupational noise (37.4%) and vibrations (33.2%) than women (18.8% and 9.6% respectively). Workplace injuries are also around 20% higher amongst men (Health and Safety Executive, 2010b).

3.2.1 **Noise**

Exposure to occupational noise above a certain threshold is known to be associated with adverse physical and psychosocial effects such as hearing loss, tinnitus (ringing in the ears), hypertension, ischemic heart disease, mental tiredness, sleep disturbance, annoyance and stress related illnesses (Passchier-Vermeer and Passchier, 2000; Persson *et al.*, 1997, 2002). The types of employment most associated with a risk of potentially health damaging noise exposure include call/contact centres, construction, demolition work, road repair, engineering, manufacturing (Health and Safety Executive, 2010c). Exposure to loud noise is particularly important in health terms in the construction industry where noise levels frequently exceed standards and where few hearing loss prevention programmes are effectively applied, resulting in high rates of significant hearing loss amongst workers (Seixas *et al.*, 2005). Exposure to health

Table 3.2 Fatal accidents at work in Europe Union (2006)

Member state	Number of accidents[a]	Standardised incidence rate[a]
Austria	129	4.2
Belgium	50	2.6
Denmark	43	2.7
Finland	25	1.5
France	395	3.4
Germany	430	2.1
Great Britain	169	1.3
Greece	58	3.8
Ireland	35	2.2
Italy	455	2.9
Luxembourg	4	1.7
Netherlands	56	1.7
Portugal	191	5.2
Spain	393	3.5
Sweden	35	1.5
EU-15[b]	2 469	2.5

[a] Excluding work related transport accidents.

[b] EU-15: The 15 pre-2004 European Union member states (Austria, Belgium, Denmark, Finland, France, Germany, Greece, Ireland, Italy, Luxembourg, the Netherlands, Portugal, Spain, Sweden and the United Kingdom).

Source: Health and Safety Executive (2010b).

damaging vibration (see below) as well as noise is linked to use of pneumatic drills and other mechanical equipment like chainsaws and cartridge operated machines (Health and Safety Executive, 2010c, 2010d).

Acoustic shock injuries are caused by a sudden, loud or piercing sound at a high decibel level via a telephone headset or handset. Call/contact centre tele phone operators are at highest risk of an acoustic shock injury. The problem may be exacerbated if call centres are so noisy that the operators need to have the volume controls on their telephones turned up higher than would be necessary in a quieter place (European Agency for Safety and Health at Work, 2006). Acoustic shock can result in damage to the inner ear, loss of hearing, tinnitus, earache and reduced tolerance to noise, headaches and nausea, dizziness and impaired balance, as well as fatigue and anxiety. Tinnitus (prolonged ringing, whistling, buzzing or humming in the ears) is another consequence of exposure to noise at work. Tinnitus can be temporary or permanent and according to Passchier-Vermeer and Passchier (2000) for those people with both noise related hearing impairment and tinnitus, 25% felt that the effects of tinnitus were more debilitating. In relation to hearing impairments, affected individuals are likely to encounter problems understanding speech even when hearing is only slightly impaired (Passchier-Vermeer and Passchier, 2000).

Occupational noise exposure is also linked to a number of psychological effects including annoyance, and feelings of stress and anxiety. Other physical health effects associated with exposure to occupational noise include an increased risk of cardiovascular disease. Although studies of the non-auditory effects of noise on health are relatively fewer in number, evidence exists for an association between occupational noise exposure and changes to blood pressure and heart rate (Lusk *et al.*, 2002). For example, a meta-analysis of 43 epidemiologic studies which investigated the relationship between noise exposure and high blood pressure (a known biological risk factor for ischemic heart disease) found a significant association for occupational noise exposure and hypertension: exposure to each additional 5 dB(A) noise produced a 14% increase in the likelihood of developing hypertension (Relative Risk = 1.14, 95% CI 1.01 to 1.29) (van Kempen *et al.*, 2002). Due to the link between noise exposure and psychosocial stress, the increased risk of cardiovascular disease is likely to be mediated through stimulation of the neuroendocrine pathways (see Chapter 4 for further details). An experimental study of the effects of noise in the workplace on salivary cortisol levels, perceived stress and annoyance found that exposure to low frequency noise (40 dBA for 2 hours at a time) increased salivary cortisol levels, stress and annoyance amongst thirty-two participants (Persson *et al.*, 2002).

3.2.2 Vibration

Hand-arm vibration syndrome was first described by Maurice Raynaud in 1862 (Chetter *et al.*, 1998) and is therefore sometimes referred to as Raynaud's disease. More commonly it is known as 'vibration white finger' syndrome (Letz *et al.*, 1992). In 1985 in the UK, hand-arm vibration syndrome became listed as an industrial injury for which compensation and disability benefits could be claimed via the Industrial Injuries and Disablement Benefits Scheme. Although prevention and control strategies have reduced the prevalence of hand-arm vibration syndrome (see Chapter 7), approximately 2 million workers in the UK are at risk of hand-arm vibration syndrome according to the Health and Safety Executive (2010d; 2010e). The syndrome affects the nerves and blood vessels in the hands and arms and is defined by multi-system involvement, with pathologies of the vascular and neurological and musculoskeletal systems being common (Chetter *et al.*, 1998; Letz *et al.*, 1992).

Exposure to vibration is also associated with development of carpal tunnel syndrome, an upper limb neuropathy, caused by compression of the median nerve travelling through the carpal tunnel, which is characterised by pain, paraesthesia and numbness (Katz and Simmons, 2002; Chetter *et al.*, 1998; Health and Safety Executive, 2010d). It is possible that the two conditions coexist (Chetter *et al.*, 1998). The effects of hand-arm vibration syndrome include blanching attacks, numbness and pain in the aforementioned areas, reduced grip strength (with obvious ramifications for worker safety), altered sensitivity and dexterity, inability to do fine work requiring delicate movement and heightened sensitivity to cold and damp conditions (Health and Safety Executive, 2010d).

Studies in the early twentieth century identified an association between Raynaud's disease and industrial work with an increased prevalence of the disease in workers who were exposed to vibration, cold conditions and high grip pressure, such as coal miners and shipyard workers (Chetter *et al.*, 1998). Hand-arm vibration is caused by the regular and frequent use of vibrating hand held tools, such as pneumatic jackhammers, drills, gas powered chainsaws and electrical tools such as grinders and polishers, power lawnmowers and chain saws (Chetter *et al.*, 1998; Health and Safety Executive, 2010d). The nature of these tools involves vibration (a rapid back-and-forth motion), which is transmitted from the tool to the hands and arms of the person holding the tool. Vibration syndrome and vibration induced white finger are the major health hazards related to the use of vibrating tools. Carpal tunnel syndrome is another health problem that has been linked to the use of smaller hand held vibrating tools. Drivers of certain types of vehicles are also at risk of exposure as vibrations are likely to be transmitted via steering devices (Åström *et al.*, 2006). It is also important to note that, although preventable, once developed hand-arm vibration syndrome is permanent and irreversible (Health and Safety Executive, 2010d).

Epidemiological evidence, including examination of the dose-response relationship, has accumulated to support the association between exposure to vibration with various disorders of the hands and arms (Adewusi *et al.*, 2010). For example, a longitudinal study of stoneworkers in quarries and mills found increased occurrence of vibration induced white finger in twenty-one active stone workers compared with workers in two control groups who had not used power tools for a period of either three (n=21) or six years (n=22) (Bovenzi *et al.*, 1994). The power tools produced vibrations of over 20m/s^2 which constitute a hazardous work environment under EU guidelines. Indeed, the study found that during the follow-up period, 38% of the active stoneworkers group reported the onset of vibration induced white finger (p<0.01).

Musculoskeletal symptoms are also thought to be linked to hand arm vibration exposures. For example, a cross-sectional study of terrain vehicle drivers (such as forest vehicles and snow mobiles) found evidence of an association between driving and musculoskeletal symptoms in the neck, shoulders and wrists (prevalence odds ratios ranged between 1.2–6.4) (Åström *et al.*, 2006). The study also found significant associations between cumulative exposure to terrain vehicle driving and symptoms of hand arm vibration syndrome (prevalence odds ratios [OR] ranged between 1.2 and 6.01).

Whole body vibration is defined as '*vibration occurring when a greater part of the body weight is supported on a vibrating surface*' (Futatsuka *et al.*, 1998: 127). It has been associated with a number of adverse health effects including lower back pain, sciatic pain and degenerative changes in the spine (Pope *et al.*, 2002). Exposure to whole body vibration tends to be associated with work involving driving over uneven surfaces where shocks or jolts are experienced and vibration is transmitted either through the driver's seat or feet (Health and Safety Executive, 2010d). This means that occupations such as bus drivers, fork lift truck operators and machine operators in quarries or workers operating earth-moving machinery are at an elevated risk of being exposed to whole body vibration (Health and Safety Executive, 2010d). Whilst difficulties exist in attributing causality of the effects of vibration on health due to the large number of confounding factors involved (such as working posture, handling of heavy materials and case history) (Futatsuka *et al.*, 1998; Pope *et al.*, 2002), evidence has accumulated to suggest that vibration causes end plate damage in the vertebrae which leads to degeneration and pain in the lumbar spine (Sandover, 1998). For example, a systematic review of 24 studies found evidence that lower back pain was more frequent in workers exposed to whole body vibration (Lings and Leboeuf-Yde, 2000). There was also some evidence of a dose-response association.

3.2.3 Workplace injuries

Non-fatal injuries are still frequent in workplaces. For example, official UK health and safety data for 2008–09 show that 131,895 non-fatal injuries to employees were reported—a rate of 502.2 per 100,000 employees. Self-reported accidents in the Labour Force Survey were higher with 246,000 injuries reported—a rate of 870 per 100,000 workers (Health and Safety Executive, 2010b). Workplace injuries in the UK resulted in a loss of 4.7 million working days in 2008–9 (Health and Safety Executive, 2010b). Table 3.2 shows comparable European data on fatal workplace injuries: Fatal accidents are significantly less common than non-fatal ones, with, for example, 169 workers killed at work in the UK in 2006—a rate of 1.3 per 100,000 workers. Rates are highest in Portugal (5.2), Austria (4.2), Greece (3.8), Spain (3.5), and France (3.4). These variations probably reflect higher participation in more dangerous occupations such as agriculture where the European Union average fatal accident rate was 8.9 per 100,000, and construction work where the European Union average fatal accident rate was 9.5 per 100,000 compared to 1.5 per 100,000 for retail and 0.9 for other service sector work (Health and Safety Executive, 2010b). The higher fatal injury rates in these countries may also reflect different regulatory regimes (section 3.5). It should be noted that deaths and injuries from commuting to work are not included in these statistics.

The most common causes of workplace injuries are slips, trips or falls, being struck by a moving object, injuries from carrying or lifting heavy loads, and falls from a height (Health and Safety Executive, 2010b). In the UK, slips and trips are the most common cause of major injuries at work, accounting for over a third of all major injuries and 20% of injuries lasting more than three days. They are the main cause of major injuries in manufacturing and in the service sectors. 95% of major slips result in broken bones and they can also be the initial cause for a range of other types of accident such as a fall from a height. Slips and trips cost £512 million per year in lost production and £133 million per year in health service costs (Health and Safety Executive, 2010b). Workplace injuries, adjusting for different working conditions, are 20% higher in men compared with women, and over 95% of workplace fatalities are amongst men, with the fatal injury rate nearly 80 times higher in men than women (Health and Safety Executive, 2010b). Job tenure is also associated with workplace injuries, with a stepwise gradient in terms of length of tenure and a decreasing risk of workplace injury: injury rates were 11.4 per 100 workers per year amongst employees with less than 6 months time in the job, compared to 5.6 for between 6 and 11 months experience, 4.2 for those with 12 months to 5 years tenure, and 3.5 per 100 workers per year amongst those who had worked the same job for more than 5 years (Health and Safety Executive, 2010b). There are also important differences in workplace injuries by occupational class status which are examined in Section 3.4.

3.3 Ergonomic work hazards

This section examines the health effects of ergonomic hazards such as physical loads, repetitive work as well as shift work. Table 3.1 shows that around 35% of workers in the European Union are exposed to heavy loads and around 30% to repetitive work for at least 25% of their working time. Shift work is also a common form of work organisation with around one in six European workers currently involved in shift work. Gender differences are smaller in terms of ergonomic factors with, for example, women (30.7%) and men (30.5%) exposed to repetitive work in almost equal amounts.

3.3.1 **Physical load**

Work involving tasks such as lifting and carrying heavy or bulky loads (often defined as loads over 25kg) is known to be a risk factor for the development of musculoskeletal disorders. Musculoskeletal disorders are defined as *'inflammatory and degenerative conditions affecting the muscles, tendons, ligaments, joints, peripheral nerves, and supporting blood vessels'* (Punnett and Wegman, 2004: 13). Disorders of the back (including lower back pain, disc degeneration and herniation) are the most common form of musculoskeletal disorder accounting for up to 60% of complaints, while neck and upper limb pain followed by knee and hip disorders make up the remainder (World Health Organisation, 2003). According to the World Health Organisation (2003), musculoskeletal disorders account for approximately one third of all sickness absences in industrialised nations. Chronic musculoskeletal disorders have adverse knock-on effects on general wellbeing and quality of life. The prevalence of musculoskeletal disorders is higher in certain occupations including nurses and allied health professionals, miners, leather tanners, and workers in air transportation, food processing and goods manufacturing (Punnett and Wegman, 2004).

The public health evidence base exploring the relationship between exposure to physical load and musculoskeletal disorders is vast, with strong evidence for a positive association between exposure to physical load and the incidence and recurrence of musculoskeletal disorders, particularly of the lower back (Parkes *et al.*, 2005). Indeed, a recent review estimated that exposure to heavy physical load accounts for between 31% and 58% of the incidence of back disorders (Punnett and Wegman, 2004). Similarly, a systematic review of risk factors for shoulder pain found that physical load factors (heavy work load, awkward postures, repetitive movements, vibration) increased the likelihood of reporting shoulder pain by up to 4 times in exposed compared to non-exposed workers (reviewed studies reported OR of 1.4 to 4.6) (van der Windt *et al.*, 2000). Some commentators suggest that there is a latency of effect in relation to musculoskeletal disorders whereby an exposure to an ergonomic hazard might precede the occurrence of musculoskeletal pain by months or even years dependent on the intensity of exposure (Punnett and Wegman, 2004).

Associated with physical load are two other related risk factors for musculoskeletal disorders: restricted postures and frequent lifting and bending. For example, in the health care sector, nurses and health care assistants are frequently exposed to ergonomic hazards such as handling, lifting and moving patients and postural awkwardness associated with tasks such as dressing or bathing patients (Menzel *et al.*, 2004). A recent review estimated that manual handling accounts for between 11% and 66% of the incidence of back disorders

(Punnett and Wegman, 2004). Increasing rates of obesity are only likely to increase the risks of manual handling for nursing personnel (Menzel *et al.*, 2004). Repetitive work and vibration are also implicated as risk factors in musculoskeletal pain and are discussed separately within this chapter. The psychosocial work environment also has a strong association with musculoskeletal disease as discussed in Chapter 4. Other risk factors in relation to musculoskeletal disorders should also not be overlooked, for example age, obesity, socio-economic class, smoking behaviour and health status at baseline (Plunnet and Wegman, 2004; European Agency for Safety and Health at Work, 2000).

3.3.2 Repetitive work

Repetitive work is known to be a stressor in the physical work environment. It is associated with a number of occupations particularly in intensive manual employment (including piece rate work) such as garment workers, assembly line workers, packaging workers, cleaners, and machinery operators (Punnett and Wegman, 2004) as well as clerical work and call centre work (Johansson, 1989). Repetitive work is also strongly correlated with psychosocial factors such as high demands (for example in the form of time pressure), low decision latitude and low skill discretion (see Chapter 4) (Bonde *et al.*, 2005). Repetitive work is also a key feature of alienating work (Johansson, 1989). Hence the adverse health effects associated with repetitive work have a complex aetiology: sometimes physical (such as wear on joints through repetitive movements), but also involving the stimulation of psychoneuroendocrine stress pathways (see Chapter 4). The association between repetitive work and stress has been long established in the public health literature. For example, two studies conducted in the 1970s of assembly workers in the Italian metal industry found significantly increased excretion levels of stress related hormones (adrenaline, catecholamines and hydrocortisone) amongst assembly line workers compared to non-assembly line workers (Timio and Gentili, 1976; Timio *et al.*, 1979).

Repetitive work has been associated with an increased prevalence of musculoskeletal symptoms involving the neck, shoulders, and upper extremities (Bonde *et al.*, 2005; Vinet *et al.*, 1989). In addition to pain and discomfort, the effects of repetitive work involving the arms and hands can include tingling, stiffness, numbness and loss of muscle strength (Health and Safety Executive, 2010e). Upper limb pain is also a particularly common consequence of repetitive work. This term refers to carpal tunnel syndrome, tenosynovitis, and pain without a known cause, and also encompasses other more vague diagnoses such as repetitive strain injury (RSI), cumulative trauma disorder and occupational overuse syndrome (Health and Safety Executive, 2010e). RSI is an increasingly common complaint not just amongst industrial workers, but also amongst clerical and white-collar office workers (such as call centre workers). RSI accounted for more than 60% of all occupational illnesses in the US in the 1990s with almost 1.9 million workers reporting symptoms in a national health survey (Yassi, 1997). RSI is not a diagnosis, but an umbrella term for disorders that develop as a result of repetitive movements (Yassi, 1997). Yassi identifies over 20 symptoms of tendon related disorders, peripheral nerve entrapment, neurovascular disorders, muscular disorders, and joint disorders which fall under the catch-all term RSI. Large increases in RSI have been recorded in the US, the UK, Australia, Japan and across Western Europe with, for example, rates tripling in the US since the 1980s and more than doubling in Canada in the same period (Yassi, 1997).

Together with repetitive work, important risk factors for upper limb pain include work involving forceful arm and hand movements and working in strenuous, painful and static postures (Fredriksson *et al.*, 2001). For example, a cross-sectional study of Swedish women assembly line workers (82 workers with exposure and 64 workers with no exposure to repetitive work tasks) found a statistically significant increase in the prevalence of neck and upper limb disorders in the group exposed to repetitive work involving a flexed neck and elevated and abducted arms (Ohisson *et al.*, 1995). The age-adjusted prevalence of diagnoses of the neck and shoulders was five times higher in the exposed group compared to the non-exposed group (age-adjusted prevalence OR = 5.0, 95% CI 2.2 to 11.0). Prevalence was even higher amongst piece rate workers (OR = 7.0, 95% CI 2.6 to 19.0) than salaried workers (OR = 3.6, 95% CI 1.1 to 11.0). In terms of diagnoses of the elbows and hands, this was more than three times higher in the exposed group compared to the non-exposed workers (OR = 3.5, 95% CI 1.2 to 10.0). A larger cross-sectional study from the US of 1,545 clerical workers also found an association between repetitive work tasks (computer based work) and musculoskeletal symptoms (neck, back, arm, hands) (Rossignol *et al.*, 1987). Employees who used a computer for more than 7 hours a day were 80% more likely to report a musculoskeletal condition than those clerical workers who did not use a computer at all (age-adjusted prevalence OR = 1.8, 95% CI 1.4 to 2.2). There is also tentative evidence to suggest that mental health conditions such as anxiety, depression and psychological tension tend to be more frequently reported by workers exposed to high-paced and repetitive work (Vinet *et al.*, 1989). This may be as a result of psychosocial stressors as well as the boredom of repetitive work. Evidence from the Whitehall Cohort Studies found that those who reported a great deal of boredom were more likely to report poor health and to die from cardiovascular disease (HR = 2.53, 95% CI 1.23 to 5.21) than those who were not bored (Britton and Shipley, 2010). Psychosocial factors and the Whitehall studies are covered in more detail in Chapter 4.

3.3.3 Shift work[1]

This section examines the health effects of shift work. There is a sizeable body of evidence spanning several decades that describes the negative effects of shift work on health and wellbeing (Akerstadt, 1990; Monk and Folkard, 1992). The definition of shift work can be complex (e.g. the UK Labour Force Survey has ten different categories) (McOrmond, 2004), however, it is generally understood to mean *any regularly taken employment outside the hours of 0700 and 1800'* (Monk and Folkard, 1992). Technologic advances, changes in the economy and the emergence of 24-hour societies (Beatson, 1995; Rajaratnam and Arendt, 2001) mean that shift work is no longer confined to the manufacturing and industrial sectors, and it is now also an important aspect of employment in the retail and service sectors. Shift work continues to be commonplace amongst healthcare and emergency-services personnel, with up to 50% of hospital staff working on shifts (Wilson, 2002). However, shift work is also socially patterned, being less common in graduates, and more common amongst manual workers (McOrmond, 2004), so it is they who most experience the adverse consequences of shift work on health and work-life balance.

The negative effects of shift work on health and work-life balance are well established (Akerstadt, 1990; Harrington, 2001; Monk and Folkard, 1992; Smith *et al.*, 1998). Reported health problems include sleep disturbances, fatigue, digestive problems, emotional problems, and stress related illnesses, as well as increases both in general morbidity and in sickness absence (Pilcher, *et al.*, 2000). These problems may derive from disruption to physiological, psychological, and social circadian rhythms (Akerstadt, 1990; Monk and Folkard, 1992). Shift work, particularly night work, disrupts the natural circadian rhythm, requiring people to be active at times when they would normally be sleeping, and vice versa (Monk and Folkard, 1992). This leads to problems with sleep (for example when natural alerting mechanisms such as the cortisol surge and temperature rise interrupt it) as well as with daytime functioning (when wakefulness at night is reduced by temperature drops and melatonin surges). Sudden changes in schedule can therefore have an effect akin to jet lag. Disruption of the circadian rhythm can also lead to disharmony within the body, as some functions (e.g. heart rate) adapt more quickly than others

---

[1] This section is reproduced from Bambra, *et al.* 2008b with permission from BMJ Publishing Group Ltd.

(typically the endogenous functions such as body temperature and melatonin production). This leads to desynchronization, which itself can result in psychological malaise, fatigue, and gastrointestinal problems. Realignment can take several weeks (Monk and Folkard, 1992).

The current literature base also suggests that cardiovascular problems such as hypertension and heart disease may be related to shift work (Bøggild, 2000). In addition, previous studies have highlighted a possible relationship between shift work and breast cancer (possibly due to circadian disruption) and the birth of premature babies (Institute for Environment and Health, 2005; Swerdlow, 2003; Mozurkewich *et al.*, 2000). Shift work may also involve increased risk of injuries and accidents as performance fluctuates (Frank, 2000; Health and Safety Executive, 2006a). For example, a review of injuries related to shift work concluded that workers on rotating shift work had a higher risk of injury than workers on fixed shifts and that there was a greater risk of injury on shifts that rotated more frequently (Frank, 2000).

Most existing research emphasizes the physiological changes that shift work induces, but shift work also involves considerable social desynchronization, involving working at times and on days that may make it difficult to maintain a balanced domestic and social life (European Foundation, 2000). This may result in 'work-family conflict', a form of role conflict whereby work and family pressures are incompatible and participation at work (or home) is made more difficult by participation at home (or work) (Bellavia and Frone, 2005; Madsen *et al.*, 2005). Work-family conflict is a particular issue for shift workers and night workers (as well as women) given the abnormal hours they work (Jansen *et al.*, 2003). It has been suggested that work-life imbalance can lead to poorer health. For example, a study of the Swedish working population found that self-reported health on the General Health Questionnaire (GHQ) was significantly worse among employees who experienced work-life imbalance (Johansson, 2002). Similarly, Netemeyer and colleagues (1996) found an association between increased work-family conflict and physical ill health as defined by an increase in the number of physical symptoms or somatic complaints reported by workers. Frone and colleagues (1997) found a strong association between work-family conflict and depression, poor physical health, hypertension as well as alcohol misuse. Other studies of mental health and sickness absence have also revealed similar relationships (Kinnunen and Mauno, 1998; Jansen *et al.*, 2006; Lidwall *et al.*, 2010).

3.4 Physical work environment and health inequalities

The health problems associated with the physical work environment are more prevalent amongst manual than non-manual workers. The physical

Table 3.3 UK injury rates per 100,000 employees by occupation and severity of injury (2008–09)

Occupation[a]	Fatal injuries	Major injuries	Over-3-day injuries	All reported injuries
(1) Managers and Senior Officials	0.3	43.7	90.7	134.7
(2) Professional Occupations	0.2	54.5	133.9	188.6
(3) Associate Professionals and Technical Occupations	0.1	72.6	309.8	382.5
(4) Administrative and Secretarial Occupations	–	35.0	88.5	123.5
(5) Skilled Trade Occupations	1.8	196.2	647.7	845.7
(6) Personal Service Occupations	0.1	127.0	529.4	656.4
(7) Sales and Customer Service Occupations	–	84.4	335.6	420.0
(8) Process, Plant and Machine Operatives	1.9	346.0	1 377.2	1 725.1
(9) Elementary Occupations	1.1	177.3	813.1	991.5
Not known	3.0	81.2	186.3	270.5
All Occupations	*0.5*	*108.9*	*411.6*	*521.0*

[a] UK Standard Occupational Classification.

Source: Labour Force Survey data available from http://www.hse.gov.uk/statistics/tables/occ1.htm

work environment thus remains an important contributory factor behind the social gradient in health. For example, as Table 3.3 shows, industrial injury rates in the UK exhibit significant occupational inequalities (measured using the Standard Occupation Classification [SOC], the basis of the UK's official measure of socio-economic class status—the Socio-economic Classification (see Chapter 1). It shows managers and senior officials and professional occupations having below average (0.5) fatal injury rates of 0.3 and 0.2 per 100,000 compared to above average rates of 1.9 and 1.1 per 100,000 for process, plant and machine operatives and elementary occupations respectively. Similarly, the reported injury rate for managers and senior officials was 134.7 per 100,000 and 188.6 per 100,000 for professional occupations, as opposed to 1725.1 and 991.5 per 100,000 for process, plant and machine operatives and elementary occupations respectively (the all occupation average is 521.0).

Physical working conditions make a clear contribution to health inequalities in terms of the relative exposure to risk: certain sectors of the economy and certain occupations within them are more associated with exposure to workplace hazards. These are disproportionately low skill occupational jobs. Table 3.4 shows European Union data comparing the prevalence of exposure to potentially

Table 3.4 Percentage of European employees reporting regular exposure to potentially hazardous physical working conditions by occupation (average across the 27 members of the European Union[a], 2005)

Occupation[b] Physical hazard[c]		1	2	3	4	5	6	7	8	9
Chemcial	Handling chemical substances	9.7	8.8	12.4	3.1	10.1	24.3	29.0	18.3	19.9
Environment	Noise	22.1	20.3	20.5	11.6	17.6	34.9	65.8	55.1	29.2
	Vibrations	15.5	9.1	11.4	5.8	8.6	38.0	67.1	51.8	25.3
Ergonomic	Heavy loads	29.7	11.2	18.6	15.2	34.1	72.7	65.0	51.9	48.7
	Repetitive work	50.9	45.1	50.2	56.9	60.7	83.2	81.1	76.5	74.9
	Shift work[d]	8.8	11.6	14.3	13.4	26.9	2.6	17.6	34.5	19.2

[a] EU-27: The 15 pre-2004 European Union member states (Austria, Belgium, Denmark, Finland, France, Germany, Greece, Ireland, Italy, Luxembourg, the Netherlands, Portugal, Spain, Sweden and the United Kingdom) plus 10 who joined in 2004 (Malta, Cyprus, Slovenia, Estonia, Latvia, Lithuania, Poland, the Czech Republic, Slovak Republic, and Hungary) and 2 who joined in 2007 (Romania and Bulgaria).

[b] International Standard Classification of Occupations (ISCO): (1) legislators, senior officials and managers, (2) professionals, (3) technicians and associate professionals, (4) clerks, (5) service, retail and sales workers, (6) skilled agricultural and fishery workers, (7) craft and related trades workers, (8) plant and machine operators and assemblers, (9) elementary occupations.

[c] Exposed at least 25% of working time.

[d] % working shifts.

Source: Based on data from the European Working Conditions Survey (European Working Conditions Observatory, 2005).

hazardous physical working conditions by occupation using the International Standard Classification of Occupations (ISCO). Whilst this classification is not a direct proxy for occupational or socio-economic class, it is similar to the UK's SOC and is similarly indicative of socio-economic class status (Mazzuco and Suhrcke, 2010). The data show that the two higher occupational groups (1, senior officials and managers and 2, professionals) have at least 50% less exposure to the majority of physical hazards compared to the bottom occupational groups (8, plant and machine operators and 9, elementary occupations). Industries with a high percentage of workers in lower socio-economic classes (such as construction or manufacturing) are also those at elevated risk of occupational injuries and accidents, restricted posture, repetitive movements and heavy lifting (Siegrist et al., 2009). Often these exposures are multiple. By way of example, one such occupation is mining where exposures to chemical hazards are multiple, including neurotoxic metals such as manganese or lead as well as coal dust and silica. In addition, the physical nature of the work, noise

and the use of vibrating machinery puts such workers at risk of musculoskeletal and hearing disorders (Marreilha Dos Santos *et al.*, 2010). They also work
shifts. Call/contact centre workers provide another example of multiple exposures as such workers are at a higher risk of acoustic shock injuries, as well as
RSI. Perhaps the workers most likely to be affected by workplace hazards are
those involved in the informal and temporary labour market which offers little
protection from both physical and psychosocial health hazards. Informal and
temporary workers are more likely to be employed in risky jobs or to be given
the least safe tasks within these jobs. Manual, unskilled and semi-skilled workers are more likely to work within the informal and temporary labour market
(Siegrist *et al.*, 2009). They are also more likely to develop ill health after exposure to hazards. For example, in the case of lead exposure, poor nutritional
conditions such as irregular food intake, high fat intake, and deficiencies in
calcium and iron, augment the physiological effects of lead uptake (Mahaffey,
1995). The associations between poverty and nutritional deficiencies thus
increase the likelihood of disease development amongst lower status workers.
These associations with routine and manual work highlight how individuals of
lower socio-economic class are at heightened risk of multiple and specific hazards in the physical work environment.

Examples of the elevated health risks experienced by lower-status workers
come in terms of musculoskeletal disease which has a considerably higher
prevalence amongst blue-collar as compared to white-collar workers. For
example, a US study of hospital workers found a linear social gradient in the
risk of lower back problems. Adjustment for psychosocial risk factors and biomechanical exposures (such as heavy lifting) largely eliminated the inequalities
in risk, suggesting strongly that differences in the physical nature of work
undertaken by different socio-economic classes are an important explanatory
factor in health inequalities (Gillen *et al.*, 2007). Other evidence of the importance of physical factors in terms of health inequalities comes from a Finnish
study of physical health functioning amongst 6,557 municipal employees
(Lahelma *et al.*, 2009). The study found that physical workload explained up to
95% of inequalities in physical functioning by occupational class and this led
the authors to conclude that improving physical working conditions amongst
lower occupational groups would help reduce health inequalities. Another
example is a study of the contribution of maternal working conditions to socio-
economic inequalities in birth outcomes (Dahlen-Gisselmann and Hemstrom,
2008). This longitudinal Swedish study of 280,000 mothers found that high
levels of physical demands and job hazards were more common amongst
manual as compared to non-manual classes, as were adverse birth outcomes.

Age-adjusted multivariate analysis showed that mothers who had the highest exposure to job hazards had increased risks of preterm births (15%), small for gestational age (19%), low birth weight (30%), very preterm (30%), very low birth weight (42%) and extremely preterm deliveries (54%), compared to mothers with the lowest exposure to job hazards. Similarly, physical work demands accounted for increased risks of preterm births (22%), small for gestational age (14%), low birth weight (28%), very preterm (36%), very low birth weight (28%) and extremely preterm deliveries (34%).

3.5 Welfare state regimes and the physical work environment

There is important cross-national variation in the physical work environment. Table 3.5 ('Percentage of employees reporting regular exposure to potentially hazardous physical working conditions in 17 European Countries') contains 2010 data on differences across 17 European countries in terms of exposures to the main work environment hazards. In terms of chemical hazards, the proportion of workers handling chemicals is highest in Finland at 24.3% and lowest in the Netherlands at 7.1%. In terms of environmental hazards, reported noise exposure is highest in Sweden at 36.4% and again lowest in the Netherlands at 18.3%; and vibration exposure at work ranges from 32.1% in Portugal to 14.2% in the UK. Exposure to ergonomic conditions is generally much higher in all countries than exposure to chemical or environmental hazards: exposure to heavy loads ranged from 42.3% in Greece to 23.2% in the Netherlands; repetitive work is highest in Germany at 41.6% and lowest in Luxembourg at 22.7%; and shift work is most common in Finland where over a fifth of the work force is involved in shift work (22.3%) and least common in Denmark (7.2%). There are also some differences by country in terms of work related health outcomes. By way of example, Table 3.2 contains data on fatal occupational injuries rates across Europe. Fatal accident rates range from 4.2 per 100,000 per year in Austria to just 1.3 per 100,000 per year in the UK.

These cross-national differences in the work environment and the related health outcomes, to some extent reflect differences in the industrial base of each country: those countries such as Finland, Greece or Spain with more people employed in high risk sectors such as agriculture, processing or construction will have higher exposure rates than those such as the UK or the Netherlands which have a higher proportion of their work force employed in the service sector. However, some cross-national differences in exposure may also reflect differences in the regulation of specific hazards. For example, despite a 1998 European Union directive governing lead exposure across member states, there are significant variations in how this directive is implemented.

Table 3.5 Percentage of employees reporting regular exposure[a] to potentially hazardous physical working conditions in 17 European Countries (2010)[b]

Country	Chemical	Environment		Ergonomic		
	Handling chemical substances	Noise	Vibrations	Heavy loads	Repetitive work	Shift work
Austria	17.5	24.3	23.9	36.6	32.2	12.4
Belgium	11.6	28.4	21.7	31.9	31.2	13.6
Denmark	7.4	31.9	15.6	30.0	27.8	7.2
Finland	24.3	35.9	19.5	38.3	31.8	22.3
France	18.8	33.0	23.5	39.6	24.2	18.9
Germany	18.4	30.4	25.3	30.0	41.6	16.6
Greece	18.8	33.0	27.9	42.3	23.4	16.3
Ireland	15.7	25.4	16.7	31.2	27.2	16.9
Italy	14.1	22.4	21.6	29.5	27.9	15.1
Luxembourg	17.2	27.5	24.1	27.6	22.7	11.7
Netherlands	7.1	18.3	15.4	23.2	35.9	7.0
Norway	12.7	28.9	17.4	33.5	33.7	18.4
Portugal	11.7	28.7	32.1	28.3	34.4	10.6
Spain	13.1	30.1	24.0	30.7	25.9	17.8
Sweden	16.4	36.4	16.4	37.5	32.7	11.0
Switzerland[c]	13.5	21.9	17.6	26.9	24.8	12.9
UK	15.2	23.6	14.2	36.0	29.3	17.3
EU-15[d]	15.7	20.0	21.6	32.0	31.3	15.9
EU-27[e]	15.3	29.0	22.5	33.5	30.5	17.0

[a] Exposed 25% of working time or more.

[b] EU-15 plus Norway and Switzerland.

[c] 2005 data.

[d] EU-15. The 15 pre-2004 European Union member states (Austria, Belgium, Denmark, Finland, France, Germany, Greece, Ireland, Italy, Luxembourg, the Netherlands, Portugal, Spain, Sweden and the United Kingdom).

[e] EU-27: The 15 pre-2004 European Union member states plus 10 who joined in 2004 (Malta, Cyprus, Slovenia, Estonia, Latvia, Lithuania, Poland, the Czech Republic, Slovak Republic, and Hungary) and 2 who joined in 2007 (Romania and Bulgaria).

Source: Based on data from the European Working Conditions Survey (European Working Conditions Observatory, 2010).

The European Directive stated that the occupational exposure limit in terms of inhaling lead should be no more than 0.15mg/m^3 per eight hour period; that the blood level should be no more than 70μg/100ml; and that medical surveillance of a worker or workplace should be carried out if lead in the air is greater than 0.075mg/m^3 over a forty hour week, or if a blood level concentration greater than 40μg/100ml is measured in any individual worker. However, as Taylor and colleagues (2007) demonstrate, national implementation across the member states of the European Union varies within these binding limits. In terms of inhalation levels these vary from 0.05mg/m^3 to 0.15mg/m^3, with Germany, Finland, and France all setting the level at 0.10mg/m^3, Denmark and Poland setting it at 0.05mg/m^3, whilst the other countries set the upper limit at 0.15mg/m^3. Similarly, nationally set blood levels ranged from 20μg/100ml in Denmark to 70μg/100ml in Belgium, Spain, Ireland, Lithuania and Portugal. There was little difference in terms of the blood levels set for medical surveillance.

Differences in the physical work environment may therefore also reflect differences within the wider welfare state and labour market regulation context, not least as workers in countries with higher union membership are able to obtain better working conditions (Benach *et al.*, 2007; Landsbergis, 2009). It is widely accepted that as a result of extensive work environment legislation, Sweden and Norway have the most regulated work environment (Schnall *et al.*, 2009). There is also evidence that the wider macro-economic climate also affects physical working conditions with, for example, injury rates increasing during periods of severe economic recession or industrial restructuring. For example, Nichols (1999) attributes the 25% increase in major industrial injuries between 1981 and 1984 in the UK to labour intensification processes introduced into manufacturing as part of the Thatcher government's industrial reform programme. Although there is a dearth of research that has examined the physical work environment from a welfare state regime perspective, Rosskam (2009) outlines a comparative typology of how countries differ in terms of protecting workers health. An index of input indicators of occupational health and safety legislation (such as International Labour Organisation conventions), process indicators (implementation and enforcement of legislation), and outcome indicators (injury rates, working hours etc) for 95 countries resulted in a clustering of countries into four types: 'Pacesetters', 'Pragmatists', 'Conventionals' and 'Much to be done'.

- 'Pacesetter' countries performed well across all three types of indicator (input, process, output).
- 'Pragmatists' performed well on output indicators but poorly in terms of input and process variables—they were able to achieve strong health and safety outcomes despite a poor legislative framework and slack implementation.
- Countries in the 'Conventional' group performed well in terms of input ratings, but poorly in terms of implementation and outcomes, suggesting that laws to protect workers' health were not translated into practice.

◆ The 'Much to be done' countries lack legislation to protect workers health and have poor occupational health outcomes.

In this typology, advanced market democracies fall into either the Pacesetter (Belgium, Denmark, Finland, France, Germany, Iceland, Italy, Luxembourg, Netherlands, Norway, Portugal, Spain, Sweden, Switzerland) or the Pragmatist groups (Austria, Australia, Canada, Greece, Ireland, Japan, New Zealand, UK, US) (Rosskam, 2009).

3.6 **Conclusion**

In this chapter, I have explored the health effects of exposures to different physical hazards in the work environment. Specifically I have examined chemical hazards, environmental factors, and ergonomic problems (including shift work). I have argued that despite changes in the nature of the economy in advanced market democracies, these physical hazards are still an important public health issue for many working age people. In the chapter, I have also suggested that differences in occupational exposures may well be of significance in terms of explaining socio economic inequalities in health. I have also examined how exposure to physical work environment hazards varies by country and how legislation can reduce the levels to which workers are exposed. This suggests that political action leading to health and safety legislation can mediate the effects of the physical work environment on health and, given differential exposure rates, socio-economic health inequalities. Above all I have shown that the aetiology of occupational disease is complex and alluded to the fact that the hazards associated with physical aspects of the workplace often interact with those in the psychosocial work environment. Many of the hazards examined in this chapter, for example noise, vibrations, ergonomic exposures, shift work and even exposures to hazardous chemicals, can all impact on health psychosocially as well as physically (Amick and Kasl, 2000). The psychosocial work environment is the topic of the next chapter.

3.7 **Further reading**

MacDonald, C. (2000) (ed.). *Epidemiology of work-related diseases* (2nd ed.). London: BMJ Books.

Nichols, T. (1999). 'Death and injury at work: A sociological approach'. In: N. Daykin and L. Doyal (eds.) *Health and Work: Critical Perspectives*. London, Macmillan.

Rosskam, E. (2009). 'Measuring the protection of workers' health: a national work security index'. In: P. Schnall, M. Dobson, E. Rosskam (eds.) *Unhealthy work: causes, consequences, cures*. New York, Baywood.

Chapter 4

The psychosocial work environment and risks to health

The nature of work has altered considerably in North America, Japan and Europe over the past two decades, with a decrease in industrial employment and an increase in the size of the service sector. For example in the UK, the manufacturing sector's share of gross domestic product has declined by nearly 50% over the last 25 years. Similarly, 7.26 million individuals were employed in the UK manufacturing sector in 1979; this figure had shrunk by 40% by 1990 (Hine and Wright, 1998). The landscape of the workplace has also shifted with the overtly physical demands (such as heavy lifting and carrying) and hazards (such as exposures to noise, vibrations, or hazardous chemicals) associated with industrial employment being displaced for the majority of the workforce by psychosocial stressors typical of jobs in the increasingly dominant service sector (Benach *et al.*, 2007). The workplace has thus moved from being understood as predominantly a material influence on health, to being a psychosocial one. The 'psychosocial work environment' is a collective way of referring to psychological and social influences on health such as time pressure, monotonous work, social reciprocity, job control and autonomy, fairness, work demands, job security, as well as social contact between co-workers and supervisors. Or, to put it another way, the psychosocial work environment is a way of describing the key elements of labour alienation (Navarro, 1982; Crinson and Yuill, 2008).

The psychosocial work environment is a meso-level factor, akin to family or community, which acts as a 'bridge' between the structural (particularly the social stratifications of welfare state capitalism) and agency (individual level cognitive and behavioural responses) determinants of health (Martikainen *et al.*, 2002). According to the psychosocial explanation of health and health inequalities (see Chapter 1), how individuals perceive their status relative to others in the social hierarchy is an important determinant of health (Bartley, 2004). Specifically, feelings of inferiority or subordination are thought to induce stress responses which can be sustained in their duration and effect. Indeed, current thinking suggests that exposures to adverse biological, psychological and social stimuli are cumulative and that the effects of these exposures amass and are compounded across the life course (Bartley, 2004). Siegrist and Marmot (2004) highlight how gaining a positive experience of self is an important motivation underpinning an individual's engagement with his or her social environment. In order to achieve a positive experience of self, the psychosocial environment must offer opportunities for autonomy, belonging, interacting, contributing and receiving feedback (Siegrist and Marmot, 2004). Likewise, positive psychosocial environments can increase self-esteem by enabling social contact and by providing arenas for positive social interaction and appropriate mechanisms for feedback and support (Siegrist and Marmot, 2004). In contrast, negative and alienating psychosocial environments in which experiences of control, inclusion and autonomy are low can result in a constricted sense of self, low self-esteem and a resulting increase in psychological stress.

Psychosocial environments exist in various places, (for example the home, the community, and the workplace) but given the wider role of the relations of production, the social importance of work to self-identity, perception and treatment by others, as well as the role of occupational status (or lack of work) within labour market based societal hierarchies, the psychosocial effects of the work environment are arguably more significant than those of other environments. Workplaces usually function in extremely hierarchical ways with a clear division by occupational status, as well as by gender and race. The workplace thus acts as a microcosm of wider societal stratifications, whilst also, through the centrality of the production process to societal infrastructure, contributing greatly to their development. Aspects of the psychosocial work environment which can help to foster feelings of self-efficacy and self-esteem (such as supportive social and managerial networks, feelings of autonomy and control over how work is undertaken and appropriate recognition and reward for contributions made) are more usually experienced by higher grade non-manual staff, with more negative, alienating psychosocial work conditions concentrated amongst manual and lower grade occupations. Women and ethnic minorities are more likely to work in adverse psychosocial work environments than men (Need *et al.*, 2005). Workplace psychosocial environments are therefore important means through which a positive or negative sense of self is created and location within the wider social hierarchy established. They are therefore significant influences on health and health inequalities.

A number of theorists have developed conceptual frameworks to explain the effects of the psychosocial work environment on health, each of which privileges a particular element of the psychosocial work environment. In public health research, the most popular contemporary explanations which have been applied to both physical and mental health (as opposed to one or the other like Warr's vitamin theory of work and mental health, Warr 1994) include the demand-control-support model (Karasek and Theorell, 1990); effort-reward imbalance theory (Siegrist, 1996), and organisational injustice theory (Elovainio *et al.*, 2002). In this chapter, I focus on these three main theoretical approaches. The chapter is divided into four main sections. The first section provides a brief overview of the biological pathways between work stress and ill health before outlining the three main theories of the psychosocial work environment. The chapter then summarises the epidemiological evidence on the impact of psychosocial risk factors at work on physical and mental health. It then examines their contribution to socio-economic inequalities in health. I conclude the chapter with an examination of how the relationship between psychosocial work factors and health varies by welfare state.

4.1 Psychosocial theories of the work environment

This section outlines the biological pathways between stress and ill health. It outlines the three main theories of the psychosocial work environment and explores how they relate to concepts of labour alienation.

4.1.1 Chronic stress and health

Assumptions about the relationship between stress and health underpin all psychosocial models of the work environment. At a biological level exposure to stress is thought to stimulate both the sympathetic-adrenomedullary and the hypothalamic-pituitary-adrenocortical systems (Bartley, 2004). Brunner (1997) uses the 'fight or flight' evolutionary response to stress to explain the biological mechanisms underpinning the body's reactions to psychosocial stressors. When the body perceives stress in the form of an adverse environmental trigger, the sympathetic-adrenomedullary pathway is stimulated with the rapid release of adrenaline and noradrenaline. These neurotransmitters orchestrate a cascade of physiological events including, amongst other changes, increases in blood pressure, heart rate and the release of energy resources (Brunner, 1997). Originally this response would have been adaptive in that it would enable the individual to retreat from the stressor or to fight back. However, such 'fight or flight' responses are not possible when exposures are longer term (for example if the stressor is poor relations with work superiors) and alternatively the response may be suppressed (as in the case of workplace bullying (Bartley, 2004)).

In addition the hypothalamic-pituitary-adrenocortical system is stimulated. In simple terms, this results in the release of cortisol, a glucocorticoid hormone, which has multiple physiological effects including the release of energy resources, suppression of the immune system and direct effects on mood

(Brunner, 1997). The process of cortisol secretion involves communication between the hypothalamus and pituitary gland (both located in the lower central part of the brain) to cause the release of adrenocorticotropic hormone in response to a stress stimulus. Adrenocorticotropic hormone subsequently induces the production and release of cortisol from the adrenal cortex (of the adrenal glands located above the kidneys) into the blood (Bartley, 2004).

Brunner (1997) highlights how activation of both the sympathetic-adrenomedullary and the hypothalamic-pituitary-adrenocortical systems is likely to be psychosocially patterned with differences in the magnitude and length of responses related to individual coping resources and differential exposures to adverse environmental factors. Prolonged activation of the autonomic nervous system and neuroendocrine cascades in this way is likely to result in reduced biological resilience and impaired homeostasis over time with measureable health consequences such as hypertension (a known risk factor for cardiovascular disease) or metabolic syndrome (a cluster of risk factors including abdominal obesity) (Chandola et al., 2006). This begins to provide some explanation for the underpinning mechanistic pathways between chronic work stress and the manifestation of physical and mental ill health. Moreover, the effects of stress are not just experienced directly via biological responses to stress triggers, but also indirectly through changes to health related behaviours such as modifications to smoking patterns, alcohol consumption, dietary intake or participation in physical activity (Martikainen et al., 2004).

4.1.2 Demand-control-support

Karasek and Theorell were amongst the first theorists to articulate how non-physical aspects of the work environment, specifically job task profiles, interact to cause stress (Karasek 1979; Karasek and Theorell, 1990). Karasek and Theorell hypothesised that jobs with high psychological demands coupled with low levels of control or decision latitude were associated with increased exposure to stress and ill health effects. Psychological demands were conceptualised in terms of time pressure, high work pace, high work load and conflicting demands, while control or decision latitude was defined as including decision authority (control over workload) and skill discretion (variety of work and skill development and utilisation). This is known as the demand-control model or the job strain model (Karasek 1979; Karasek and Theorell, 1990). According to Karasek's model, jobs characterised by excessive psychological demands in combination with low control are 'high stress' jobs because they do not enable individual autonomy and are often conducted in high pressure contexts which can lead to an increased risk of stress related morbidity. Conversely, work with high demands but also high control is termed 'active work' as the worker is able to manage his or her own workload and has a high degree of choice and autonomy over how the work is undertaken. Karasek and Theorell (1990) suggest that strain and learning are related so that opportunities to learn new skills mitigate the stress inducing effects of high strain in active jobs. Conversely, 'passive jobs' characterised by low demands and low control are likely to have fewer opportunities for learning.

In the late 1980s Johnson and colleagues extended the demand-control model to include the influence of social support as a mediating factor in the relationship between high demands, low control and ill health (Johnson *et al.*, 1988). It was suggested that the presence of social support from co-workers and supervisors in the workplace might in some way moderate or act as a buffer to reduce ill health effects (Stansfeld *et al.*, 1997). The term high 'iso-strain' is used to refer to working conditions defined by high demands, low control and low social support.

Low status occupations in both the industrial and service sectors tend to be associated with high strain and iso-strain (Marmot *et al.*, 2006). Karasek and Theorell (1990) observe that high psychological demands, low decision latitude and limited autonomy are frequent in work marked by an assembly-line approach both in industrial and non-industrial settings. The distribution of low control and low support has been shown to follow the social gradient (with high strain and iso-strain being found in low status workers) although the same it is not true for high job demands (Bosma *et al.*, 1997; Siegrist *et al.*, 2009). Data from European surveys illustrate that since 1990, both work intensity and job demands have increased whilst at the same time, levels of job control have decreased: the psychosocial work environment is becoming increasingly stressful (Benach *et al.*, 2007).

Critics of the demand-control and demand-control-support models have suggested that certain psychosocial factors are more important than others (e.g. control is more important than demand) (Siegrist and Marmot, 2004; Godin and Kittel, 2003). Commentators have also criticised the overly structuralist nature of the demand-control-support model and have highlighted the possibly mediating effects of individual level factors, such as mastery or self-efficacy, on the pathway between psychosocial stressors and physical or psychological morbidity (Marmot *et al.*, 2006). These criticisms have resulted in the promotion by some of the effort-reward imbalance model in relation to health.

4.1.3 Effort-reward imbalance

The effort-reward imbalance model represents an alternative hypothesis which is centred on the concept of social reciprocity in the work contract

(Marmot *et al.*, 2006). Social reciprocity is defined as the *'mutual co-operative investments based on the norm of return expectancy, where efforts are assumed to be equalised by respective rewards'* (Siegrist, 2005: 1033, following Gouldner, 1960). Social reciprocity is at the heart of the work contract: certain tasks or obliga tions are performed in exchange for equitable rewards. The premise of the effort-reward imbalance model is that psychosocial stress results from a mismatch between the efforts made by workers and the rewards they receive from their employer in terms of pay, esteem, job security and career opportunities (Siegrist, 1996). Working with inequitable rewards when balanced against the efforts exerted is thought to induce prolonged stress responses which can lead to adverse health outcomes (Siegrist *et al.*, 2009). In contrast, where the balance between efforts and rewards is perceived to be more equitable (i.e. when sufficient rewards are received), positive emotions are elicited leading to sustained health and wellbeing. For Siegrist and colleagues (2004), the work contract is marked by a lack of clarity regarding the accepted equilibrium between efforts exerted and rewards received. They also observe that this burden of asymmetry between efforts and rewards tends to be disproportionately shouldered by lower socio-economic classes who lack flexibility due to low skill level or lack of mobility.

A discord between efforts and rewards can be observed at both structural (extrinsic) and individual (intrinsic) levels (Siegrist, 2005). Sigerist (2005) identifies a number of examples where structural or extrinsic causes of failed reciprocity can occur including limited mobility, lack of opportunities for skills development, confinement to fixed-term contracts and a dearth of alternative labour market opportunities, particularly when unemployment levels are high. Equally, certain psychological characteristics including overcommitment, a high need for approval, inappropriate perceptions of demands and poorly developed coping strategies are cited as reasons for failed reciprocity at the individual or intrinsic level (Siegrist, 2005). In some instances, workers may sacrifice short-term rewards, for example by accepting 'unfair' job arrangements such as fixed-term contracts, in order to gain longer term rewards such as career advancement (Siegrist, 2005). However, the model demonstrates that a failure to equalise efforts and rewards over time results in high stress levels and subsequent stress related ill health.

4.1.4 Organisational injustice

The organisational injustice model is a more recently developed theory of the psychosocial work environment. It focuses on issues of fairness, justice and equity in the workplace. This is a significant extension of the demand-control-support and effort-reward imbalance models of the relationship between the psychosocial environment and health, particularly because it captures the importance of equity and fairness at work (National Institute for Health and Clinical Excellence, 2009a). The emergence of atypical forms of employment (including flexitime, part-time working and fixed-term contracts) and the changing demographic of the workforce have increased interest in the notion of organisational justice (Foresight Mental Capital and Wellbeing Project, 2008). In some ways, this model can be seen as applying more political concepts to the workplace.

Organisational justice is composed of three aspects: procedural justice (relating to formal decision-making procedures), distributive justice (the fairness and equity of decisions), and relational justice (the fairness of supervisors' actions and decisions) (Kivimäki *et al.*, 2003a). Much of the literature to date on the relationships between organisational justice and health focuses on relational justice. According to Head and colleagues (2007) relational justice '*involves the extent to which supervisors consider employees' viewpoints, are able to suppress personal biases, and take steps to deal with subordinates in a fair and truthful manner*'. High levels of perceived justice in the workplace invoke '*a sense of psychological security*' (National Institute for Health and Clinical Excellence, 2009a: 36) and cooperation, while low levels are thought to result in de-motivation, lack of stability, increased stress and elevated risks for both physical and mental ill health (Head *et al.*, 2007: 433). Although aspects of the organisational injustice explanation of work stress coincide with the other models of psychosocial stress, as Elovainio *et al.* (2002: 105) explain, the concept of organisational injustice helps to identify other important constructs which shape the psychosocial work environment such as "*organisational consistency, accuracy, ethicality, managerial decision-making, procedures used, and discrimination in organizations*" which may have significant influences on the pathway between work stress and ill health.

4.1.5 **Work, stress, and alienation**

These are the three mainstream theoretical models for conceptualising the effects of the psychosocial work environment on health. The models are not mutually exclusive, as whilst each model offers a plausible explanation of how factors in the psychosocial work environment impact on health outcomes, there is some overlap between each of the different frameworks, and taken together they identify what can be described as 'toxic' elements of the psychosocial work environment (Siegrist *et al.*, 2009): specifically, low control, low reward and injustice at work. Individually these all have negative impacts on health but in combination their effects are magnified (Siegrist *et al.*, 2009). However, none of the models link the structures of the work environment into the broader social and material context and none reflect on the psychosocial work environment in terms of labour alienation (Crinson and Yuill, 2008).

The political economy concept of alienation actually forms an essential backdrop to understanding how the psychosocial work environment produces stress, which in turn leads to poor physical and mental health (Coburn, 1979; Navarro, 1982; Crinson and Yuill, 2008). The psychosocial work environment literature has placed too much reliance on psychological and evolutionary models. This is not sufficient as the material basis of these psychosocial experiences has also to be considered (Crinson and Yuill, 2008). Alienation is the result of the appropriation of surplus labour value (profit making) within capitalist economies. Alienation includes the separation of the worker from the product of work (labour product alienation), from control over the process of work (labour process alienation), from his own skills and knowledge (self-alienation), and from his fellow workers (fellow being alienation):

> 'What constitutes alienated labour? First, that the work is external to the worker—that it is not part of his nature; and that consequently he does not fulfil himself in his work, but denies himself, has a feeling of misery rather than wellbeing, does not develop freely his mental and physical energies, but is physically exhausted and mentally debased'.

> Marx (1963: 124)

In terms of the mainstream discourse of the psychosocial work environment, alienation can be considered as: effort-reward imbalance, low control at work, lack of organisational justice, lack of creativity, the high demands and lack of variety resulting from monotonous or repetitive work, and a lack of social support from colleagues and supervisors. Alienation thus impacts on health at both the physical (direct) and psychosocial (indirect) levels in terms of the cumulative physical damage to the health of the worker as a result of the physical production process, and also the psychosocial impacts on health generated by the stress which results from the inequalities innate within the system of production (Crinson and Yuill, 2008). Taking a political economy perspective means that workplace psychosocial models can be used to explain health outcomes within the wider material context in which it is not just the distribution of psychosocial stressors which matters but how they are related to the system of production (Muntaner and Lynch, 1999; Lynch *et al.*, 2000).

4.2 The Psychosocial work environment and health

In this section, an overview is given of the empirical literature which has linked models of the psychosocial work environment with various stress related physical (most notably cardiovascular disease and musculoskeletal conditions) and mental (psychological morbidity) health conditions.

4.2.1 Demand-control-support and health

The demand-control-support model was the first to be applied to health outcomes (particularly by the Whitehall studies—Box 4.1), and as such there is a

Box 4.1 The Whitehall studies

The Whitehall studies (I and II) are longitudinal cohorts of British civil servants which aimed to investigate risk factors for ill health. The first Whitehall cohort was set up by Geoffrey Rose and Donald Reid, two British epidemiologists who were interested in examining risk factors for cardio-respiratory disease and diabetes. The original cohort included 18,000 male civil servants who were followed from 1967. This study presented convincing evidence for the first time to disprove the commonly held belief that higher status workers encountered elevated stress levels and as such higher rates of ill health such as coronary heart disease. For coronary heart disease mortality at 10 year follow-up, the relative risk was 2.2 in low grade clerical workers and 1.6 for intermediate grade staff when compared with 1.0 for senior level administrative workers (Marmot *et al.*, 1984; Marmot and Brunner, 2005). A similar social gradient was observed for all-cause mortality, and non-coronary heart disease mortality (Marmot and Brunner, 2005). Based on follow-up data over a period of 25 years it was shown that the differences in cause-specific mortality observed could not simply be explained by risk factors such as cholesterol, smoking, systolic blood pressure, glucose intolerance and diabetes (van Rossum *et al.*, 2000). Indeed, it was demonstrated that these risk factors accounted for only one third of the difference in mortality between high and low grade workers (Marmot *et al.*, 1984; van Rossum *et al.*, 2000). At this point psychosocial explanations gained popularity in accounting for the observed differences in health (Marmot *et al.*, 1984; Marmot and Brunner, 2004).

The Whitehall study II, set up between 1985 and 1988, included women in the cohort of 10,308 non-industrial civil servants aged 35–55 years and aimed to unpack *the social gradient* in morbidity and mortality further by examining social and occupational influences on health (Bosma *et al.*, 1998; Marmot and Brunner, 2005). Participants ranged from low occupational grade clerical workers to middle ranked executives through to senior administrator grade staff. Data relating to material and social circumstances, health behaviours, and mental and physical health were routinely collected at five year intervals (Marmot and Brunner, 2005). Data on psychosocial factors were also obtained.

greater empirical evidence base relating to Karasek's model and its derivatives. This is reflected in the overview of studies provided in this section and in the next on health inequalities. A clear issue with the demand-control-support model is that whilst there is compelling evidence in relation to the multivariate model relationships (e.g. iso-strain or job strain) with health outcomes, only job control seems to have a significant univariate relationship with adverse health outcomes. There is little compelling evidence of univariate associations with health between high demands or low support. Job control arguably emerges as the most important psychosocial work environment determinant. Further, the evidence on the role of social support as a potential buffer against the negative health effects of low control is equivocal (Egan *et al.*, 2007; Bambra *et al.*, 2007b). This is evident in the summaries provided below.

Coronary heart disease and associated risk factors

Cardiovascular diseases including heart disease and stroke are the major cause of death in industrialised countries (Landbergis *et al.*, 2009). An extensive international literature regarding the association between the demand-control-support model (specifically the issue of job strain) and coronary heart disease has amassed over the past two decades. A number of systematic reviews have been conducted on this topic, many of which strengthen the hypothesis that job strain is likely to be important in the aetiology of coronary heart disease. For example, a systematic review of prospective cohort studies, conducted in various occupational settings, found that of ten studies assessing the association between job strain and coronary heart disease, six reported statistically significant associations (Hemmingway and Marmot, 1999). The relative risk of coronary heart disease ranged from 1.5 to 4.95 for adverse psychosocial work characteristics (high demands, low control or job strain). In an update to this systematic review, a strong or moderate association between psychosocial work factors and coronary heart disease was found in the majority of prospective studies included in the review (Kuper *et al.*, 2003). A third systematic review (Belkic *et al.*, 2004) examined a range of study designs: longitudinal, case controlled and cross-sectional studies, and found consistent evidence of an association between exposure to job strain and cardiovascular disease in men; the evidence for women was less convincing.

In terms of primary data, several studies have drawn upon the Whitehall II cohort (see Box 4.1) to investigate the association between aspects of the demand-control-support model and coronary heart disease (Bosma *et al.*, 1997; Kuper and Marmot, 2003). For example, Bosma and colleagues (1997) followed the cohort over a 5 year period and found that low control in the workplace increased the risk of subsequent coronary disease in both men and women.

The odds ratio (OR) for a coronary event for workers with low control was 1.93 (95% confidence interval [CI] 1.34 to 2.77) when compared with those with high control. The evidence presented suggested that low control was more important than other work related psychosocial factors in increasing the risk of coronary heart disease (high job demands, social support and job strain were not shown to be associated with new coronary disease). The association between low control and new coronary heart disease was not explained by traditional coronary risk factors (e.g. smoking, BMI, alcohol use, serum cholesterol, hypertension and exercise) or occupational grade (Marmot *et al.*, 2006).

Evidence has also accumulated to support the association between job strain (low control, high demands) and coronary heart disease (Kuper and Marmot, 2003). In one particular study, exposure was assessed by self-reported psychosocial work characteristics over a mean follow-up period of 11 years and the outcome was defined as validated incident coronary heart disease (Kuper and Marmot, 2003). After adjusting for occupational grade, socioeconomic status and traditional coronary heart disease risk factors, job strain was the strongest predictor of incident coronary heart disease (hazard ratio [HR] 1.38 95% CI 1.10 to 1.75) (Kuper and Marmot, 2003). The effect of job strain was strongest in younger workers. High job demands predicted future coronary heart disease in both men (grade adjusted HR 1.27 95% CI 1.00 to 1.60) and women (grade adjusted HR 1.51, 95% CI 1.10 to 2.05) but low decision latitude predicted coronary heart disease in men only (age-adjusted HR 1.55, 95%CI 1.26 to 1.90, p=0.0001). There was no modifying effect of social support at work (Kuper and Marmot, 2003).

Studies from outside of the UK also tend to support the hypothesis that job strain is associated with coronary heart disease. For example, data from a prospective cohort study (mean follow-up 25.6 years) conducted in Finland found that, after adjusting for age and sex, job strain doubled the risk of cardiovascular mortality for workers free of 'overt disease' at baseline: the relative risk (RR) was 2.2, 95% CI 1.2 to 4.2 (Kivimäki *et al.*, 2002). Similar findings were reported in a large international case control study of myocardial infarction and psychosocial risk factors (the INTERHEART study). Analysis of 11,119 cases and 13,648 controls from 52 countries showed that permanent stress at work more than doubled the risk of myocardial infarction (OR 2.14, 95% CI 1.73 to 2.64) after adjusting for age, sex, geographic region, and smoking (Rosengren *et al.*, 2004).

Health behaviours such as smoking, physical activity and dietary intake are known to be important in the aetiology of cardiovascular disease (as well as other diseases) (Bambra *et al.*, 2009a, 2010b). In acknowledgement of the role of health behaviours in preventable chronic disease and the putative effect of the psychosocial work environment on health behaviours, Lallukka and associates (2008) conducted a cross-national comparative study to examine the association between job strain and adverse health behaviours (unhealthy food habits, physical inactivity, heavy drinking, smoking and obesity). Analysis of data from three comparable cohort studies (white collar workers aged between 45 and 60 years) based in England, Finland and Japan, uncovered a mixed picture of evidence. For example, the combination of low job demands and low control was associated with physical inactivity in English men (fully adjusted OR = 1.64, 95% CI 1.18 to 2.27) and Finnish women (fully adjusted OR 1.31, 95% CI 1.05 to 1.62). In Japan, job strain was associated with smoking behaviour in men (fully adjusted OR 1.56, 95% CI 1.01 to 2.41). Lallukka and colleagues (2008) hypothesised that the complex patterning of associations observed is likely to be related to the varying social, cultural and workplace contexts.

Brunner and colleagues (2007) worked with the Whitehall II cohort to explore the effect of cumulative iso-strain (high demands, low control and low social support) on obesity as measured by body mass index (BMI) and waist circumference. A dose-response relationship was observed for both obesity indicators over a period of 19 years, with greater exposure to stress being associated with increased odds of general obesity (BMI $\geq$30 kg/m^2) and central obesity (waist circumference >102 cm in men and >88 cm in women) (Brunner et al., 2007). Effect estimates were only slightly reduced after exclusion of individuals defined as obese at baseline and adjustment for established confounders, such as health behaviours and socio-economic status (Brunner et al., 2007). The same authors also observed a dose-response relationship between exposure to chronic stress (measured by iso-strain) and the metabolic syndrome (Chandola et al., 2006). The metabolic syndrome refers to a combination of risk factors for coronary heart disease and type II diabetes which includes abdominal obesity, plus any two of the following indicators: raised triglycerides, reduced high density lipoprotein-cholesterol, raised blood pressure, raised fasting plasma glucose (Alberti et al., 2005). Using data from the Whitehall II cohort (with a mean follow-up period of 14 years), Chandola and colleagues (2006) showed that cumulative exposure to iso-strain (the presence of iso-strain at three or more time points) more than doubled the odds of developing metabolic syndrome. The association remained statistically significant after adjusting for employment grade and self-reported health behaviours including smoking status, absence of daily fruit and vegetable consumption, heavy alcohol use, and lack of exercise (OR for men and women combined 2.39, 95% CI 1.36 to 4.21). Likewise the association remained after excluding individuals obese at baseline. Importantly the data exhibited a social gradient, with men of the lowest occupational grade having twice the odds of developing metabolic syndrome of those in the highest grade. When the authors adjusted for iso-strain the gradient was reduced by 11%.

Musculoskeletal conditions

A smaller evidence base relates to the association between the demand-control-support model and musculoskeletal disorders such as lower back pain and upper limb pain. Given the complex aetiology of these conditions and the inextricable links between physical and psychosocial stressors, the evidence for these associations is less substantive in comparison with the literature on coronary heart disease. Despite this observation, it is widely acknowledged that the psychosocial work environment has an important role to play in musculoskeletal disease. For example, researchers agree that physical or biomechanical stressors can only partially explain the high prevalence of musculoskeletal symptoms in certain occupations (Bongers *et al.*, 1993). Indeed, it is estimated that for symptoms of the back, the aetiologic fraction explained by physical load is only between 11% and 58% (Burdorf and Sorock, 1997).

Existing systematic reviews are inconsistent in terms of finding positive associations between psychosocial risk factors in the work environment and lower back pain. For example, Bongers and colleagues (1993) concluded that although it was difficult to separate out the contribution of physical load, there was some evidence to suggest a positive association between musculoskeletal disease and demand-type psychosocial variables (such as monotonous work, perceived work load and time pressure) as well as low control and lack of social support. The authors also suggested that stress was likely to be a mediating factor in the aetiology of musculoskeletal disorders. These findings were supported to some extent by Burdorf and Sorock (1997) who identified evidence to suggest that low job decision latitude and job dissatisfaction were predictors of lower back pain, but they were unable to demonstrate these associations consistently. Similarly, Hoogendoorn and colleagues (2000) reported an association between low levels of social support and low job satisfaction and lower back pain. However, in a later systematic review, Hartvigsen and colleagues (2004) found little evidence for a positive association between organisational aspects of work and social support in the workplace and lower back pain.

Mental health

Not only are psychosocial work characteristics known to be associated with physical morbidity and health behaviours, the combination of high demands (including high work pace and conflicting demands) and low control and support at work has also been shown to predict mental ill health (Stansfeld, 2002). Stansfeld and colleagues (1999) drawing on the Whitehall II cohort (see Box 4.1) conducted a prospective study (1985–1993) which used the 30-item

General Health Questionnaire (GHQ) to examine the longitudinal association between psychosocial work stressors and development of psychiatric disorders. After adjustment for age, employment grade and baseline GHQ score, high demands, and to a lesser extent low decision authority and low social support in the workplace at baseline were associated with an increased likelihood of psychiatric disorders at follow-up. For example, for men high demands at work were associated with a 33% increased risk of ill health (fully adjusted OR = 1.33, 95% CI 1.1 to 1.6) and a 26% elevated risk for women (fully adjusted OR = 1.26 95% CI 1.1 to 1.7). The authors also examined the effect of *changes* in psychosocial work characteristics on mental ill health and found that for both women and men, changes to job demands had a significant impact on the development of morbidity, with a beneficial change significantly reducing risk (fully adjusted OR men = 0.82, 95% CI 0.7 to 1.0; fully adjusted OR women = 0.72, 95% CI 0.5 to 1.0) and a negative change in job demands increasing the risk of psychiatric disorder (fully adjusted OR men = 1.66, 95% CI 1.4 to 2.0; fully adjusted OR women = 1.31, 95% CI 1.0 to 1.7).

Drawing on data from the GAZEL cohort study (a longitudinal study of 20,624 workers in the French National Electricity and Gas Company, followed since 1989) Paterniti and colleagues (2002) also reported a moderate association in both men and women between high job demands and low social support at work and depression as measured by the Centre for Epidemiologic Studies Depression (CES-D) scale. Low control, however, was predictive of increased depression score for men only. A Swedish study also examined the impact of the psychosocial work environment on emotional exhaustion (Hanson *et al.*, 2008). The study followed a cohort of 1,511 men and 1,493 women from the Swedish Longitudinal Occupational Survey of Health (SLOSH) over a three year period and found that high job demands were important predictors of emotional exhaustion in both men (fully adjusted OR = 2.09, 95% CI 1.52 to 2.88) and women (fully adjusted OR = 1.79, 95% CI 1.36 to 2.35). Similar associations were found with regard to low decision authority (fully adjusted men OR = 1.36, 95% CI 0.98 to 1.88; fully adjusted women OR = 1.41, 95% CI 1.07 to 1.86). However, in terms of social support the findings for men and women differed: lack of support from superiors was an independent predictor of emotional exhaustion in men (fully adjusted OR = 1.65, 95% CI 1.19 to 2.31), whilst lack of support from co-workers predicted it in women (fully adjusted OR = 1.92, 95% CI 1.25 to 2.93).

4.2.2 Effort-reward imbalance and health

A number of prospective cohort studies have shown that effort-reward imbalance or failed reciprocity increases the risk of various stress related diseases. Most of the literature to date examines the association between effort-reward imbalance and cardiovascular disease and evidence for the association is particularly compelling for men rather than women. Evidence from the Whitehall II studies (see Box 4.1) demonstrated an elevated risk of new coronary heart disease for workers with high efforts (defined as competitiveness, work related over-commitment and hostility) and low rewards (defined as poor progression prospects and a blocked career trajectory). The fully adjusted OR for men and women combined was 2.15, and the effect was found to be statistically significant (95% CI 1.15 to 4.01). Similar findings were reported in a Finnish study (Kivimäki *et al.*, 2002). After adjusting for the main confounders (including occupational, physiological and behavioural factors) the risk ratio for workers with an imbalance between efforts (pace of work and physical and mental load) and rewards (low salary, lack of social approval, and few career opportunities) and cardiovascular mortality was 2.4 (95% CI 1.3 to 4.4).

In relation to general health outcomes, cross-sectional data from the GAZEL cohort illuminated a statistically significant association between effort-reward imbalance and self-reported health for both men (fully adjusted OR = 1.80, 95% CI 1.37 to 2.37) and women (fully adjusted OR = 1.94, 95% CI 1.27 to 2.96) (Niedhammer *et al.*, 2004). Over-commitment was also a significant risk factor for both men (OR = 1.46, 95% CI 1.25 to 1.71) and women (OR = 1.81, 95% CI 1.41 to 2.32). Longitudinal prospective data from the study was less conclusive as at 12 month follow-up, effort-reward imbalance was not a significant predictor of poor self-reported health for men or women, and over-commitment was only significant for men (fully adjusted OR = 1.67, 95% CI 1.32 to 2.12). A comprehensive literature review of 45 studies examining the relationship between effort-reward imbalance and a range of psychological and physical health outcomes found that there was growing empirical support for the extrinsic effort-reward imbalance model: high efforts in combination with low rewards increase the risk of poor health (van Vegchel *et al.*, 2005).

Stansfeld and colleagues (1999) were the first to provide longitudinal evidence from the Whitehall II cohort on the association between effort-reward imbalance and mental ill health. They examined various measures of the psychosocial work environment and mental health status as assessed using the General Health Questionnaire (GHQ). After adjusting for age, employment grade and baseline GHQ score, effort-reward imbalance was shown to increase the risk of psychiatric disorder in both men (fully adjusted OR 2.64, 95% CI 2.0 to 3.5) and women (fully adjusted OR = 1.48, 95% CI 0.9 to 2.3). These associations persisted even when GHQ cases at baseline were excluded from the analyses.

In an examination of Siegrist's model of job stress and depression in a Japanese manufacturing plant, Tsutsumi and colleagues' (2001) small study (n=190) found that effort-reward imbalance (fully adjusted OR 4.13, 95% CI 1.39 to12.28) and over-commitment (fully adjusted OR − 2.56, 95% CI 1.01 to 6.47) were independently associated with depressive symptoms as measured using the Center for Epidemiologic Studies Depression scale (CES-D). Similar findings in relation to associations between the effort-reward model and the CES-D scale were reported in a cross-national study of psychosocial work factors and depression (Pikhart et al., 2004). Using cross-sectional data from three cities across Central and Eastern Europe (Russia, Poland and Czech Republic), Pikhart and colleagues (2004) found that effort-reward imbalance was strongly associated with depression scores. There was a dose-response relationship with an increase of one standard deviation in effort-reward imbalance associated with a 2.0 point increase (95% CI 1.5 to 2.4) in the depression score. This association persisted after controlling for age, sex and country.

These observations are consistent with a Belgium study of effort-reward imbalance and health (Godin et al., 2005). This prospective study of 1986 employees across four different worksites reported that consistent effort-reward imbalance (at both baseline and 12 month follow-up) was negatively associated for both men and women with depression (fully adjusted OR men = 2.8, 95% CI 1.3 to 5.7; OR women = 4.6, 95% CI 2.3 to 9.0) and anxiety (fully adjusted OR men = 2.3, 95% CI 1.1 to 4.8; OR women = 4.5, 95% CI 2.1 to 9.8). Over-commitment was also found to be predictive of depression in both men (fully adjusted OR = 2.4, 95% CI 1.4 to 4.1) and women (fully adjusted OR = 1.8, 95% CI 1.0 to 3.0) but it only predicted the onset of anxiety in men (fully adjusted OR 2.5, 95% CI 1.5 to 4.4). Godin and colleagues (2005) also highlighted that associations with mental ill health are generally stronger for the extrinsic (structural), as opposed to intrinsic (individual) components of the effort-reward imbalance model.

4.2.3 Organisational injustice

An emerging body of work suggests that relational injustice at work is related to cardiovascular morbidity and mortality (Elovainio et al., 2006a; Kivimäki et al., 2003a, 2005). For example, using data from the Whitehall II cohort (see Box 4.1), Kivimäki and colleagues (2005) found that men who reported a high level of perceived justice at work had a 35% lower risk of incident coronary heart disease when compared with men reporting a low or medium level of justice in the workplace: fully adjusted Hazard Ratio (HR) = 0.65 (95% CI 0.47 to 0.89). This study also found that organisational injustice remained an independent predictor of coronary heart disease when other psychosocial work factors such as job strain and effort-reward imbalance were taken into account (fully adjusted HR = 0.70, 95% CI 0.51 to 0.94). Similar associations were found in relation to both men and women in a study of 804 factory workers using mortality data from the Finnish national mortality register (Elovainio *et al.*, 2006b): employees reporting high justice at work had a 39% lower risk of cardiovascular death than their counterparts experiencing low or intermediate justice (fully adjusted HR = 0.61, 95% CI 0.36 to 1.00).

The relationships between organisational justice and other health conditions such as inflammation, sickness absence, and mental ill health, as well as health behaviours have also been investigated (see Ferrie *et al.*, 2006; Elovainio *et al.*, 2002, 2010; Kivimäki *et al.*, 2003a). For example, with regard to psychiatric morbidity, Ferrie and colleagues (2006), using data from the Whitehall studies, examined the effect of organisational justice on mental health. They found that employees experiencing low levels of organisational justice at baseline were significantly more likely than those reporting high levels of organisational justice to experience psychiatric morbidity as measured by the GHQ at follow-up of five years or more (age-, grade- and physical illness-adjusted OR men = 1.52, 95% CI 1.27 to 1.82; OR women = 1.64, 95% CI 1.27 to 2.13). Further analysis showed that experiencing a reduction in organisational justice between baseline and follow-up was associated with an increase in immediate and long-term risk of psychiatric morbidity (adjusted OR men = 1.81, 95% CI 1.48 to 2.21; OR women = 1.74, 95% CI 1.31 to 2.30), while an increase in justice was associated with a reduction in risk (adjusted OR men = 0.75, 95% CI 0.60 to 0.94; OR women = 0.74, 95% CI 0.55 to 1.01).

These Whitehall study findings reflect those of a Finnish study of 3,773 hospital workers by Kivimäki and colleagues (2003a) which also examined associations between psychiatric morbidity, as measured by the General Health Questionnaire, and organisational justice (justice of decision-making procedures, and justice of interpersonal treatment). It found that after adjustment for baseline characteristics, low versus high procedural justice was associated with a 60% higher risk of minor psychiatric morbidity amongst men (Rate Ratio [RR] = 1.6, 95% CI 1.0 to 2.6) and a 40% higher risk amongst women (RR = 1.4, 95% CI 1.2 to 1.7). This study also examined associations with self-rated health and sickness absence. For sickness absence, low justice in terms of decision-making resulted in a 41% higher risk in men (RR = 1.4, 95% CI 1.1 to 1.8), and a 12% higher risk in women (RR = 1.1, 95% CI 1.0 to 1.2). In terms of self-reported health there was an increased risk of 40% in both sexes. With respect to interpersonal justice, low justice increased the risk of sickness absence (RR men = 1.3, 95% CI 1.0 to 1.6; RR women = 1.2, 95% CI 1.2 to 1.3) and minor psychiatric morbidity (OR = 1.2 in both sexes) but the association with self-rated health status was non-significant (combined OR = 1.08, 95% CI 0.89 to 1.31). These figures largely persisted after control for other risk factors (for example, job control, workload, social support, and hostility). The study also found significant associations between low procedural justice and an increased prevalence of smoking in women (OR = 1.19, 95% CI 1.01 to 1.40) and heavy alcohol consumption in men (OR = 1.57, 95% CI 1.12 to 2.20). Low relational justice was associated with an increased likelihood of obesity in women (OR = 1.30, 95% CI 1.08 to 1.57).

4.3 The psychosocial work environment and health inequalities

The distribution of adverse psychosocial working conditions is socially patterned with jobs at the lower end of the socio-economic class scale more likely to entail a higher exposure to adverse conditions than those towards the higher end. Table 4.1 contains data on the prevalence of different aspects of the psychosocial work environment by occupational group (based on the International Standard Classification of Occupations, ISCO) across 27 European countries (data taken from the European Working Conditions Survey, 2005—for details about the survey see Box 3.1 in Chapter 3). It shows that in terms of social support at work (colleague and supervisor support), there are few differences by occupation, with the lowest occupational groups, plant and machine operators and assemblers (ISCO 8) and elementary occupations (ISCO 9), and the highest occupational groups, legislators, senior officials and managers (ISCO 1) and professionals (ISCO 2), reporting broadly similar levels of social support. For example, 47.5% of those working in elementary occupations reported that they could get assistance from superiors if asked, compared to 48.3% of legislators, senior officials and managers. However, in terms of the measures of job demands (repetition, tight deadlines, machine paced, monotonous) and control at work (control over tasks or speed of tasks, consulted about changes), there are stark differences by occupational status between the highest and lowest occupations. For example, in terms of demands at work, monotonous work was around 50% higher amongst plant and machine operators and assemblers (58.2%) and elementary occupations (55.8%) when compared to legislators, senior officials and managers (34.9%), and professionals (28.2%). Similarly, in terms of control at work, workers in the two highest occupational groups were almost twice as likely to report that they were consulted about changes to the organisation of work as those in the two lowest occupational groups: 67.3% of legislators, senior officials and managers, and 61.2% of professionals compared to 35.4% of plant and machine operators and assemblers, and 36% of elementary occupations.

Table 4.1 Psychosocial work environment in Europe by occupation (percentage of employees, European Union average[a], 2005)

Occupation[b]		1	2	3	4	5	6	7	8	9
Support	Colleagues[c]	64.2	70.5	74.4	71.1	65.4	56.2	70.3	64.2	58.1
	Superiors[d]	48.3	60.4	64.3	63.4	55.7	33.2	54.1	53.6	47.5
Control	Control tasks[e]	85.2	76.0	71.0	63.8	61.5	84.4	49.3	34.7	54.6
	Control speed[f]	82.2	80.7	73.8	68.3	63.3	87.9	63.5	49.2	62.3
	Consulted[g]	67.3	61.2	53.4	48.0	43.7	31.9	38.4	35.4	36.0
Demand	Repetition[h]	29.2	27.2	35.1	39.4	42.3	39.4	48.5	47.3	44.6
	Tight deadlines[i]	65.6	60.1	64.0	61.8	49.1	64.9	77.2	68.5	48.7
	Machine paced[j]	15.0	7.9	12.4	13.0	9.4	18.4	33.7	49.6	19.7
	Monotonous[k]	34.9	28.2	32.3	45.2	42.1	54.8	49.8	58.2	55.8

[a] EU-27: The 15 pre-2004 European Union member states (Austria, Belgium, Denmark, Finland, France, Germany, Greece, Ireland, Italy, Luxembourg, the Netherlands, Portugal, Spain, Sweden and the United Kingdom) plus 10 who joined in 2004 (Malta, Cyprus, Slovenia, Estonia, Latvia, Lithuania, Poland, the Czech Republic, Slovak Republic, and Hungary) and 2 who joined in 2007 (Romania and Bulgaria).

[b] International Standard Classification of Occupations (ISCO): (1) legislators, senior officials and managers, (2) professionals, (3) technicians and associate professionals, (4) clerks, (5) service, retail and sales workers, (6) skilled agricultural and fishery workers, (7) craft and related trades workers, (8) plant and machine operators and assemblers, (9) elementary occupations.

[c] Superiors: % reporting they can get assistance from superiors if asked.

[d] Colleagues: % reporting they can get assistance from colleagues if asked.

[e] Control tasks: % reporting they have some control over the order of their work tasks.

[f] Control speed: % reporting they have some control over the speed of their work.

[g] Consulted: % reporting that they are consulted about changes in work organisation.

[h] Repetition: % reporting that their job involves short repetitive tasks of less than 10 minutes 25% of the time or more.

[i] Tight deadlines: % working to tight deadlines 25% of the time or more.

[j] Machine paced: % reporting that their work pace is determined by automated machines.

[k] Monotonous: % reporting that their work involves monotonous tasks.

Source: Based on data from the European Working Conditions Survey (European Working Conditions Observatory, (2005)).

Similarly, in 1994 a special version of the annual Health Survey for England was carried out which looked at cardiovascular disease and its known risk factors—including the psychosocial work environment variables of job control and social support (Figure 4.1). This nationally representative survey found that amongst men and women aged 16 or over, 'low control over work' was reported by 47% of men and 46% of women in the lowest socio-economic class (Registrar General's Occupational Class V) as opposed to just 6% and 14% respectively by those in the highest socio-economic class (Registrar General's Occupational Class 1). A similarly stark social divide was evident in terms of 'low task variety' but less so in terms of 'severe lack of social support'.

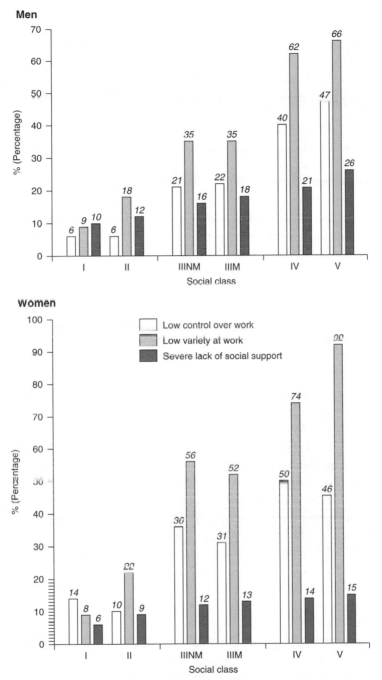

Fig. 4.1 Low job control and task variety, and severe lack of social support in relation to sex and social class.
Source: Based on Health Survey for England 1994 data as cited in Marmot and Wilkinson, 2001.

The data also showed important gender inequalities with women of all social classes (apart from the lowest social class—V) reporting much higher rates of exposure to poor psychosocial environments in terms of both job control and task variety. However, women consistently reported better levels of social support. Higher grade workers experience more control, more creativity, higher utilisation of their skills, and have a more supportive environment: in other words, higher level workers experience less alienation (Crinson and Yuill, 2008).

One of the most important findings of the Whitehall studies (see Box 4.1) is the observation that occupational grade is inversely associated with incidence of coronary heart disease (Marmot *et al.*, 1997b) and related health conditions (Brunner *et al.*, 1997; Marmot *et al.*, 1991). For example, coronary heart disease mortality at ten year follow-up, the relative risk was 2.2 in low grade clerical workers and 1.6 for intermediate grade staff when compared with 1.0 for the reference group of senior level administrative workers (Marmot *et al.*, 1984; Marmot and Brunner, 2005). A similar social gradient was observed for all-cause mortality, and non-coronary heart disease mortality (Marmot and Brunner, 2004). Similarly, the age-adjusted incidence of heart disease was 50% higher in the lower grade employees. Adjustment for standard risk factors (e.g. smoking, body mass index [BMI], hypertension) reduced the inequality by 40% in men and 26% in women. However, adjustment for psychosocial work environment factors (specifically demand-control-support and effort-reward imbalance) reduced the inequality between occupational grades by 64% in men and 51% in women (Marmot *et al.*, 1997b).

Risk of musculoskeletal disease is also higher amongst low versus high grade workers (Landsbergis, 2010). For example, in a study of Finnish civil servants, risk of self-reported musculoskeletal disease was 40–50% higher among manual workers than among managers and professionals (Aittomaki *et al.*, 2007). These differences are not entirely explained by differences in physical load, with psychosocial working conditions playing an important role in the aetiology of musculoskeletal disease and in inequalities in the distribution and development of the disease (Gillen *et al.*, 2007). Similarly, socio-economic inequalities in psychological disorders are also strongly associated with inequalities in exposures to harmful psychosocial work environments. For example, data from the Whitehall studies has demonstrated that the prevalence of depressive symptoms ranged from 9% in the highest occupational group to 22% in the lowest amongst men, and from 11% to 17% amongst women (Stansfeld *et al.*, 2003). These socio-economic inequalities were reduced by 66% and 43% once adjustment was made for adverse psychosocial working conditions (high demands, low support, effort-reward imbalance).

People in lower socio-economic class positions, who are already paid less for their work, are therefore more likely to be exposed to the negative impacts on their health and well-being of hazardous psychosocial working conditions. Thinking more broadly about the psychosocial theory of health inequalities, people from lower socio-economic classes are also less likely to have control over wider aspects of their lives (for example their housing choices will be limited by their incomes). Lack of control at work is thus part of a wider experience of disempowerment. In contrast, good, or health promoting, psychosocial work environments are more likely to be experienced by people with higher socio-economic class status, adding to the control which they already have over their wider lives as a result of their income (largely derived from work). For certain types of occupation, usually the routine and manual ones undertaken by people from lower socio-economic class backgrounds, exposure to an adverse psychosocial work environment (be it low reward and/or low control) is often exacerbated by exposure to physical, ergonomic and chemical hazards in the workplace. This can obviously multiply the resulting negative effects on their health, although few studies have examined the longer term effects of such cumulative exposures (Siegrist et al., 2009).

The psychosocial work environment is thus an important contributory factor in the existence of socio-economic health inequalities, but the role of the work environment must also be understood within the wider social and economic environment experienced by individuals (Siegrist et al., 2009). This results in discussions about whether the experience of psychosocial work stress mediates the relationship between socio-economic class and health or conversely whether psychosocial work stress acts as an effect modifier in the relationship (Marmot et al., 2006). Evidence for both explanations has been documented (Marmot et al., 2006). For example, low control was shown to account for approximately half of the social gradient in coronary heart disease (Marmot et al., 1997b). Equally, in terms of the effect modification hypothesis, other studies have shown that low socio-economic class status is associated with increased susceptibility by demonstrating higher effect sizes in workers with low socio-economic class status compared with those with higher status on exposure to the same psychosocial stressors (Marmot et al., 2006). These two perspectives have different policy implications, with mediation implying that a general improvement in the work environment could reduce health inequalities across the population, whilst the effect modification approach would suggest that interventions should target the most vulnerable population groups first (Siegrist et al., 2009).

4.4 Variation in the psychosocial work environment by welfare state regime

Levels of workplace stress vary by country, as do the associations between workplace stress and health (Salavecz et al., 2010). This is because workplace stress does not develop in a vacuum and, as the concept of alienation makes clear, it is critical to take account of wider society level economic, political and social context when thinking about how work environments impact on health (Siegrist and Theorell, 2006). To this end, it is necessary to consider wider structural influences on the workplace and how macro-level changes can impact on the organisation of work. The macro social, political and economic environment, particularly the labour market and levels of social protection, influences the psychosocial work environment, as well as the other social determinants of health. One clear example of how wider social and economic structures can influence the work environment comes in the form of economic recession and company downsizing, where studies have shown that instability within macro labour markets can reduce the quality of the psychosocial work environment with demands increasing and control decreasing (Siegrist and Theorell, 2006). Similarly, the wider context within which the psychosocial work environment is experienced can either exacerbate or reduce its consequences for health. For example, the relationship between job insecurity or job loss and poor health is less in those countries with more extensive social security systems which improve the ability of individuals to cope with stressful events (Bartley and Blamce, 1997). Recent epidemiological work has applied this perspective to the work environment by comparing whether relationships between stressful psychosocial work environments and health differ by country and welfare state regime. It has shown a lower prevalence of work related stress in countries with more comprehensive welfare states (where the psychosocial work environment is more regulated such as Sweden or Norway), and that the effects on health and health inequalities of adverse psychosocial work environments are also lessened in these countries (Dragano *et al.*, 2010; Sekine *et al.*, 2009).

Dragano and colleagues (2010) used data from the Survey of Health, Ageing and Retirement in Europe (SHAPE) and the English Longitudinal Study on Ageing (ELSA) to examine the links between welfare state regime type (Anglo-Saxon, Bismarckian, Scandinavian and Southern—see Chapter 2 for descriptions), stressful work environments (measured as low control and effort-reward imbalance) and the development of mental ill health (measured by depressive symptoms using the Centre for Epidemiological Studies Depression scale [CES-D] and the EURO-D depression scale) amongst older employed adults (9,917 men and women aged 50–64) in twelve European countries (England, Sweden, Denmark, Germany, Netherlands, Belgium, France, Switzerland, Austria, Italy, Spain, Greece). The study found that levels of workplace psychosocial stress were highest in the Southern European welfare states (i.e. levels of low control at work and effort-reward imbalance were highest in the Southern countries) and that in multi-level models, welfare state regime type accounted for almost 75% of the differences between countries in terms of workplace stress. With respect to health, the study found that participants in any country who reported high levels of workplace stress, had an increased risk of depressive symptoms: effort-reward imbalance twelve country pooled odds ratio OR = 2.12 (95% CI 1.83 to 2.46); low control pooled OR = 1.81 (95% CI 1.53 to 2.14). However, there were significant variations in the level of this association by welfare state regime type, with the odds ratios highest in the Anglo-Saxon welfare state regime and lowest in the Scandinavian one: effort-reward imbalance Anglo-Saxon OR = 2.64 (95% CI 2.03 to 3.43), Southern OR = 2.14 (95% CI 1.47 to 3.11), Bismarckian OR = 1.96 (95% CI 1.53 to 2.50), Scandinavian OR = 1.69 (95% CI 1.07 to 2.66); low control Anglo-Saxon OR = 2.29 (95% CI 1.69 to 3.11), Bismarckian OR = 1.75 (95% CI 1.33 to 2.28), Southern OR = 1.67 (95% CI 1.12 to 2.50), Scandinavian OR = 1.48 (95% CI 0.89 to 2.45). The health effects resulting from stressful work environments are less pronounced in older workers in welfare states with higher levels of social protection.

Another comparative study by Sekine and colleagues (2009) examined the contribution of psychosocial work environment characteristics to health inequalities. Using data on physical and mental functioning (measured using the Short Form SF-36) of British (an example of a Liberal/Anglo-Saxon welfare state), Finnish (a Social Democratic/Scandinavian welfare state) and Japanese (considered to be either Conservative/Bismarckian or Confucian) civil servants aged 40–60 years, it tested whether socio-economic inequalities (measured using employment grade) in adverse psychosocial working conditions (measured using the demand-control-support model) and poor health were smaller in the context of the more supportive Finnish welfare state. The study found that work characteristics were socially patterned, with lower grade employees generally having significantly lower levels of control. However, inequalities in work characteristics were highest in the British cohort. Low job control was reported by 77.8% of lowest employment grade and 11.3% of highest grade British men (a difference of 66.5 percentage points), 47.3% and 10.5% respectively of Japanese men (a difference of 36.8 percentage points), and 63.0% and 8.4% respectively of Finnish men (a difference of 54.6 percentage points). Similarly, low job control was reported by 76.6% of lowest employment grade and 9.6% of highest grade British women (a difference of 67 percentage points), 46.5% and 0% respectively of Japanese women (a difference of 46.5 percentage points), and 52.9% and 7.7% respectively of Finnish women (a difference of 45.2 percentage points).

There were also significant socio-economic inequalities in physical functioning for both men and women in all three countries, with the lowest employment grades consistently experiencing poorer physical functioning: British men age-adjusted odds ratio OR = 1.74 (95% CI 1.34 to 2.25), Japanese men OR = 1.73 (95% CI 1.24 to 2.42), and Finnish men OR = 2.01 (95% CI 1.49 to 2.71), British women age-adjusted odds ratio OR = 1.89 (95% CI 1.43 to 2.50), Japanese women OR = 5.44 (95% CI 1.25 to 23.8), and Finnish women OR = 2.23 (95% CI 1.84 to 2.71). The patterns for mental functioning were similarly socially distributed for British and Japanese men, although the trends were unclear for women: British men age-adjusted odds ratio OR = 1.15 (95% CI 0.88 to 1.51), Japanese men OR = 1.95 (95% CI 1.36 to 2.80), British women age-adjusted odds ratio OR = 0.88 (95% CI 0.67 to 1.15), Japanese women OR = 1.17 (95% CI 0.44 to 3.11). The Finnish data, however, demonstrated the reverse gradient with men and women in lower employment grades reporting better mental functioning: Finnish men age-adjusted OR = 0.76 (95% CI 0.57 to 1.01) and Finnish women OR = 0.71 (95% CI 0.58 to 0.87). The authors attributed these differences in the mental health effects of the work environment in Finland to the influence of the wider welfare state context. Sekine and colleagues (2009) assert that the smaller inequalities in work characteristics in the Finnish cohort:

> 'May be attributable to the universal and egalitarian policies of Social Democratic countries because . . . policies such as extensive welfare and social services, full employment policies, wealth redistribution through tax and transfer systems are considered to result in less inequalities in working conditions and health'.

Sekine *et al.* (2009)

4.5 **Conclusion**

In this chapter I have outlined and compared different models of the psychosocial work environment. I have summarised the empirical literature which examines the effects of the psychosocial work environment on health and health inequalities. The chapter has highlighted significant inequalities in exposure to adverse psychosocial working conditions, with levels of job control lowest and psychological demands highest for the lowest occupations. Workers in the lowest socio-economic classes are therefore at a higher risk of developing stress related diseases including coronary heart disease. The chapter has looked at variations by welfare state in the psychosocial work environment and in its relationship with health. This has shown that 'toxic' work environments are less prevalent and the negative health effects of the psychosocial work environment are weaker in the Social Democractic welfare states where legislation enhances worker participation and control. This legislation was largely the result of successful collective action by workers (through their trade unions and political representatives) to improve their environments

(Benach *et al.*, 2007). In this chapter, I have suggested that one of the mechanisms through which the psychosocial work environment impacts on stress and subsequently on health and health inequalities is as a result of the process of labour alienation. The negative health effects of work are more apparent when workers are treated unfairly—which is the result of being considered as mere production costs within an individualistic economic relationship between employer and worker. Workplace health is better when the work environment is fairer and work itself is considered as an important aspect of individual and collective self-realisation. The latter requires partnerships between workers, employers, the state and society: corporatism.

4.6 **Further reading**

Karasek, R.A. and Theorell, T. (1990). *Healthy Work: Stress, Productivity, and the Reconstruction of Working Life.* New York, Basic Books.

Marmot, M., Siegrist, J., and Theorell, T. (2006). 'Health and the psychosocial work environment'. In: M. Marmot and R. G. Wilkinson (eds.) *Social Determinants of Health,* Oxford: Oxford University Press.

Peterson, C. (1999) *Stress at Work: A Sociological Perspective.* New York, Baywood.

Chapter 5

Recession, unemployment, and health

Unemployment has always been an important determinant of health as the vast majority of the population in advanced economies rely upon employment for their income. The development of capitalism in the nineteenth and early twentieth centuries was marked by economic booms and busts in which unemployment peaked and troughed in line with the expansion and contraction of the economy. Unemployment in this pre-welfare state period had severe economic and health impacts, particularly in the Great Depression of the 1930s. In the Fordist politics of the post-war period, a commitment to full (male) employment therefore became one of the cornerstones of the Keynesian post-war consensus in the advanced capitalist economies (albeit to a lesser extent in the US). Governments took on responsibility for unemployment rates and intervened in the economy (for example by increasing state employment) to iron out the impact on employment rates of the inevitable fluctuations of the capitalist economic cycle. However, the economic crises of the 1970s and the resulting ascendancy of more neo-liberal economic models to a large degree ended this political consensus (see Chapter 2). The subsequent increase in the individualisation of social and economic life has seen unemployment shift from being considered as an important political—and therefore collective—issue, to being merely an economic—individual—one: the 'right to work' has shifted from meaning a collective commitment to full employment, to the right to be unhindered in selling one's individual labour power in a deregulated labour market (Beynon and McMylor, 1985).

In this new post-Fordist political and economic environment, unemployment can be considered as an important means of wage discipline, keeping wage levels down as competition for work and job insecurity increase. The unemployed can therefore be described, in political economy terms, as part of a 'reserve army of labour'. In the post-war period, to a greater or lesser extent, the unemployed have been 'maintained' by the welfare state (Ginsburg, 1979). However, the welfare state itself acts as another mechanism for the discipline of labour through the level of social security benefits paid to those out of work, and the organisation of access to these benefits (Dominelli, 1991). The welfare benefits system, by default, sets the unofficial minimum thereby lowering the price of labour power (Ginsburg, 1979). Benefit levels are set so that they do not impinge on the ability of employers to attract workers to low-paid jobs (Dominelli, 1991). Similarly, through the conditions that are attached to benefits, such as evidence of recent employment or active job search, the welfare system restricts the support given to non-compliant workers. In a different way, the stigma that is associated with unemployment and welfare receipt also acts as a discipline upon the labour force (Katz, 1986). This ethos encourages people to take jobs that are low-paid or which require them to work in poor conditions. The discipline of labour is therefore psychosocial as well as material.

In this chapter, I examine the relationships between economic recessions, unemployment and health. The chapter is divided into four main sections. The first section examines the effects of economic recessions on health. The second section summarises the literature on the relationship between unemployment and health. The effects of recessions on health inequalities, as well as the importance of unemployment to health inequalities are then examined. Variation by welfare state in the health effects of recessions, as well as in the relationship between unemployment and health are then examined.

5.1 **Economic recessions and population health**

National economic wealth (i.e. gross domestic product [GDP]) has long been considered as the major global determinant of population health, with the vast differences in mortality between the developed and developing countries accounted for in terms of differences in economic growth. Indeed, the World Health Organisation Commission on the Social Determinants of Health (2008:1) concluded that *'a toxic combination of bad policies, economics, and politics'* was responsible for global health inequalities. Changes in the economy therefore potentially have important implications for population health and inequalities in health.

Recessions are characterised by instability (in terms of inflation and interest rates) and sudden reductions in production and consumption with corresponding increases in unemployment. For example, the recession of the late 2000s was characterised by unemployment rates in 2010 of 8.5% in the UK and the US, 10% in France and 20% in Spain. Evidence suggests that economic recessions have detrimental health effects for those losing jobs or in fear of losing their jobs (Neumayer, 2005). At an individual level, unemployment is associated with an increased likelihood of morbidity and mortality (as described in the next section). Similarly, downsizing and redundancy, and the increased job insecurity of the remaining labour force are all independently associated with negative health impacts including increased rates of mental health, depression, and mortality (Bartley *et al.*, 2006). There are also wider negative effects on population health of recessions, e.g. on general mental health (Novo *et al.*, 2001) and on child mental health (Solantaus *et al.*, 2004). The health effects of recession are unequally distributed across the population socially and geographically, thereby potentially exacerbating health inequalities (Kondo *et al.*, 2008).

Whilst economic growth over the twentieth century has been credited with improved living conditions and subsequent better public health, there is no reason to assume that the periods of economic growth between recessions have had a positive public health effect. For example, a study of mortality trends in the twentieth century in the US found that the secular improvement in mortality accelerates during economic recessions and slows or reverses in periods of economic growth (Tapia Granados, 2005a). However, other commentators have suggested that it is only very rapid economic growth which leads to increased mortality and that overall the effect of economic growth is positive (Brenner, 2005). Nor is it possible to assume that economic growth (and any resulting health effects) is evenly distributed across areas, within countries or within populations. The health effects of economic growth may therefore be experienced differently by different areas and populations, and the cumulative effect of economic trends over time may also vary. There is therefore something of a debate over the health effects of economic recessions, with commentators split between those who argue that economic recession is bad for health and those who propose that economic downturns can have a positive effect on population health (Moore, 2009). The latter argue that during recessions, leisure time increases as job pressures and work hours decrease, motor vehicle accidents lower and reductions in income lead to a reduction in hazardous health behaviours. However, the evidence shows that significant relationships between economic recessions and population health vary according to the health indicator in question (Riva *et al.*, 2011).

5.1.1 Recessions and mortality

The work of Brenner in the US was the first to suggest a negative relationship between economic recession and all-cause mortality: recessions are 'bad' for mortality. In an initial exploration of economic changes and mortality in New York State (1900–1967), Brenner (1971) found that increases in unemployment rates were associated with an increase in ischemic heart disease mortality. Two further studies led by Brenner which compared economic change and cardiovascular disease mortality in Britain (1955–1976) and health and social well-being in Sweden (1950–1980), found a similar relationship between economic downturn and increased mortality (Brenner and Mooney, 1982; Brenner, 1987a). A comparative study of the relationship between economic growth, alcohol consumption and heart disease mortality in nine industrialised countries seemed to have consolidated findings on the correlation between unemployment and heart disease mortality rates (Brenner, 1987b). Other researchers found support for Brenner's thesis. For example, Bunn found an association between increases in the unemployment rate and ischemic heart disease mortality in Australia (Bunn, 1979). Some more recently conducted studies have also found a negative recession effect. For example, Gerdtham and Johannesson (2005) found that recession increased all-cause mortality in Swedish men although the findings were non-significant for Swedish women. Similarly, Economou and colleagues (2008) analysed the relationship between unemployment and mortality in 13 European countries. They also found that all-cause mortality increased as the economy worsened. However, Brenner's work has been heavily criticised due to aspects of his methodology (for an overview see Gravelle *et al.*, 1981). When his methods were interrogated, the subsequent analysis failed to replicate his findings (Wagstaff, 1985).

This, in combination with subsequent empirical research (especially by Ruhm), has led to the emergence of something of a new academic consensus around the effects of recessions: recessions are 'good' for mortality (Moore, 2009; Riva *et al.*, 2011). Graham and colleagues (1992) as well as Ruhm (1995, 2000) were the first to suggest that it is economic growth, not recession that is detrimental to health. Graham and colleagues, examining death rates in the US (1972–1991), demonstrated that death rates slow when the economy deteriorates. They found that a 1% increase in the unemployment rate reduced death rates by 4.6 per 100,000. Similarly, Ruhm (2000) found that a 1% reduction in unemployment rates in the US increased cardiovascular disease mortality by 0.75%. Ruhm (1995) also found that deaths from motor vehicle accidents also decreased as the economy deteriorated with a one standard deviation increase in the unemployment rate associated with 3% reduction in daytime fatal accidents (from 23.0 to 18.9 per 100,000) and 7% for night time accidents (from 4.16 to 4.04 per 100,000). Similar results were reported by Tapia Grandos (2005a). Other studies of the relationship between all-cause mortality and recessions have also found recessions to have a positive effect on all-cause mortality. For example, Neumayer's (2004) study of all-cause mortality amongst the German population found an inverse relationship with the unemployment rate for both men and women. Tapia Granados (2005b) also found similar results for Spain, although the relationship was slightly stronger for men.

An interesting study of economic growth and health in Sweden in the nineteenth and twentieth centuries found that the positive association between economic growth and improvement in population health gradually weakened over time to the extent that it was completely reversed by the end of the twentieth century at which point economic growth began to have a negative impact on health (Tapia Granados and Ionides, 2008). A comparative European study by Stuckler and colleagues (2009) found no association between recession (as measured by an increasing unemployment rate) and all-cause mortality.

However, when suicide is examined, the weight of evidence suggests a strong negative effect of recessions. For example, Stuckler and colleagues' pan-European study (2009) found a significant relationship between increases in unemployment rates and suicides amongst men and women aged under 65, with the greatest effect seen for men aged 30–44 and women aged 15–29. A 1% increase in the unemployment rate was associated with a 0.79% (95% confidence interval [CI] 0.16 to 1.42) rise in suicides amongst those aged under 65. Gerdtham and Johannesson (2005) also found suicide among men (but not women) to increase significantly in times of economic recession in Sweden, with Tapia Granados (2005b) reporting a similarly gendered finding for Spain. Ruhm (2000) also reported these results for the US as whilst suicides amongst women were only weakly related or unrelated to economic change, suicide rates amongst men escalated during economic downturns.

5.1.2 Morbidity and health behaviours

Various studies show deteriorations in various indicators of psychological health during economic recessions; including distress and dissatisfaction (Tausig, 1999), sleep difficulties and psychosomatic complaints (Hyyppä and Alanen, 1997), depression and anxiety (Hagquist *et al.*, 2000), and mental health (Solantaus *et al.*, 2004). In terms of limiting long-term illness and self-reported general health, again studies indicate that these decline during economic recessions (Leeni and Berntsson, 2001). There is some counter evidence which suggests that some chronic conditions and acute morbidity may actually decrease during economic recessions (Ruhm, 2003), as well as evidence that babies born during economic recessions are healthier (Dehejia and Lleras-Muney, 2004). In terms of health behaviours, a USA study by Ruhm (1995) found that increases in levels of local (state) unemployment were associated with reductions in alcohol consumption. However no such relationship between alcohol consumption and national employment rates was found. Other studies have identified decreases in alcohol consumption amongst the heaviest drinkers (Ruhm and Black, 2002). Additionally it appears that economic recessions lower spirit consumption more than that of wine or beer and the decreases in spirit consumption occur among the heaviest consumers (Ruhm and Black, 2002; Johansson *et al.*, 2006). For example, in the US an increase in the local unemployment rate was found to lower the consumption of spirits by 1.1% compared to 0.4% for beer and wine (Ruhm and Black, 2002). Johansson *et al.* (2006) also found alcohol consumption to rise in line with increases in economic growth potentially as a result of increases in personal income. Studies have also found that tobacco consumption decreases during economic recession, especially amongst the heaviest smokers (Ruhm, 2000; Novo *et al.*, 2000). For example, Ruhm (2000) found that economic recession was associated with a decrease in smoking, with a 1% increase in local unemployment resulting in a reduction of at least 1% in the number of smokers. Novo and colleagues (2000) found reductions in tobacco amongst those aged under 21 during a period of recession. However, the relationship with any reduction in personal income is unclear (Ruhm, 2005). There is also some evidence that recessions result in increases in physical activity levels as well as increases in the proportion of people in the healthiest weight range (Ruhm, 2000).

5.1.3 Overview of recession and health research

In summary then, the majority of recent studies have concluded that all-cause mortality as well as deaths from cardiovascular disease and motor vehicle accidents decrease during economic recessions. However, there is clear evidence that economic recessions increase deaths from suicides amongst men. Psychological ill health, limiting long-term illness and poor self-rated health all appear to increase during economic recessions, although Ruhm's work (2003) suggests that this is not universal. The evidence base also suggests that health behaviours improve during economic recessions, especially amongst heavy alcohol and tobacco consumers. Given the debate about Brenner's methods, it is worth highlighting some general methodological limitations of the economic recession and health evidence base (Moore, 2009). Firstly, the specific indicator of economic recession used can produce very different results. Unemployment is the most commonly used indicator but it says very little about the distribution of wealth within a country or its subsequent inequalities. Secondly, the lag period between the recession period and the time at which the health outcome is measured (particularly for mortality studies) may have an important effect on the results of studies. Thirdly, the spatial level of analysis can lead to different results (e.g. if it is local rather than national unemployment rates which are the indicator of recession). In overall terms then, it is not currently possible to conclude one way or another as to whether the relationship between economic recession and health is positive or negative.

5.2 **Unemployment and health**

The overall effects of recessions on mortality and morbidity may be debatable. However, one clear way in which recessions negatively impact on public health (and potentially increase health inequalities) is through the increase in the rate of unemployment. The International Labour Organisation defines someone as unemployed if they are without a job, but have actively looked for one within the last four weeks. Studies have consistently shown that unemployment increases the chance of poor health (Bambra and Eikemo, 2009). Empirical studies from the recessions of the 1980s and 1990s have shown that unemployment is associated with an increased likelihood of morbidity and mortality (Bartley *et al.*, 2006). There are clear relationships between unemployment and increased risk of poor mental health and suicide (Platt, 1986; Montgomery *et al.*, 1999a; Blakely *et al.*, 2008), higher rates of all-cause and specific causes of mortality (Morris *et al.*, 1994; Scott-Samuel, 1984; Moser *et al.*, 1984; Martikainen and Valkonen, 1996), self-reported health and limiting long-term illness (Bartley and Lewis, 2002; Korpi, 2001), and, in some studies, a higher prevalence of risky health behaviours (particularly amongst young men), including problematic alcohol use and smoking (Montgomery *et al.*, 1999b; Luoto *et al.*, 1998). The negative health experiences of unemployment are not limited to the unemployed only but also extend to their families and the wider community (Moser *et al.*, 1984). For example, figures from a 1984 study suggested that for every '*2,000 men seeking work 2 (1.94), and among their wives 1 (0.98), will die each year as a result of unemployment*' (Moser *et al.*, 1984: 1324). Unemployment therefore also has serious implications for health service planning with, for example, increased pressures on mental health services (Watkins, 1986).

Links between unemployment and poorer health have conventionally been explained through two inter-related concepts: the psychosocial effects of unemployment (e.g. stigma, isolation and loss of self-worth) and the material consequences of unemployment (e.g. wage loss and resulting changes in access to essential goods and services). The psychosocial explanation of the health effects of unemployment draws upon the 'latent deprivation theory' which asserts that being employed imposes a structure for time use, enforces some level of activity, provides opportunities for contact with others, a sense of social status and opportunities to work in unison towards collective goals (Jahoda 1982: 59). The unemployed are, according to Jahoda (1982), deprived of these latent functions of employment and thus they experience psychological distress which may in turn led to physical ill health. Materialist critics of the psychosocial explanations of unemployment and health, such as Fryer (1986), have argued that it is actually the loss of the income from employment and the control over life which an income gives, as well as the relative poverty experienced by the unemployed, which accounts for the deterioration in health.

Studies which have examined the loss of social status and the 'shaming' aspects of unemployment, such as Eales (1989) or Rantakeisu and colleagues (1997), found that around one in four unemployed men had experienced feelings of shame related to unemployment and that these feelings of shame were strongly related to depression, anxiety and minor affective disorders. Similarly, an Italian study of factory workers who were made redundant in the early 1990s recession found that mental health declined even though the material situation of the workers did not deteriorate as they were given 100% of their wages for the first six months of unemployment (Rudas et al., 1991). Longer term though, the unemployed suffer from a greatly reduced income and many unemployed people live in relative poverty. For example, the benefit income of an unemployed adult, excluding housing costs, aged over 25 in the UK in 2010 is £65.45 per week (it is only £51.85 for those aged under 25) which is almost 50% below the poverty line disposable income of £115 per week for a single adult (Department for Work and Pensions, 2010a; Poverty site, 2010). In addition, these subsistence level payments are another means of disciplining the unemployed and ensuring that even low paid work remains attractive (Ginsburg, 1979). Commentators have also drawn attention to the contributory role of ill health itself as a factor behind unemployment. This 'health selection' hypothesis suggests that people who are in work and experiencing illness are more likely to lose their jobs than those who are healthy, and that this effect will probably be exacerbated in times of economic recession.

5.2.1 Unemployment, mental health, and suicide

Unemployment is associated with a more than two-fold increase in the likelihood of poor mental health. A longitudinal UK study of young men examined the relationship between unemployment and depression and anxiety (Montgomery et al., 1999a). It analysed data for 3,241 men taken from the 1958 British Birth Cohort. Baseline measures were taken when the men were aged 23 and the follow-up was at age 33, with the outcome being the onset of depression between these ages. The study compared the onset of depression or anxiety between those who had experienced recent unemployment (those who were unemployed at any point in the year before) and those who had not. It found that, after adjustment for potential confounding factors (pre-existing tendency to depression, social class, education, region), the relative risk (RR) of developing symptoms resulting in consultation for the recently unemployed was 2.10 (95% CI 1.21 to 3.63). Excluding those men with a pre-existing tendency to depression (as measured by the Malaise Inventory at age 23) increased this to 2.30 (95% CI 1.44 to 3.65). In addition, the study looked at the effects of accumulated unemployment (more than three years unemployment) since age 23. It found that in general, long-term unemployment of over three years did not significantly increase the risk of consulting a health professional about depression or anxiety (fully adjusted RR = 1.63, 95% CI 0.95 to 2.79) compared to those who had not experienced unemployment. However, once those young men with a pre-existing tendency to depression were excluded, long-term unemployment doubled the likelihood of depression and anxiety (fully adjusted RR = 2.04, 95% CI 1.17 to 3.54).

One of the most important areas of research into the recessions of the 1980s and 1990s examined the relationship between unemployment and suicide (Platt, 1986). Studies generally found a more than two-fold increased risk of suicide (Lewis and Sloggett, 1998; Kposowa, 2001) and attempted suicide (parasuicide) amongst the unemployed (Platt, 1986). Parasuicide rates are over 10 times higher in unemployed young men than those in employment (Dorling, 2009). For example, a paper by Blakely and colleagues (2003) used data from 2.04 million respondents to the 1991 New Zealand census. It linked census data with mortality records and examined deaths from suicide amongst those aged 16–64 years from 1991 to 1994. It found that death by suicide was more than twice as likely amongst the unemployed than those in employment (age-adjusted OR women = 2.46, 95% CI 1.10 to 5.49; age-adjusted OR men = 2.63, 95% CI 1.87 to 3.70). No patterning of suicide by socio-economic class was detected. When controlling for rates of mental ill health (using population estimates of the prevalence of mental ill health), the RR of death by suicide amongst unemployed men compared to employed decreased to 1.88 (95% CI 1.35 to 2.43). This suggests that 47% of the excess suicide deaths amongst unemployed working age men were attributable to confounding by mental illness. There has been debate about whether the associations between suicide and unemployment are direct—that unemployment is a traumatic life event which increases vulnerability to suicide; indirect—unemployment increases exposure to other risk factors for suicide (e.g. poor mental health, financial strain); or non-causal—that people with an increased risk of unemployment are also those with an increased risk of suicide (and vice versa) (Blakely *et al.*, 2003).

5.2.2 **Unemployment and mortality**

Other causes of death are also more common amongst the unemployed. A prospective cohort study of 6,191 middle-aged British men (aged 40–59 in 1978) examined the impact of loss of employment during the early 1980s recession on mortality (Morris *et al.*, 1994). Baseline questionnaires were sent out 1978–80 and five year mortality data was obtained from death registers. It found that men who experienced unemployment (n=1,779) during the five year follow-up were twice as likely to die as those who remained continuously employed (all-cause mortality RR = 2.13, 95% CI 1.71 to 2.65). Controlling for smoking, weight and alcohol consumption as well as socio-economic class reduced the RR slightly to 1.95 (95% CI 1.57 to 2.43). These risks were consistent across different causes of death, with the unemployed more than twice as likely to die from cancers (fully adjusted RR = 2.07, 95% CI 1.45 to 2.97) and cardiovascular diseases (fully adjusted RR = 2.13, 95% CI 1.57 to 2.89) as the employed. However, once those who were unemployed on the grounds of illness were excluded, the relative risk of death amongst the *'healthy unemployed'* (n= 923) decreased substantially to 1.49 (95% CI 1.10 to 1.96) for all-causes, to 1.59 (95% CI 1.00 to 2.51) for cancers and 1.64 (95% CI 1.10 to 2.43) for cardiovascular diseases. Although this is still an excess mortality of at least 49%, it brings into play questions about selection versus causation in the relationship between unemployment and ill health.

It also perhaps draws attention to the wider context within which unemployment is experienced. In a period when unemployment is higher (during recessions), it is likely that the relationship between unemployment and health will be weaker as more people are drawn on a short-term basis into the pool of the unemployed. Certainly, the findings of a Finnish study suggest that the association between unemployment and mortality weakens as the general employment rate increases. This prospective study, by Martikainen and Valkonen (1996), examined the Finnish population aged 25–59 years (2.5 million people) and linked census and labour market information from 1990 with mortality records for 1991 to 1993. After controlling for age, marital status and socio-economic class factors, it found that whilst all men and women who had experienced unemployment had an increased risk of death compared to those who were employed, the increased risk was much lower amongst those who were unemployed for the first time in a period of high unemployment (1992, unemployment was 22% amongst men and 15.3% amongst women) compared to those who initially experienced unemployment in a period of low overall unemployment (1990, unemployment was 7.6% amongst men and 6.0% amongst women). Men unemployed for the first time in 1990 had an increased mortality risk of 2.11 (95% CI 1.76 to 2.53) compared to 1.35 (95% CI 1.16 to 1.56) in 1992, and amongst women the risks were 1.61 (95% CI 1.09 to 2.36) in 1990 and 1.30 (95% CI 0.97 to 1.75) in 1992. The unemployed who were later re-employed had a higher mortality than those who were continually employed, but a lower mortality than those who remained unemployed.

These relationships were replicated by a 2010 Finnish panel study of mortality after downsizing (Maki, 2010).

5.2.3 Unemployment, self-reported health, and limiting long-term illness

The negative relationship between unemployment and health is also reflected in studies of self-reported health and limiting long-term illness (LLTI). For example, a twenty year longitudinal study of limiting long-term illness amongst UK men (Bartley and Lewis, 2002) found a substantially increased risk amongst the unemployed. Data were examined relating to 60,000 men aged 15–40 at the start of the twenty year study period (1971) and thus aged 35–60 at the end (1991). The study found a large degree of continuity in the unemployed population with over 25% of those unemployed in 1971, 30% of those unemployed in 1981 and 46% of those unemployed in both 1971 and 1981, also unemployed in 1991. In terms of health, the study found that the odds of reporting a LLTI in 1991 increased in a graded manner depending on the number of times someone had experienced a period of unemployment in the previous twenty years: men who were unemployed in 1971 or 1981 were almost twice as likely (OR 1.88, 95% CI 1.70 to 2.10) as those who had been continuously employed to report LLTI; men who were unemployed in both 1971 and 1981 were three times more likely to report LLTI (OR = 3.04, 95% CI 2.18 to 4.24). Adjustment for low socio-economic class only reduced these increased odds of LLTI to 1.68 (95% CI 1.51 to 1.87) and 2.50 (95% CI 1.79 to 3.50) respectively, showing that unemployment had an independent relationship with increased odds of developing a LLTI. Similar findings were reported in relation to self-reported health by a Swedish study (Korpi, 2001).

5.2.4 Unemployment and health behaviours

There is some longitudinal data which suggests that unemployment also increases the likelihood of hazardous health behaviours such as smoking or excess alcohol consumption. This is particularly the case amongst young men. For example, a study of 2,887 men from the 1958 British Birth Cohort found an increased risk of smoking and problem drinking amongst those who were unemployed (Montgomery et al., 1999b). After adjustment for potential confounding factors (socio-economic and behavioural factors before the onset of unemployment), the RR of smoking for those aged 33 who had been unemployed in the last year was 2.92 (95% CI 2.13 to 4.01), for heavy drinking it was 1.73 (95% CI 1.18 to 2.54), and having a drink problem was 2.90 (95% CI 1.99 to 4.21). In addition, the study looked at the effects of accumulated unemployment (more than three years unemployment) since age 16. It found that long-term unemployment of over three years increased the risk of smoking (fully adjusted relative odds [RO] = 2.11, 95% CI 1.42 to 3.12), and problem drinking (fully adjusted RO = 2.15, 95% CI 1.39 to 3.33) compared to those who had never experienced unemployment. Similarly, a Finnish study of alcohol use found that associations between high levels of alcohol consumption and unemployment were only consistent across periods of both high and low national unemployment levels amongst poorly educated, single, unemployed men (OR = 1.6, 95% CI 1.1 to 2.4) (Luoto *et al.*, 1998).

5.2.5 Unemployment and health in the twenty-first century[1]

This research literature from the previous recessions of the 1980s and 1990s therefore suggests that the increased unemployment resulting from the current economic recession will have negative public health effects and result in a corresponding increase in the use of health services. However, significant changes in the constitution of economic life mean that the magnitude of the unemployment related health effects of the 2008 recession may be under-estimated if we only rely on research data from the recessions of previous eras. There are key differences between then and now, especially in terms of the structure of the welfare state and the organisation and experience of work (Bambra, 2010a).

Changes to the welfare system: reform and recommodification

The welfare systems of most developed economies have experienced considerable reform since the last two economic recessions (see Chapter 2). This has meant that access and entitlement to out of work cash benefits and welfare services have decreased considerably. For example, the population coverage of unemployment benefit in the UK decreased from 90% in 1980 to 77% in 1999, in Germany it decreased from 100% to 84% and in Norway, from 100% to 79% (Eikemo and Bambra, 2008). The replacement value of unemployment benefit has also decreased in the UK from 45% of average wages in 1980 to just 16% in 1999; in Germany it decreased from 68% to 37%, and in Norway from 70% to 62% (Eikemo and Bambra, 2008). Further, the welfare safety net for women is often smaller than that for men (Bambra and Eikemo, 2009). The extent to which the welfare state can act as a buffer against the negative social and health consequences of economic recession has therefore been diminished.

Further, there is an increased use of welfare to work policies, requiring the unemployed to partake in compulsory employability and skills training in

---

[1] This section is reproduced from Bambra (2010a) with permission from BMJ Publishing Group Ltd.

order to receive benefits (Rhodes, 1997). The likely success of such schemes in returning people to employment seems limited within a contracting labour market. In fact, from a health perspective, they may well be counterproductive in terms of their stigmatising effects and the division of the poor into deserving and undeserving (Bambra, 2008; Bambra and Smith, 2010). Certainly, an Australian study of welfare to work schemes amongst young people in the 1990s found them to be almost as detrimental to mental health as being unemployed (Morrell *et al.*, 1998). Indeed, the economic recession and the resulting rise in unemployment have not put a stop to the continued individualisation of responsibility for unemployment or indeed, for poor health. Previous recessions suggest that the stigmatising of benefit recipients as 'scroungers' will only increase, particularly in the UK, Australia and the US (Campbell, 1984). This means that although unemployment benefit has long been characterised by stigma and means-testing (Campbell, 1984; Orwell, 1937 [1981]) the cash benefits now provided to people when they are out of work are of considerably less value in real terms than they were in the rest of the post-war period and a lot more is required in order to be entitled to them. Given the links between material poverty and poor health, and between social stigma and poor health, this may have important negative influences on the relative health of the unemployed (Watkins, 1986; Bartley *et al.*, 2006). This may increase health inequalities between those with and without work (Kondo *et al.*, 2008).

It is also important to note that this 'new' unemployment coexists with structural worklessness in the form of long-term sickness absence and disability pension receipt (see Chapter 6). Across Europe, disability pension receipt has increased significantly over the past 25 years and in some post-industrial areas of Europe, rates are as high as 18% of the working age population (Bambra and Norman, 2006). The vast majority of new disability claims are made on the basis of mental health. Mental health problems also develop as co-morbidities amongst those who are initially out of the labour market due to chronic physical health problems (such as musculoskeletal conditions) (Organisation for Economic Cooperation and Development, 2009). It therefore seems likely that the new wave of unemployment will impact on mental health more than on physical health. It is possible that the coexistence of high levels of health and disability related worklessness may actually decrease the stigma attached to unemployment as worklessness of various forms becomes 'normalised' within certain deprived post-industrial communities. As Orwell commented in *The Road to Wigan Pier*:

> 'When people live on the dole for years at a time they grow used to it, and . . . though it remains unpleasant, it ceases to be shameful . . . It makes a great deal of difference when things are the same for everybody' (Orwell, 1937 [1981]: 78).

This will not of course decrease the health effects of the material deprivation experienced by unemployed individuals and workless communities. Further, the social exclusion of workless communities (as opposed to unemployed individuals within them) may well increase in the longer term and lead to the further stigmatisation of such places with resulting rises in geographic inequalities in health and economic development.

Changes to the world of work: precarious employment, job insecurity, and health

The nature of work has altered considerably over the past few decades, with a decrease in industrial employment and an increase in the size of the service sector, as well as an increase in the use of abnormal working hours. Simultaneously, women's employment rates have also substantially increased in most Western economies (e.g. in the UK they have increased from 56% in 1971 to 70% in 2007). This has been accompanied by a rise in flexible, precarious employment: increasing numbers of people working on either temporary contracts or no contracts, with limited or no employment or welfare rights. In this new economy, skills, working hours, contracts, conditions, pay and location are all more flexible (Beatson, 1995; Marmot *et al.*, 1999). The formerly standard full-time, permanent contract with benefits has been superseded by a number of atypical forms of employment characterised by lower levels of security and poorer working conditions (both physical and psychosocial) (Benach *et al.*, 2002). Rather than being a transitory stage in an individual's employment history, these atypical forms of labour are becoming the norm for many workers in the labour force of advanced capitalist economies (Virtanen *et al.*, 2002). Temporary, insecure, work accounts for an average of around 15% of paid employment across the European Union (an average of 16.4% in the EU-15 countries and an average of 14.0% in the EU-27 countries, Massarelli, 2009). This amounts to 19.1 million full-time temporary workers: the so-called 'precariat' (Massarelli, 2009). Across all European countries (except Germany), temporary work is considerably higher amongst women than men (Table 5.1). The gains to employers from such job insecurity include increased performance and productivity, lower wages and lower associated costs such as pensions or sickness benefits: or put more simply—higher profits. However, these benefits to capital are accompanied by adverse consequences for labour, with insecure workers having lower levels of physical and mental health.

Precarious or contingent employment is characterised by a lack of security and stability (Benach and Muntaner, 2007; Hadden *et al.*, 2007). Examples include informal work, temporary or fixed-term work, contract work, casual work, piece work, home working, part-time work and other less regulated forms

Table 5.1 Job insecurity in 17 European countries[a]

Country	Share of employees with limited duration contract (%)[b]		
	Total	Men	Women
Austria	9.0	8.9	9.1
Belgium	8.3	6.6	10.2
Denmark	8.3	7.6	9.1
Finland	15.0	11.2	18.7
France	14.2	13.0	15.4
Germany	14.7	14.7	14.6
Greece	11.4	9.9	13.7
Ireland	8.4	7.2	9.8
Italy	13.3	11.5	15.6
Luxembourg	6.3	5.6	6.2
Netherlands	18.2	16.6	19.9
Norway	9.1	7.1	11.1
Portugal	22.8	21.7	24.2
Spain	29.3	27.6	31.4
Sweden	16.1	13.4	18.7
Switzerland	13.2	13.2	13.1
UK	5.4	4.9	6.0
EU-15[c]	*16.4*	*15.4*	*17.5*
EU-27[d]	*14.0*	*13.3*	*14.9*

[a] EU-15 plus Norway and Switzerland.

[b] 2008 European Union Labour Force Survey Data (Massarelli, 2009).

[c] EU-15: The 15 pre-2004 European Union member states (Austria, Belgium, Denmark, Finland, France, Germany, Greece, Ireland, Italy, Luxembourg, the Netherlands, Portugal, Spain, Sweden and the United Kingdom).

[d] EU-27: The 15 pre-2004 European Union member states plus 10 who joined in 2004 (Malta, Cyprus, Slovenia, Estonia, Latvia, Lithuania, Poland, the Czech Republic, Slovak Republic, and Hungary) and 2 who joined in 2007 (Romania and Bulgaria).

Source: European Union Labour Force Survey Data (Massarelli, 2009).

of labour (World Health Organisation Commission on the Social Determinants of Health, 2008). Benach and Muntaner (2007) regard precarious employment as the lack of labour market regulation. According to Hadden and colleagues (2007) there is an employment continuum, with the quality of job security provided by a standard (full-time, year-round, unlimited duration, with benefits) employment contract at one end and a high degree of precariousness at the other. Precarious employment is also a multidimensional construct covering temporality, powerlessness, lack of benefits and low income (Hadden *et al.*, 2007).

Precarious employment is becoming more commonplace in developed economies with trends toward less well regulated labour markets and the disempowerment of workers, job seekers and unions (World Health Organisation Commission for Social Determinants of Health, 2008: 73). Precarious employment represents around 15% of all forms of paid employment across the European Union (Benavides *et al.*, 2000). Women and immigrants tend to be over-represented in temporary forms of work (Marshall, 1989). Precarious employment is usually associated with low income, long and unsociable working hours and often high strain and stress (Quinlan *et al.*, 2001). It therefore impacts on health and well-being through material, psychosocial and behavioural pathways, by affecting amongst other aspects, income, social interaction, and opportunities for physical activity.

Analysis of data from the European Survey of Working Conditions (see Box 3.1 in Chapter 3) found that a number of adverse physical and mental health indicators were associated with precarious employment (Benavides *et al.*, 2000). Specifically, precarious employment was associated with stress, fatigue, backache and muscular pains, job dissatisfaction and absenteeism. These trends were noted for all European countries and worse health outcomes were reported for full-time as opposed to part-time workers. Similarly, a systematic review of the occupational health and safety effects of precarious employment found that the majority of included studies demonstrated an association between precarious employment and poor occupational health outcomes (Quinlan *et al.*, 2001). The types of adverse health and well-being outcomes associated with precarious work included exposure to hazardous materials, fatigue, injuries, musculoskeletal disorders as well as psychological and physical well-being. There is also longitudinal evidence from the Whitehall II studies (see Box 4.1 in Chapter 4) on the negative association between perceived job security and a number of health indicators including self-reported health, minor psychiatric morbidity, physiological measures (blood pressure) and health related behaviours (Ferrie *et al.*, 2002). Kivimäki and colleagues (2003b) have also reported a negative association between temporary employment and overall, as well as cause-specific, mortality. In this Finnish longitudinal study conducted over a ten year period, overall mortality was shown to be more than 20% higher in temporary employees when compared with those employees on a permanent contract. Further, mortality from alcohol related causes was increased for both men and women temporary workers when compared with permanent workers (men hazard ratio [HR] = 2.0, 95% CI 1.4 to 2.9; women HR = 1.7, 95% CI 1.1 to 2.5). Mortality from smoking related cancer was higher amongst male temporary workers only (HR = 2.8, 95% CI 1.3 to 6.0).

In terms of mental health, a Finnish cross-sectional survey (Virtanen *et al.*, 2002) compared health outcomes for workers on fixed compared to permanent contracts.

It found that psychological distress was greater for women on fixed-term contracts (age-adjusted OR = 1.26, 95% CI 1.09 to 1.45) than those on permanent contracts. Further, in terms of job security, high perceived security was associated with high levels of self-rated health, low levels of psychological distress and low levels of chronic disease (Virtanen *et al.*, 2002). Another cross-sectional study, from South Korea, demonstrated strong associations for women between precarious employment (part-time work, temporary work, and work with less than a one-month contract) and mental ill health (measured by depression and suicidal thoughts) (Kim *et al.*, 2006). For women, precarious employment was significantly associated with both depression and suicidal thoughts after adjusting for socio-economic class and health behaviours (depression OR = 1.66, 95% CI 1.02 to 2.69; suicidal thoughts OR = 1.62, 95% CI 1.19 to 2.22). For men, however, the associations between depression, suicidal thoughts and precarious employment did not remain significant after adjusting for confounders. Artazcoz and associates (2005) also examined the effects of different forms of precarious employment on mental health in Catalonia, Spain. They found a greatly increased likelihood of developing poor mental health amongst women (age-adjusted OR= 3.87, 95% CI 1.52 to 9.85) and men (OR = 4.30, 95% CI 1.96 to 9.44) who were temporary workers compared to those with permanent contracts (Artazcoz *et al.*, 2005). Likewise, working with no contract was associated with poor mental health amongst manual workers (OR men = 6.34, 95% CI 1.89 to 21.22; OR women = 3.27, 95% CI 1.54 to 6.94) (Artazcoz *et al.*, 2005).

Further, it is recognised that poor quality work with little security can be as health damaging as unemployment (Benach and Muntaner, 2007). For example, a cross-sectional study of 2,497 middle-aged Australian workers found that poor quality jobs with low security, low marketability and high job strain were associated with poorer health when compared to work with few or no stressors (Broom *et al.*, 2006). However, respondents whose work was marked by three or more adverse conditions reported health that was no better than those who were unemployed. By way of illustration, poor self-rated health was significantly higher amongst workers with three adverse employment conditions when compared with those workers with only one adverse condition (age-adjusted OR 2.44, 95% CI 1.08 to 5.49). Further, workers with three or more adverse conditions had substantially higher odds of developing depression (OR 7.27, 95% CI 3.64 to 14.51) than those who were unemployed (OR 4.11, 95% CI 2.15 to 7.86). Many workers on atypical contracts can cycle from precarious work into unemployment, thus augmenting the negative consequences for health (Furlong and Cartmel, 2004).

These new employment forms also impact on the experience and distribution of unemployment, as those with the least protection will be at most risk of unemployment, often without redundancy packages. These are likely to be women, the young, and immigrants—what in political economy terms is referred to as the *reserve army of labour* or the 'precariat' (see Chapter 6). These are also the workers who have the least entitlement to public welfare benefits, and when they do it will be to the lower value, more stigmatising means-tested benefits which do not provide enough material support to protect against the ill health effects of unemployment (Rodriguez, 2001). They are also less likely to have community based social support. Previous research suggested that the health effects of unemployment were greater for men than for women. Explanations of this were based on the vital importance of paid work for men's self-identity (Campbell, 1984; Orwell 1937 [1981]) and/or the fact that men are less likely to seek health and social support (Dorling, 2009). In contrast, women's traditional social roles (notably motherhood or homemaking) acted as buffers to the mental health effects of job loss as they gave alternative sources of identity. As the labour market is becoming increasingly feminised and gender roles shift, this might no longer be the case (if indeed it ever was) as work becomes an increasingly important part of most women's self-identity. This time, the negative health effects of unemployment may be more equally experienced by women as well as men. Further, workers currently experiencing a daily existence of low paid, high strain, temporary employment, may be ill prepared for, and least resilient to, the additional negative health premium of unemployment. So in such cases, whilst unemployment may temporarily release people from the negative health effects of insecure employment, it does not provide an adequate safety net to be a healthy alternative. Further, even for those who remain in work, perceived job insecurity increases during periods of economic recession. The health effects of such insecurity may well be stronger in a period when the material social safety net for the unemployed has been eroded.

5.3 Recessions, unemployment, and health inequalities

This section examines the effects of recessions on health inequalities. It also examines the contribution of socio-economic differences in unemployment rates to the social gradient in health.

5.3.1 Recessions and health inequalities

There have only been a few studies that have examined the effects of recessions on health inequalities. The findings of these studies are rather mixed as one Japanese study found that recession increased relative occupational inequalities in self-rated health amongst men (Kondo *et al.*, 2008), whilst a Finnish study found that the recession slowed down the trend towards increased inequalities in mortality (Valkonen *et al.*, 2000), and a series of Scandinavian studies of morbidity concluded that there were no significant effects of the 1990s recession on inequalities in morbidity in these countries (Lahlema *et al.*, 2002). The effect of economic recessions on health inequalities is underexplored and as such currently unclear (Riva *et al.*, 2011).

The Japanese recession of the 1990s lasted ten years and in Japan, this period is referred to as the 'lost decade'. The effect of this prolonged recession on health inequalities was studied by Kondo and colleagues (2008). Using a repeat cross-sectional design, pooled national data from the Japanese working age population (aged 20–60 years old) was taken for 168,801 people from 1986–1989 (pre-recession) and 150,016 people from 1998–2001 (towards the end of the recession). Self-perceived health was compared by occupational status. After the recession, the proportion of people reporting poor health decreased across all occupational groups (by between 11.0% and 21.2%). Multivariate analysis showed no significant association between occupational status and health before the crisis (i.e. no significant health inequalities). This was also the case for women after the crisis. However, after the economic crisis, amongst men, non-manual clerical and service workers were 16% more likely to report poor health compared with executive and managerial workers: the socio-demographically-adjusted OR of reporting poor health increased from 1.00 (0.89 to 1.13) pre-recession to 1.16 (1.02 to 1.32) post-recession, a statistically significant temporal change of $p=0.04$. Unemployed men were more than twice as likely to report poor health as executive and managerial workers at both time points (pre-recession OR = 2.87, 2.48 to 3.32; post-recession OR = 2.18, 1.85 to 2.58). Unemployed women were also more likely to report poor health across the period but at a lower level (pre-recession OR = 1.62, 1.26 to 2.09; post-recession OR = 1.87, 1.37 to 2.54). So, whilst the likelihood of reporting poor health decreased across all occupational groups, relative health inequalities between men in the top and middle occupational groups increased.

In contrast, a Finnish study of socio-economic inequalities amongst middle-aged men and women found that the recession reduced occupational inequalities in mortality (Valkonen *et al.*, 2000). The longitudinal study which used linked census and mortality records examined men and women aged 35–64 and covered 122,250 deaths divided into three time periods of 1981–1985 (pre-recession), 1986–1990 (economic boom) and 1991–1995 (severe recession). The deaths of manual workers were compared to non-manual workers in these time periods. Over the whole time period, (1981 to 1995), total mortality declined by 26% amongst men and 17% amongst women. However, these reductions were greater in the non-manual class than the manual class: the absolute class difference in death rates amongst men increased from 318 per 100,000 in the period 1981–1985, to 401 in 1986–1990, and then reduced to 392 in the recession period 1991–1995. In relative terms the differences increased from 49.5% to 75.3% and 85.8%. Amongst women, the absolute difference in death rates increased across the period from 60 per 100,000 in 1981–1985, to 95 per 100,000 in 1986–1990, to 113 per 100,000 in the recession period 1991–1995. In relative terms, the differences increased from 21.2% to 36.2% to 47.7%. The authors concluded that the recession slowed down the rate at which inequalities in mortality were increasing since the 1980s.

A comparative study of working age (16–64) morbidity conducted in Finland (Manderbacka *et al.*, 2001), Norway (Dahl *et al.*, 2001), Sweden (Lundberg *et al.*, 2001) and Denmark (Lahlema *et al.*, 2002) found that both relative and absolute educational inequalities in self-reported health remained stable during the 1980s and 1990s (Lahelma *et al.*, 2002). The latter was a period in which Finland and Sweden in particular experienced significant recession and welfare state reform (including tax increases, cuts in public spending per capita on welfare services, decreased value of benefits). The Finnish study found that the patterning and size of relative socio-economic inequalities (measured using education and occupational class) in ill health remained generally stable (although there were some slight decreases in educational inequalities amongst men). Similarly, the Swedish study found that overall prevalence of ill health and educational and occupational inequalities in limiting long term illness and self-reported health remained stable across the study period. The Norwegian and Danish studies also found negligible changes in health inequalities despite economic and social upheaval. The authors of the studies concluded that health inequalities in the Social Democratic countries were not strongly influenced by changes in income and labour market inequalities because the strong welfare state arrangements, although subject to reform in the 1990s, were still comparatively generous and buffered against the structural pressures towards widening health inequalities (Lahlema *et al.*, 2002).

5.3.2 Unemployment and health inequalities

Unemployment is associated with poverty and social exclusion, and it tends to be concentrated in lower socio-economic classes (Arber, 1987; Rodriguez, 2001): Employment rates are consistently higher amongst more educated groups. For example, according to English census data, in 2001 in London, 90.1% of men and 81.5% of women with a university degree were employed compared to just 69.2% of men and 51.8% of women with no qualifications. Ill health related job loss also has a social gradient, with adverse employment consequences more likely for those in lower socio-economic (i.e. lower educated) classes (Bartley and Owen, 1996). Unemployment is potentially therefore a very important social determinant of health inequalities.

The importance of unemployment to health inequalities was demonstrated in a recent study which used data on employment status, socio-economic class, and self-rated heath for people of working age (25–59) who had ever worked from a 3% sample of the 2001 English census (349,699 women and 349,181 men) (Popham and Bambra, 2010). This study found that, regardless of socio-economic class, people experiencing unemployment or other forms of worklessness were universally more likely to have poor self-reported health. However, for both men and women, not being in paid employment accounted for up to 81% of the inequalities in the prevalence of self-rated poor health between the most affluent and the least affluent socio-economic classes in the English working age population (for men ranging from 57% to 81%, for women 50% to 74%). As an example, 5.6% of men living in owner occupied housing reported that they did not have good general health compared to 19.1% of men in social rented housing, an age-adjusted difference of 13% points. After further adjustment for employment status this difference reduced to 2.5% points, a reduction of 81%. Adjusting for employment status reduced the prevalence of poor self-reported health in all socio-economic classes thereby substantially reducing the social gradient.

This study suggests that policies to reduce health inequalities, not just between the most affluent and the poorest, but across the whole social gradient may need to focus on increasing the proportion of people in paid employment. This translates as not just the need to get people into work or to help people maintain employment in times of adversity (such as ill health), but also an increase in the demand for labour particularly in regions with high unemployment rates amongst the lower skilled (Coombes and Raybould, 2004). It is not clear though whether the relationship between unemployment and health inequalities results from the material deprivation experienced by the unemployed, or from their feelings of stigma and isolation.

5.4 **Welfare state regimes, recessions, and unemployment**

As described in detail in Chapter 2, developed countries vary greatly in terms of their labour market frameworks and welfare state regimes, and various studies have shown that population health indicators (including self-reported health, life expectancy as well as infant mortality rates) and socio-economic inequalities in health also vary by type of welfare state. National welfare state arrangements thereby moderate the effects of labour market position on health.

This potentially includes mitigating against the negative health effects of recessions as well as the experience of unemployment.

5.4.1 Welfare states and recessions

There is some tentative evidence to suggest that the health effects of recessions vary by welfare state context (Moore, 2009; Riva et al., 2011). For example, a study by Gerdtham and Ruhm (2006) on the relationship between unemployment rates and mortality in 23 of the Organisation for Economic Cooperation and Development (OECD) countries found that countries with low welfare state expenditure had larger fluctuations in mortality than those with more generous provision. A study of different responses to the Asian economic crisis concluded that social safety nets and public expenditure were important in mitigating the health effects of economic crises (Hopkins, 2006). Similarly, a European study by Stuckler and colleagues (2009) concluded that public investment in active labour market programmes could also reduce the effects of recessions on suicide. It found that whilst every 1% increase in unemployment was associated with a 0.79% (95% CI 0.16 to 1.42) rise in suicides amongst those aged under 65, every $10 per person per year increased investment in active labour market programmes reduced the effect of unemployment increases on suicides by 0.038% (95% CI −0.0004 to −0.071) (Stuckler et al., 2009). Further, expenditure of more than $190 per person per year on active labour market programmes (as in Scandinavia), meant that increases in the unemployment rate did not increase suicide rates. For example, in Sweden between 1991 and 1992, unemployment rose from 2.1% to 5.7% but suicide rates actually fell. The wider welfare state and labour market context are therefore potentially important mediatory factors in the health effects of recessions.

5.4.2 Welfare states, unemployment, and health[2]

Social protection (particularly wage replacement rates) during unemployment varies by welfare state regime. To a large degree this reflects the historical influence of differing political traditions, with those countries experiencing more post-war years of Social Democratic rule providing more generous systems of support (Esping-Andersen, 1990). Table 5.2 breaks down the various characteristics of social protection during unemployment by five different welfare state regimes: Scandinavian, Anglo-Saxon, Bismarckian, Southern and Eastern. In essence, there are three interrelating principles underpinning provision: universalism,

---

[2] This section is reproduced from Bambra and Eikemo (2009) with permission from BMJ Publishing Group Ltd.

Table 5.2 Characteristics of unemployment protection in 23 European countries, ranked by welfare state regime

Welfare regime (1–5, high-low)	Country	Funding system	Qualifying period[a]	Initial net replacement rate (% of net, average wages)[b]	Unemployment insurance benefit duration (months)[c]	Waiting Period (days)[d]
1. Scandinavian	Denmark	Subsidised voluntary insurance	12 months in last 3 years	70	48	0
	Finland	Voluntary subsidised insurance and social assistance system	43 weeks in last 2 years	70	23	7
	Norway	Social insurance	Annual earnings in last year equal to 75% of base amount	68	48	5
	Sweden	Subsidised programe of basic insurance and voluntary income-related insurance	6 months in last 12 years	75	28	5
2. Bismarckian	Austria	Social insurance	28 weeks in last 12 months	63	9	0
	Belgium	Social insurance	468 days in last 27 months	61	No limit	0
	France	Social insurance and social assistance	6 months in last 22 years	75	23	8
	Germany	Social insurance and social assistance	12 months in last 2 years	69	12	0

	Luxembourg	Social insurance	26 weeks in last 12 months	80	12	0
	Netherlands	Social insurance and social assistance	26 weeks in last 39 weeks	74	24	0
3. Anglo-Saxon	Switzerland	Social insurance	12 months in last 2 years	77	24	5
	Ireland	Social insurance and social assistance	39 weeks in last 12 months	49	15	3
	United Kingdom	Social insurance and social assistance	Contributions equivalent to 25 and 50 times the lower earnings limit must have been paid in the last 2 years	54	6	3
4. Southern Europe	Greece	Social insurance	125 days in last 14 months	55	12	6
	Italy	Social insurance	2 years of insurance contributions with 52 weeks contributions in last 2 years	54	6	7
	Portugal	Social insurance and social assistance	540 days in last 24 months	83	24	0
	Spain	Social insurance	12 months in last 6 years	67	21	0

(continued)

Table 5.2 (*continued*) Characteristics of unemployment protection in 23 European countries, ranked by welfare state regime

Welfare regime (1-5, high-low)	Country	Funding system	Qualifying period[a]	Initial net replacement rate (% of net, average wages)[b]	Unemployment insurance benefit duration (months)[c]	Waiting Period (days)[d]
5. Eastern Europe	Czech Republic	Social insurance	12 months in last 3 years	56	5	6
	Hungary	Social insurance	12 months in last 4 years	49	9	7
	Poland	Social insurance	Earnings in 18 months prior to claim must be at least equivalent to the minimum wage	59	12	0
	Slovenia	Social insurance	12 months in last 18 months	56	8	–

[a] For unemployment insurance benefits.

[b] Net replacement rate = (benefit income when unemployed – tax on benefit income)/(earned income + benefit income when employed – tax on earnings and benefits) × 100; it is assumed that the unemployed worker is 40 years old and has an uninterrupted employment record of 22 years Benefits included in calculation: Unemployment insurance, unemployment assistance, social assistance, family benefits, housing benefits.

[c] Months at equivalent to the initial rate for the Czech Republic, the Slovak Republic and Spain where the benefit level declines overtime (e.g. for Spain, where the nominal replacement rate declines from 70% to 60% after six months, the months equivalent initial rate is calculated as six months plus 6/7ths of 18 months). In most countries after the insurance period ends the unemployed person is entitled to claim social assistance (which may be means-tested).

[d] Table reproduced from Bambra and Eikemo (2009) with permission of BMJ Publishing Group Ltd.

social insurance and means-testing (Diderichsen, 2002). Systems based on universal provision do not make reference to previous contributions or means-testing and are offered to all citizens on an entitlement basis as long as specific demographic, social or health criteria are fulfilled. Often flat rate benefits are paid. Under social insurance systems, entitlement to benefits is dependent on previous contributions and in most cases subsequent benefit levels reflect previous earned income. Under means-testing, entitlement is restricted on the basis of income and the (often minimal) financial support is targeted at those in most need, usually after they have exhausted all other means (e.g. personal savings or social insurance) (Rhodes, 1997).

Welfare provision for the unemployed is governed by these three principles in varying ways. For example, with differing degrees of generosity, universalism is more prominent within the Scandinavian welfare states (high population coverage) and the Anglo-Saxon regime (fixed benefit rates for all), whilst social insurance is the key component of provision within the Bismarckian, Southern and Eastern European welfare states. Means-testing is more commonly a characteristic of the Anglo-Saxon welfare states, however it is also used for social assistance payments in other welfare state regimes. For example, in the UK (Anglo-Saxon) unemployment benefit is only payable (for a maximum of six months) to those who fulfil the minimum National Insurance contribution requirement within the two years before claiming (Table 5.3). Most claimants do not meet these criteria and are therefore reliant on means-tested social assistance benefits (Eurostat, 2000). However, this mixed approach is also evident in Sweden where there is a social insurance based benefit (Unemployment Insurance Benefit) based on past contributions and which pays a benefit as a proportion of previous wages, as well as a means tested social assistance scheme (Unemployment Assistance Benefit) which pays a (lower) flat rate (Eurostat, 2000). Similarly, a three-tier system is operated in Germany (Bismarckian): those with a full contribution record receive the full unemployment insurance benefit (Arbeitslosengeld), those with a smaller contribution criteria, receive a means-tested insurance benefit (Arbeitslosenhilfe) whilst those who do not have a sufficient contribution record must rely upon the Sozialhilfe social assistance scheme (Eurostat, 2000). This link between benefit levels and employment related insurance contributions is an example of the labour discipline inherent within the welfare state as it maintains a connection with previous market performance (Ginsburg, 1979).

Unemployment protection in each welfare state regime therefore represents a complex mix of these differing principles. However, there are clear differences by welfare state regime—due to the influence of differing political traditions—in terms of how these principles are put into pratice, particularly in

Table 5.3 Prevalence rates, rate differences and age standardised odds ratios (95% CI) of the relationship between unemployment and health by welfare state regime (European Social Survey 2002 and 2004)

Welfare state regime		Limiting long-term illness (LLTI)				Poor/fair general health (PH)			
		Prevalence Employed %	Prevalence Unemployed %	Rate Difference (unemployed–employed)	OR for Rate Difference (95% CI)	Prevalence Employed %	Prevalence Unemployed %	Rate Difference (unemployed–employed)	OR for Rate Difference (95% CI)
Men	Scandinavian	17.5	30.3	13.5	1.96 (1.47–2.61)	18.4	35.4	17.0	2.27 (1.72–3.01)
	Bismarckian	13.7	25.1	12.0	2.21 (1.74–2.79)	20.1	39.9	19.8	2.72 (2.21–3.35)
	Anglo-Saxon	11.1	16.4	5.7	1.67 (0.99–2.81)	12.7	29.6	16.9	2.97 (1.92–4.60)
	Southern	6.8	12.5	6.2	2.07 (1.34–3.18)	21.9	34.5	12.6	1.82 (1.35–2.46)
	Eastern	17.6	27.4	10.8	1.89 (1.43–2.52)	33.1	50.9	17.8	2.15 (1.67–2.76)
Women	Scandinavian	19.4	35.3	17.0	2.28 (1.71–3.03)	17.8	35.3	18.7	2.99 (2.34–4.00)
	Bismarckian	14.8	23.5	9.4	1.87 (1.48–2.37)	21.9	34.7	13.8	2.06 (1.67–2.55)
	Anglo-Saxon	10.0	23.1	13.7	2.73 (1.50–4.95)	13.6	27.5	14.8	2.78 (1.63–4.73)
	Southern	7.8	11.8	4.5	1.52 (1.03–2.25)	30.5	39.3	10.1	1.66 (1.31–2.11)
	Eastern	18.1	24.4	7.0	1.65 (1.24–2.19)	38.4	49.0	12.0	1.76 (1.38–2.25)

terms of the generosity of benefits paid to the unemployed (replacement rates), the qualifying period and conditions, duration of benefit payments and the waiting period before entitlement is activated. In each of these respects, the Scandinavian welfare states are generally more generous than the other welfare state regimes (Table 5.2), particularly in comparison to the Anglo-Saxon and Eastern European regimes.

Differences in the social protection offered to the unemployed could therefore be an important mediatory factor in the relationship between poverty, unemployment and health (Bartley *et al.*, 2006). In a recent paper with Eikemo (Bambra and Eikemo, 2009), I examined the extent to which relative health inequalities between unemployed and employed people varied across 23 European countries and in terms of the different approaches to social protection taken by the five European welfare state regimes (Scandinavian, Anglo-Saxon, Bismarckian, Southern and Eastern). The study used data from the 2002 and 2004 waves of the cross-sectional European Social Survey (37,499 respondents, aged 25–60). Employment status was measured as the main activity in the last seven days. Health variables were self-reported limiting long term illness (LLTI) and fair/poor general health (PH).

We found that in all countries, unemployed people reported higher rates of PH than those in employment (see Table 5.3). There were also clear differences by welfare state regime. Relative inequalities between employed and unemployed were largest in the Anglo-Saxon (men: OR_{PH}=2.97, 95% CI 1.92 to 4.60; women: OR_{LLTI}=2.73, 95% CI 1.50 to 4.95 and OR_{PH}=2.78, 95% CI 1.63 to 4.73) Bismarckian (men only: OR_{LLTI}=2.21, 95% CI 1.74 to 2.79 and OR_{PH}=2.72, 95% CI 2.21 to 3.35), and Scandinavian (women only: OR_{LLTI}=2.28, 95% CI 1.71 to 3.03 and OR_{PH}=2.99, 95% CI 2.31 to 4.00) regimes, and smallest in the Southern (men: OR_{PH}=1.82, 95% CI 1.35 to 2.46; women: OR_{LLTI}=1.52, 95% CI 1.03 to 2.25 and OR_{PH}=1.66, 95% CI 1.31 to 2.11) and Eastern (women only: OR_{LLTI}=1.65, 95% CI 1.24 to 2.10 and OR_{PH}=1.76, 95% CI 1.38 to 2.25) welfare state regimes.

Our study shows that the relationship between unemployment and health is consistent across European countries, with the unemployed in each country reporting worse self-reported health than the employed. It seems therefore, that even though the levels of social protection offered to the unemployed vary by welfare state (and welfare state regime), in all countries, a relationship exists between unemployment and poorer self-rated health. This suggests that current wage replacement rates, even in the more generous welfare states, are not sufficient to overcome the financial effects of unemployment on health. On the other hand, it may indicate the importance for health of the non-financial losses associated with unemployment (e.g. social isolation) (Bartley *et al.*, 2006, Rudas *et al.*, 1991). However, the study identified important differences in the magnitude of the relationship by welfare state regime. Specifically, relative inequalities were found to be largest for men and women in the Anglo-Saxon countries. Wage replacement rates for the unemployed are the lowest in these welfare states, and benefits are means-tested and subject to strict entitlement rules. The unemployed in the Anglo-Saxon welfare states are therefore at a great financial disadvantage in comparison to those in employment and this may well explain the magnitude of inequality as financial strain has been found to be an important factor in the relationship between unemployment and ill health (Kessler *et al.*, 1987). Furthermore, means-tested benefits are associated with stigma and so the non-financial problems of unemployment may be greater in the Anglo-Saxon welfare states (Diderichsen, 2002). A comparative study by Rodriguez (2001) found that in the UK, Germany and the US, the likelihood of reporting poor health was significantly higher amongst unemployed people in receipt of means-tested benefits than those in receipt of entitlement benefits (see Chapter 7). The higher inequalities in the Anglo-Saxon countries are in keeping with broader based studies of welfare state regimes and health indicators which have found that overall population health tends to be worse in the welfare states of the Anglo-Saxon regime (see Chapter 2).

5.5 Conclusion

In this chapter, I have explored the health effects of cyclical capitalist economic recessions, concluding that they seem to positively impact on some health outcomes (particularly mortality and health behaviours) whilst extremely negatively affecting others such as suicide rates. I have also reflected on the large indirect negative health effects of recessions in terms of how they increase the unemployment rate. I have summarised the vast and well established empirical literature on the negative relationship between unemployment and health, as well as the various theories which attempt to explain it. The chapter has also highlighted the importance of unemployment to health inequalities. This literature suggests that increasing employment, particularly amongst low skilled groups or in areas of high unemployment, has the potential to reduce socio-economic inequalities in health. The chapter has also examined how the health effects of recessions and the relationship between unemployment and health vary by welfare state regime, and argued that higher levels of social protection, as found within Social Democratic welfare states, buffer the negative health effects of unemployment, and potentially also the negative effects on health of recessions. This has shown that politically driven public policy responses are important in terms of determining the health effects of recessions and the health of the unemployed.

5.6 **Further reading**

Bartley, M., Ferrie, J. and Montgomery, S. (2006) 'Health and labour market disadvantage: unemployment, non-employment, and job insecurity'. In: M. Marmot and R. G. Wilkinson (eds.) *Social Determinants of Health*. Oxford, Oxford University Press.

Showler, B. and Sinfield, A. (1981) (eds.) *The Workless State: a study of unemployment*. Robertson, Oxford.

Smith, R. (1985) 'Bitterness, shame, emptiness, waste': an introduction to unemployment and health, *British Medical Journal; 291*:1024–1027.

Chapter 6

Health related worklessness

The previous chapter examined how one form of worklessness—unemployment—is associated with an increased risk of ill health and mortality. This chapter examines the opposite relationship, in which the development of ill health can result in long-term worklessness. 'Health related worklessness' is thus a term used to refer collectively to people who are out-of-work on a long-term basis (over four weeks) due to a chronic illness or disability (National Institute for Health and Clinical Excellence, 2008). A 'disability' in this context is defined as an illness or impairment that limits the usual activities of daily living, including work ability (Organisation for Economic Cooperation and Development, 2009: 11). Across advanced market democracies, poor health is a significant risk factor for unemployment, as well as remaining unemployed. For example, a study using European Community Household Panel Data from the 1990s found that people who developed chronic health problems whilst in employment were twice as likely to become workless within a four year period as those who remained healthy (Schuring *et al.*, 2007). These effects were also noted in a study of health and worklessness in the US (McDonough and Amick, 2001). Over the same period, women in poor health and men in poor health were 60% and 40% less likely to enter paid employment than men in good health (Schuring *et al.*, 2007). In combination with other labour market disadvantages such as low educational level, poor health further increases the risk of worklessness and there are substantial inequalities in health related worklessness (Bartley and Owen, 1996; van der Wel, 2011).

In most advanced market economies, long-term health related worklessness therefore carries an entitlement to receipt of financial support from the welfare state in the form of sickness and disability pensions or, in the case of the UK, incapacity related benefits (as described in Box 6.1). Rates of receipt of these health related benefits have increased across all advanced market economies. For example, in the UK the numbers claiming health related benefits have increased from 0.5 million recipients in 1975 to 2.6 million in 2007. By 2007, around 7% of the UK working age population was in receipt of health related benefits, accounting for 11% of UK social security expenditure, at a cost of around £8 billion per annum and amounting to 1.8% of gross domestic product (GDP)

Box 6.1 The main UK health related social security benefits (2010)

Incapacity Benefit replaced Invalidity Benefit in 1994. It is a non-means-tested social security cash benefit, paid to people in the UK who are medically certified as being incapable of work due to illness or disability and who have contributed sufficient National Insurance payments. Incapacity Benefit is similar in remit to the long-term sickness and disability insurance schemes of other Western countries, such as the US's Social Security Disability Insurance and the disability pensions of Germany and Sweden. There are three rates of Incapacity Benefit including two short-term rates: a lower rate which is paid for the first 28 weeks of sickness, and a higher rate for weeks 29 to 52. The third, a long-term rate, applies to people who have been sick for more than a year and comprises the largest number of claimants. Incapacity Benefit can be received up to pensionable age.

Employment and Support Allowance was introduced in 2008 to replace Incapacity Benefit. It has a two-tier system of benefits. Those judged (via a medically administered Work Capability Test) unable to work or with limited work capacity due to the severity of their physical or mental condition will receive a higher level of benefit with no conditionality. Those who are deemed 'sick but able to work'—the work related activity group—will only receive an additional Employment Support premium if they participate in employability initiatives. Failure to participate in such programmes will result in the removal of the Employment Support component and recipients will then only be entitled to the basic Employment and Support Allowance (paid at the same rate as unemployment benefit—Jobseeker's Allowance). Since 2010, receipt of Employment and Support Allowance for the 'work related activity' group is limited to a maximum of 1 year.

Source: Reproduced from Bambra and Smith (2010) reprinted by permission of the publisher Taylor & Francis Ltd.

(Gabbay *et al.*, 2011). In 2007, 5.8% of the working age population of advanced market democracies (Organisation for Economic Cooperation and Development [OECD] countries) received such benefits (Table 6.1), with an average of 1.2% of GDP spent on long-term disability pensions as well as 0.8% of GDP on short-term sickness absence, usually paid by employers (Organisation for Economic Cooperation and Development, 2009). The probability of returning to work after being in receipt of long-term health related- benefits is just 2% annually (Organisation for Economic Cooperation and Development, 2003)

Table 6.1 Percentage of the working age population in receipt of health related benefits across OECD countries (2007)

Country	Percentage
Australia	5.4
Austria	4.6
Belgium	6.0
Canada	4.3
Czech Republic	7.1
Denmark[a]	7.2
Finland	8.5
France[b]	4.9
Germany	4.4
Greece	4.6
Hungary	12.1
Ireland	6.3
Italy[a]	3.2
Japan[a]	2.0
Korea	1.5
Luxembourg[c]	4.9
Mexico	0.7
Netherlands	8.3
New Zealand	3.8
Norway	10.3
Poland	7.2
Portugal	4.7
Slovak Republic[a]	6.3
Spain	3.8
Sweden	10.8
Switzerland	5.4
United Kingdom	7.0
United States[a]	5.9
OECD[a]	5.8

[a] 2006.

[b] 2004.

[c] 2005.

Source: Data taken from Organisation for Economic Cooperation and Development (2009).

with most recipients who have been workless for six months or more having only a 20% chance of returning to work within five years (Wardell and Burton, 2006). The employment rates of people with disability or chronic illness are also much lower, at an average of only 40% across the OECD (in the Netherlands only 10% of disabled people have work as their main source of income as compared to 50% in Sweden [Schuring *et al.*, 2007]), and people with health problems are also more than twice as likely to work part-time (Organisation for Economic Cooperation and Development, 2009). Poverty, social exclusion as well as downward social mobility are also important issues (Acheson, 1998; Myung *et al.*, 2010).

Health related worklessness varies by gender, age, occupation, employment sector, and region (Barham and Begum, 2005). The most common causes of long-term sickness absence among manual workers are acute medical conditions followed by back pain, musculoskeletal injuries, stress and mental health problems. Among non-manual workers the most common causes are stress, acute medical conditions, mental health problems (such as depression and anxiety), musculoskeletal injuries and back pain (Black, 2008), although these are often present as co-morbidities and further complicated by social and employment issues (Bambra, 2010b). In the UK, mild to moderate mental health problems are now more prevalent than musculoskeletal diseases as the prime causes of long-term sickness absence and work incapacity (Shiels *et al.*, 2004). Internationally the pattern is similar, with mental health problems accounting for a third of new disability claims across OECD countries. Mental health is also a more frequent diagnosis amongst younger claimants, amongst those who have never worked and amongst women (Brown *et al.*, 2009; Organisation for Economic Cooperation and Development, 2009). This may well be as a result of more demanding work requirements leading to a greater prevalence of stress related conditions — work intensity increased by 7% across the OECD between 1995 and 2005 (see Chapter 4), as well as problems which individuals with mental health problems face when attempting to find or retain work (Organisation for Economic Cooperation and Development, 2009). Studies of health related worklessness in the UK have found substantial regional variation, with rates highest in areas which have experienced rapid de-industrialisation and the loss of manufacturing jobs (Norman and Bambra, 2007; Brown *et al.*, 2010).

Concern over the rising numbers of people in receipt of health related benefits has meant that health related worklessness has a high political profile in most European countries. However, to date, health related worklessness has been largely ignored by public health researchers, policy makers and practitioners. This is despite the importance of health related worklessness in terms of health equity (Schuring *et al.*, 2007), as well as the central role that health practitioners play in terms of certifying sickness absence (Section 6.2.3). Health related worklessness has therefore tended to be framed as a social policy and labour market problem rather than a public health or medical concern (Williams, 2010). This means that much of the academic research has been conducted by social policy specialists, particularly in the UK. This chapter therefore starts by outlining the key material from this field with a particular focus on health related worklessness in the UK. The first section examines health related worklessness within the UK social security system. Four key issues in current social policy debates about health related worklessness are then examined: 'hidden unemployment', 'cultures of worklessness', the 'medicalisation of sickness absence', and the 'reserve army of labour' thesis. The chapter then examines socio-economic inequalities in the employment consequences of ill health. The final section takes a more international approach by comparing health related worklessness by welfare state regime.

6.1 **Health, worklessness, and the welfare state**[1]

This section summarises the historical development of social policy in the UK with regard to health related worklessness, outlines the current social security system in relation to people who are workless on the grounds of ill health or disability, and then draws on political economy perspectives of the welfare state to analyse the changes.

6.1.1 **The history of health related welfare**

Historically in the UK and other advanced market economies, disability and chronic illness are associated with poverty and social exclusion (Acheson, 1998; Bartley and Lewis, 2002; Oliver and Barnes, 1998). This is largely because work is the main source of income for the majority of the population and people with disabilities and chronic illnesses have disproportionately low employment rates. Since 1945, UK government action in terms of changing this situation can be categorised into three distinct phases: 'passive welfare', 'active welfare' and what can be viewed as the emergence of 'workfare'. This matches the broader development of advanced welfare states as previously outlined in Chapter 2.

---

[1] Parts of this section are reproduced from Bambra and Smith (2010) reprinted by permission of the publisher Taylor & Francis Ltd.

Passive welfare (1940s to 1990s)

The first phase of public policy towards the employment of people with a disability or chronic illness was framed by the Disabled Persons Employment Act of 1944 which set up supported employment programmes (such as Remploy), medical rehabilitation services, and the post-war employment quota (Figure 6.1). In the 1970s, these measures were supplemented with a number of specific health related out-of-work cash benefits, such as Invalidity Benefit in 1971 (renamed Incapacity Benefit in 1994). Cash benefits claimed on the basis of ill health were higher than those paid on the basis of unemployment in recognition of the long-term nature of ill health and the additional costs that it can involve. During the social security reforms of the 1980s and early 1990s, additional restrictions were placed on these cash benefits (e.g. the introduction of

1944	**Disabled Persons (Employment) Act** Set up the post-war disability employment quota of 3% for employers with over 20 staff. Some vocational services initiated and special, initially sheltered, employment started ('Remploy').
1970	**Chronically Sick and Disabled Persons Act** Improved access to local authority public buildings and services
1971	**National Insurance Act** Invalidity benefit set up
1973	**Employment and Training Act** Introduced employment rehabilitation centres and resettlement officers **Social Security Act** Attendance Allowance introduced—subsidises the costs of home care/assistance
1975	**Social Security Benefits Act** Introduced the Mobility Allowance—a cash benefit paid for transport costs **Social Security Pensions Act** Non-Contributory Invalidity Pension (later known as Severe Disablement Allowance)
1980	**Social Security Act** Reduced benefit levels
1991	**Disability Living Allowance and Disability Working Allowance Act** Disability Living Allowance combined the Attendance and Mobility allowances, Disability Working Allowance—wage top-up for low-paid workers (replaced with a tax credit in 1999) **Placement, Assessment and Counselling Teams (PACTs)** Vocational preparation and placement services (renamed Disability Service Teams in 1999)

Fig. 6.1 'Passive welfare' for health related worklessness in the UK (1944 to 1991).
Source: Adapted from Bambra *et al.* (2005b).

the 'all work' test in 1994). However, a radical shift of policy, fuelled by growing Treasury concerns about the costs of disability related benefits (HM Treasury, 1998), alongside pressure from disability campaign groups in relation to social exclusion (Barnes, 1991, 2002; Danieli and Wheeler, 2006), occurred in the mid-1990s. The Disability Discrimination Act of 1995 (and subsequent amendments) abolished the post-war disability employment quota in favour of a more rights based approach to the employment of disabled people (Floyd and Curtis, 2000; Oliver and Barnes, 1998). This Act saw the beginning of a distinction in social policy between people with a legally recognised disability and those with a chronic illness (Warren, 2005).

Active welfare (1990s to 2000s)

Although the UK welfare state has always contained a certain element of active welfare (for example Beveridge himself was an 'activist' and many of the initial post-war cash benefits, such as pensions, were only available to those who had previously paid social insurance contributions [Fulcher and Scott, 2003]), in more recent decades this element has become more prominent and far reaching. In the second phase of government action, people with a disability or long-term condition have been represented as a key group of working age benefit recipients and, as such, they have been the targets of a number of diverse active labour market interventions (HM Treasury, 2003). For example, the Disability Working Allowance, the New Deal for Disabled People, and the Access to Work programme (Figure 6.2). These interventions have generally tried to overcome the different barriers which people with a disability or chronic illness face when trying to enter employment, including: lack of experience or skills; uncertainty from employers; problems with physical access to work; and concerns over pay, hours and conditions (Gardiner, 1997; Goldstone and Meager, 2002). However, the majority of interventions have been supply-side focused, with little account taken for actual labour market demand. Participation by people in receipt of benefits has been on a voluntary basis (Bambra *et al.*, 2005b; Bambra, 2006c). Houston and Lindsay (2010) note that 'activation' has also emerged as one of the dominant themes of reform across other European welfare states with benefits and services for people of working age becoming more focused on re-connecting recipients with the labour market and requiring recipients to be 'active' in seeking employment. Active labour market policies are outlined in more detail in Chapter 7.

Towards 'workfare' (2003 onwards)

Despite a rapid increase in these kinds of intervention since the 1990s, the employment rate for people with disabilities or a chronic illness has remained very low, at around 49%, compared with 81% for those without (Bambra and

1994	**Social Security (Incapacity for Work) Act** Introduced the All Works Test and Incapacity Benefit. **Access to Work Programme** *Provided financial assistance towards practical aids, workplace adaptation, fares to work and personal support.*
1995	**Disability Discrimination Act** Since 1996, it has been unlawful to discriminate in recruitment, promotion, training, working conditions, and dismissal on the grounds of disability or ill health (restricted to employers with over 20 employees, reduced to 15 in 1998). Abolished the 3% employment quota of 1944.
1998	**New Deal for Disabled People Pilots** A package of different interventions including the Personal Adviser service, the Innovative Schemes, and smaller projects such as the Job Finders Grant.
1999	**Tax Credit Act** Introduced the Disabled Person's Tax Credit – a wage top-up for people with disabilities in low-paid employment (merged into the Working Tax Credit in 2002). **Disability Rights Commission** Monitored implementation of the Disability Discrimination Act from 2000 onwards **Welfare Reform and Pensions Act** Incapacity Benefit became means-tested, Severe Disablement Allowance was age-restricted, and the Personal Capacity Test replaced the All Works Test. **ONE Pilot** People applying for benefits were given an adviser to discuss work options. Compulsory after 2000.
2000	**WORKSTEP programme** Assists with transition from segregated supported work into mainstream employment
2001	**Special Educational Needs and Disability Act** Extended the provisions of the Disability Discrimination Act to education providers (provisions in force from 2002) **New Deal for Disabled People National Extension** Introduced Job Brokers (public, PVS vocational advisers) **Job Centre Plus** Services of the Employment Service and the Benefits Agency were combined.
2002	**Tax Credits Act** Disabled Persons Tax Credit merged into the Working Tax Credit for all low-paid workers **Permitted Work Rules** Allows benefit claimants to undertake paid work for up to 16 hours per week.

Fig. 6.2 'Active welfare' for health related worklessness in the UK (1994 to 2002). Source: Adapted from Bambra *et al.* (2005b).

Smith, 2010). In the 2000s, there were still around 2.7 million people in receipt of health related benefits in the UK. This group has thus remained at the centre of the welfare reform agenda, with the benefits of (re)employment for health and well-being increasingly being emphasised in policy circles (Black, 2008). In 2003 Work Focused Interviews were a compulsory part of the Pathways to Work programme for new benefit recipients and most significantly, in 2008, Incapacity Benefit was replaced with the two-tiered Employment Support Allowance (see Box 6.1). This built on the previous reforms enacted in 1999, when health related claims became dependent on social insurance contributions and the Personal Capacity Test was introduced. However, the addition of such an element of conditionality for people in receipt of health related benefits is fairly new within the UK context and signals a break with the voluntary nature of previous participation in employment interventions. It is in some respects, therefore, the dawn of a third phase of policy towards the employment of people with a disability or chronic illness, and one which could be considered as a move towards making these recipients subject to a form of 'workfare' (Figure 6.3).

Workfare originated in the US, where it has a long history through such schemes as the Community Work and Training programme (1962–1967), the Work Incentive programme (1967), the Community Work Experience programme; and the Family Support Act (1988) (Burghes, 1987). Perhaps most well known are the Clinton-era reforms of 1996 when the Personal Responsibility and Work Opportunity Reconciliation Act introduced sanctions and benefit limits for millions of poor Americans, particularly lone mothers and their children: the so-called '99ers' (as benefit receipt is limited to 99 weeks). Economically this Act has been considered a success, as welfare rolls halved in the first five years from 12.2 million in 1996 to 5.3 million in 2001. However, the social and economic costs for individuals are far more problematic, with only around 10–20% of those leaving welfare rolls actually getting work that pays above the federal poverty line. Similar reforms were announced in the UK in 2010, with compulsory work-for-benefit, as well as a 'claimant contract' with benefit sanctions, to be key aspects of the new Universal Working Age Benefit which will replace Jobseeker's Allowance, Employment and Support Allowance and Income Support by 2015 (Department for Work and Pensions, 2010b). The term 'workfare' is used to refer to those welfare reforms that have linked participation in employment programmes to income maintenance. Workfare is thus the obligation on welfare recipients to 'earn' their benefit via participation in training as well as compulsory 'work-for-benefit' (Burghes, 1987).

The Employment and Support Allowance requires all but the most severely sick or disabled recipients to be work-ready by, for example, taking part in rehabilitation or retraining. All existing Incapacity Benefit recipients will

2003	**Disability Discrimination Act 1995 (Amendment) Regulations 2003** Incorporates the Disability provisions of recent EU Employment Directives, removed small employer exemption. Came into force in October 2004. **Pathways to Work Pilots** 'Return to work' credit for new claimants leaving Incapacity Benefit, Condition Management Programmes, and mandatory Work Focused Interviews.
2004	**Pathways to Work Extension 1** Job Preparation Premium paid to those on Incapacity Benefit undertaking return to work activity, extended to IB claims started in last two years.
2005	**Disability Discrimination Act 2005** Extends service provisions to transportation. Definition of disability broadened to cover more people with HIV, cancer and multiple sclerosis. New duty placed on public authorities to promote equality of opportunity for disabled people. **Pathways to Work Extension 2** Pilot measures extended to cover around 1/3 of the UK **Job Retention and Rehabilitation pilot** Examines retention in work comparing employment-focussed support and health-based support.
2007	**Welfare Reform Act** Announced the phase-out of Incapacity Benefit and introduced the Employment and Support Allowance from 2008 (see Box 6.1). Established Work Capability Assessment to assess entitlement to Employment and Support Allowance.
2010	**Equality Act** Merged previous anti-discrimination legislation relating to age, disability, gender, race, religion and belief, sexual orientation and gender reassignment into one piece of legislation. Set up the Equality and Human Rights Commission (which incorporated the Disability Rights Commission amongst others) **Comprehensive Spending Review** Entitlement to Employment and Support Allowance (Work-related activity premium) restricted to a maximum of 12 months. Compulsory 'Work Programme' introduced with providers paid by results. **Welfare Reform White Paper** Outlined plans for a new Universal Credit to replace Jobseeker's Allowance, Employment and Support Allowance, Income Support etc. It will be rolled out by 2015. A new 'claimant contract' applies sanctions of 3 months, 6 months and up to 3 years benefit removal for those recipients who refuse job offers.

Fig. 6.3 Towards 'workfare' for health related worklessness in the UK (2003 onwards).
Source: Updated from Bambra *et al.* (2005b) and Bambra (2006c).

be re-evaluated and moved onto Employment and Support Allowance or Jobseeker's Allowance. In addition, a new 'fit note' has replaced the old General Practitioner administered 'sick note' with the intention of keeping people in work once a health problem emerges to reduce long-term sickness absence and welfare rolls (Department for Work and Pensions, 2009). A Department for Work and Pensions report *Building Bridges to Work* explicitly stated that:

> 'The old-style, passive, incapacity benefits have been replaced by the new, active Employment and Support Allowance' in a bid to create a 'something for something' approach that aims to widen 'the right to support and deepens the responsibility to take up this support: individuals have the responsibility to move towards and into work, in return they should get the help they need to do so'.
>
> Department for Work and Pensions (2010c: 7 & 21)

Employment and Support Allowance has several important features. Firstly, the new medical test is intended to tighten up eligibility and thereby cut the inflow of new recipients onto health related benefits. Indeed, the proportion of new applicants rejected by the new medical test has increased considerably from 39% under the old Incapacity Benefit regime tests, to 69% under the new regime (Department for Work and Pensions, 2009). Secondly, Employment and Support Allowance has introduced a new distinction between those recipients who might be expected to work ('work related activity' group) and those whose condition is so severe that there is relatively little prospect of them engaging in paid work ('support' group).

Under the new benefits regime, those deemed 'fit for work' will be immediately transferred onto the lower paying Jobseeker's Allowance (Box 6.2), those deemed to be too 'incapacitated' for work will be placed on the Employment and Support Allowance with a 'support' premium and with no conditionality, whilst those considered 'sick but able to work' will be placed on Employment and Support Allowance with a 'work related activity' premium (see Box 6.1).

Box 6.2 Weekly UK welfare benefit rates (2010)

£115 UK Poverty Line
£91.40 Incapacity Benefit (long-term rate)
£91.40 Employment and Support Allowance (Work related activity premium)
£96.85 Employment and Support Allowance (Support Premium)
£65.45 Employment and Support Allowance (Basic Allowance)
£65.45 Job Seekers Allowance
£65.45 Income Support

Source: Reproduced from Bambra (2010) with permission from BMJ Publishing Ltd.

Failure to engage in compulsory 'work related activity' will result in a loss of this premium and placement on the Employment and Support Allowance basic rate. The reforms announced in 2010 mean that the 'work related activity' group will also see their entitlement to Employment and Support Allowance limited to one year. After a year they will have no right to benefits (not even Jobseeker's Allowance) and will therefore become reliant on family support, charities or means-tested assistance (e.g. Income Support). It is expected that more than half of the 2.7 million Incapacity Benefit recipients will be placed into this group. Thus, for the great majority of recipients, Employment and Support Allowance is only a temporary benefit that will 'activate the aspirations' of recipients and encourage them to look for and take up paid work, and shift the 'culture' of incapacity benefits from 'invalidity to employability' (Department for Work and Pensions, 2008). Finally, in terms of delivery, Employment and Support Allowance will see an expansion in the contracting-out of work related activation to private and voluntary sector service providers on a 'pay by results' basis (i.e. the number of recipients moved into employment) (Freud, 2007). This mode of delivery is not unique to Employment and Support Allowance, but the large numbers involved means that contractors are delivering services to benefit recipients on an unprecedented scale.

There is little doubt that these reforms will succeed in reducing the levels of public expenditure spent on health related welfare benefits in the short-term, as those placed onto Jobseeker's Allowance will face an immediate drop in income of about a third and the 'work related activity' group of Employment and Support Allowance recipients will see at least an equivalent reduction in their incomes after a year (Box 6.2). Many commentators, however, have questioned the likely success of these reforms in terms of actually increasing the employment rates of people with ill health or a disability. For example, in the context of economic recession, Fothergill (2010) has argued that shifting large number of recipients onto the Employment and Support Allowance via the Work Capability Assessment is a mistake. Many existing Incapacity Benefit recipients have poor health, poor skills, and have experienced extended periods out of the labour market, thus rendering their chances of finding employment in a highly competitive environment of low labour demand marginal. Further, Grover and Piggott (2010) have warned that Employment and Support Allowance is effectively a form of 'social sorting', separating people with a sickness or disability into subgroups of claimants dependent upon medicalised perceptions of the legitimacy of their condition and therefore of their entitlement to state support (see Section 6.2.3).

These welfare reforms are not unique to the UK and are fairly common in the welfare states of all advanced market democracies (Organisation for Economic

Cooperation and Development, 2009). For example, in Switzerland, reforms made in 2008 have meant that people on health related benefits are now obliged to participate in work related activities and there are clear sanctions for non-compliance. Similarly, in Luxembourg, people with partial work capacity are now obliged to enrol in training and reintegration measures. The Netherlands has reassessed all recipients under the age of 50 with significant reductions in benefit receipt. Sweden has also implemented less draconian reforms whereby long-term disability benefit recipients can engage in small amounts of paid work without benefit reductions, they can also engage in higher levels of work with only proportionate reductions to their benefits. However, if they cease work, they can resume their full disability benefit at any time without a new assessment (Organisation for Economic Cooperation and Development, 2009).

6.1.2 The political economy of health related welfare

Adding conditionality, in the form of compulsory involvement in active labour market programmes, is novel in terms of UK health related benefits. However, it is in keeping with the reform of other UK benefits (such as the reforms to unemployment benefit of the 1980s and 1990s) and changes to health related benefits elsewhere, such as in Australia, the US and other countries in the European Union (Stone, 1984; Organisation for Economic Cooperation and Development, 2003, 2009; Kemp 2006). These reforms are often presented as being initiated on the grounds of reintroducing recipients to the labour market or providing an incentive for people who are out of work to look for and return to work (Henning-Bjorn *et al.*, 2004). However, the application of political economy theories provides some alternative explanations. Most notably in terms of labour discipline and moving those with ill health from the 'deserving' to the 'undeserving' poor.

Reasserting labour discipline

The reforms to health related welfare benefits can also be conceptualised as a way of reasserting labour discipline and instilling the work ethic. There are four salient aspects of the labour discipline thesis: Firstly, commentators such as Ginsburg argue that the social security benefits system disciplines the labour force by attaching conditions to benefits which 'ensure that the intransigent worker cannot so easily turn to the welfare state for support' (Ginsburg, 1979). This aspect of the labour discipline thesis is evident in the UK reforms as recipients of the Employment and Support Allowance will have to take part in employability schemes in order to receive full benefits. Secondly, following Piven and Cloward (1971/1993), the reforms can be seen as part of a wider welfare state retrenchment, as welfare provision acts as a means of 'regulating the poor'. Hence, provision tends to be expanded during times of political unrest and subsequently reduced once a measure of social peace has been restored. For example the civil unrest in the US in the 1960s was associated with a subsequent expansion of the welfare state which, once social order was restored, was followed up by a series of cut backs under the 1980s Reagan administration. Given that the UK has recently experienced a period of relative 'peace', it might be expected that welfare benefits would now be cut back. Thirdly, Katz (1986) argues that the stigma associated with benefit receipt also acts as a discipline upon the labour force, with dependency on state benefits considered not only a misfortune but a moral failure. The tiered approach of the new Employment and Support Allowance system to recipients may heighten this aspect of labour discipline, with those deemed 'sick but able to work' feeling particularly stigmatised. Finally, as Byrne's work has shown (2005), the reforms to welfare provision of the last two decades in the UK and elsewhere (particularly the Clinton-era in the US) have not been about ending benefit dependency but about linking benefit receipt more closely to work. So for example, the Clinton administration's Earned Income Tax Rebate and Earned Income Tax Credit as well as the Blair and Brown UK governments' Working Family Tax Credit or Child Tax Credit have increased the income of working families substantially, but only whilst they are in-work—out-of-work cash benefits have not been increased and in some cases have been decreased (e.g. lone parents). Similarly, as has long been argued in regard to the political economy of the welfare state (see Gough, 1979), in-work benefits act as wage subsidies to low paying employers as they are funded via horizontal redistribution within the working class rather than vertically via income redistribution and corporate taxes (Byrne, 2005: 156). The welfare reforms can thus be seen as the somewhat logical extension of the use of the benefits system to assert the work ethic. The reforms similarly reinforce divisions of who is (working poor) and who is not (non-working poor) deserving of state support.

No longer deserving

The separation of health based claims into two distinct categories is, on the one hand, a logical consequence of the philosophy of *'work for those who can, welfare for those who cannot'* approach to welfare reform (Blair, 2002), and an acknowledgment that previous, more passive approaches have often exacerbated the labour market exclusion experienced by people with a disability or chronic illness. However, on the other hand, the division into two levels of benefits is inevitably tied into notions of the 'deserving' and 'undeserving' poor (Katz, 1989; van Orschot, 2006). Health related cash benefits are amongst the last in the UK system to be the subject of extensive reform and, until recently, did not attract as much popular stigma as other types of benefits (most notably lone parent benefits). This is also the case in other countries, where people in receipt of benefits due to ill health or disability have been viewed and treated as more 'deserving' or morally worthy than those in receipt of other types of benefit (Stone, 1986; van Orschot, 2006). Indeed, as Stone argued in 'The Disabled State' (1986), in many Western countries, disability was for a long time considered to be a special administrative category in the welfare state and one which came with distinctive entitlements in the form of social aid and exemptions from certain obligations of citizenship, such as the duty to work (Stone, 1986: 4). Drawing on Stone (1986), welfare reform in this area can thus be seen as a clear move away from the more accommodating perspective of the period of 'passive welfare', and the beginning of a potentially disturbing political discourse which dictates that certain types of illness or disability are less deserving of unconditional public support than others.

People with a disability or chronic illness are thus variously categorised and re-categorised within the 'deserving' and 'undeserving' poor dichotomy. The relations of production which arose from capitalist industrialisation established a discourse of 'able-bodiedness' which excluded the impaired and the chronically ill from the workplace and the discourse of employability in general (Oliver, 1990; Stone, 1986; Finkelstein, 1980; Gleeson, 1991). However this has been renegotiated at various times and on different terms. For example, the context of the Second World War forced employers to employ groups who were not traditionally regarded as employable, such as disabled people. Disability and ill health were also transformed by the experience of the war as perceptions of 'disability' shifted because impairment was now more visible, prevalent and also more socially acceptable as these impairments were being acquired by those traditionally cast as those most worthy of employment: young adult males who had served in the armed forces (Stone, 1986). The Disabled Persons Employment Act of 1944, which followed the recommendations of the Tomlinson Committee on the rehabilitation of disabled people, thus established the long-term sick and disabled as the 'deserving' poor. It did not attempt to promote wider equality in the labour market where the social contract was to provide full employment for able-bodied male workers (see Chapter 1).

What is clear in the welfare reforms implemented since the 1990s has been the renegotiation of this 'deserving' and 'undeserving' dichotomy. This was influenced by a number of factors. Firstly, from the late 1980s onwards, disabled people mounted increasingly visible and successful campaigns to gain equal rights legislation (as had been passed in the 1970s with regard to sexual and racial equality). This influenced the enactment of the 1995 Disability Discrimination Act which is similar in remit to those in the US, Australia and Sweden (Bambra and Pope, 2007). Since 2006, all EU member states are obliged to adopt similar legislation (Organisation for Economic Cooperation and Development, 2009). The Disability Discrimination Act, whilst limited in many ways (for an overview see Roulstone and Warren, 2006), was an important landmark as the state had conceded that disabled people faced widespread discrimination and disadvantage in the labour market, workplace and wider society (Box 6.3). The Disability Discrimination Act is also significant, as its very existence clearly differentiates 'disability' from 'sickness' (e.g. long-term health conditions which are limiting but not disabling).

This group who could be termed the 'sick but not disabled' are arguably now more marginalised as they have no recourse to anti-discrimination legislation and have thus been moved out of the 'deserving' and into the 'undeserving' poor. The diminished status of the 'sick but not disabled' who are workless has implications regarding citizenship. It means that their citizenship is also 'lesser' than that of those classified as 'disabled' under the Disability Discrimination Act. Their lack of any special legislative protection means they are potentially subject to greater surveillance by the state via the welfare system, which is able to make receipt of benefits increasingly conditional. This conditionality involves the collusion of certain parts of the medical profession with, for example, tests of the legitimacy of the health claims of Incapacity Benefit recipients administered by doctors employed by private sector healthcare groups on behalf of the Department for Work and Pensions—an example of Finkelstein's (1980) 'administrative model of disability'. The construction of disability has long been an important feature of the welfare state as it places fewer obligations on those deemed 'disabled' (Stone, 1986). As Stone comments, the state determines what injuries, diseases, and incapacities those defined as non-disabled have to endure as part of their normal working lives (Stone, 1986: 4). In this context, it is worth considering that this deserving/ undeserving dichotomy and the redrawing of the lines around what is and what is not incapacity may well magnify stigma attached to claims based on 'hidden' (i.e. mental illness) as opposed to 'visible' illnesses (i.e. physical illness). Arguably everyone who is not in employment and dependent upon the state for their subsistence is subject to increased surveillance and subsequently has diminished citizenship. However the long-term 'sick but not disabled' are in a particularly disadvantageous position, as they are without the 'rights' attributed to 'disability', and are statistically far less likely to return to the labour market than the unemployed. Consequently they endure state surveillance for longer whilst also being subjected to medical administration.

Box 6.3 Definition of disability from the UK Disability Discrimination Act (1995)

The 1995 UK Disability Discrimination Act (DDA) made discrimination on the grounds of physical or mental disability or limiting long-term illness illegal: since the implementation of the DDA from 1996 onwards it has been unlawful to *'discriminate against disabled persons in connection with employment, the provision of goods, facilities and services, or the disposal or management of premises'*.

Employers are required to make 'reasonable adjustments' to work and premises to cater for people with a disability.

Under the Act, disability is defined as: *'a physical or mental impairment that has a substantial and long-term adverse effect on his/her ability to carry out normal day-to-day activities'*:

♦ *Physical impairment*—this includes weakening or adverse change of a part of the body caused through illness, by accident or from birth such as blindness, deafness, heart disease, the paralysis of a limb or severe disfigurement.

♦ *Mental impairment*—this can include learning disabilities and all recognised mental illnesses.

♦ *Substantial*—this does not have to be severe, but is more than minor or trivial.

♦ *Long-term adverse effect*—that has lasted or is likely to last more than 12 months.

♦ *A normal day-to-day activity*—that is, one that affects one of the following: mobility; manual dexterity; physical co-ordination; continence; ability to lift, carry or otherwise move everyday objects; speech, hearing or eyesight; memory or ability to concentrate, learn or understand; or perception of the risk of physical danger.

Source: Reproduced from Bambra and Pope (2007) with permission from BMJ Publishing Ltd.

6.2 Key debates about health related worklessness

Given the increased rates of sickness and disability related social security claims in the UK and other European countries, worklessness is now much discussed in academic, policy and media spheres (for examples, see Crisp, 2008; Webster, 2006; Ritchie *et al.*, 2005). Many issues have therefore emerged and chief amongst these are: concerns as to whether ill health related workless-ness is actually 'hidden unemployment' (Beatty *et al.*, 2000); whether inter-generational and structural worklessness over the last 30 years has created 'cultures of worklessness' (Fletcher, 2007); whether the medicalisation of sickness absence and the legitimacy of the 'sick role' is part of the problem (Black, 2008); and whether those out of work due to illness actually form a 'reserve army of labour' (Russell, 2002). This section explores these issues in more detail.

6.2.1 Hidden illness and hidden unemployment

The reforms to health related benefits outlined in Section 6.1.1 need to be understood in the context of political debates about the relationship between unemployment and health (Bambra, 2008; Bambra and Smith, 2010) and the relationship between benefit receipt, health and employment (Bambra and Norman, 2006). Although in order to qualify for most health related benefits across the OECD, medical certification by a general practitioner or benefits system doctor is required, welfare systems have long been criticised as provid-ing a means of avoiding work, and thereby obscuring true unemployment levels (Beatty *et al.* 1997, 2000, 2007; Fieldhouse and Hollywood, 1999). Certainly, the rapid increase in health related benefit claims across the OECD in the 1980s and 1990s coincided with similar decreases in the numbers in receipt of unemployment benefits. This in itself is potentially indicative of substitution between the two types of benefit schemes, perhaps linked to the earlier reform of unemployment benefits (Organisation for Economic Cooperation and Development, 2009).

In the UK, this perception is also fuelled by the fact that the geographical distribution of incapacity related benefit claims in the UK is skewed towards the de-industrialised areas of the North East of England, the West of Scotland and South Wales: the spatial patterning of health related worklessness thus reflects *'the loss of jobs in manufacturing and mining, which has not only been large overall, but has also clearly been concentrated in the cities and coalfields'* (Webster, 2000: 124). This is shown clearly in the map of England and Wales (Figure 6.4) and Table 6.2, which lists the 'best' and 'worst' 10 local authorities in England and Wales in terms of Incapacity Benefit standardised ratios. The best local authorities are mainly semi-rural non-deprived commuter and 'stock-broker' belt areas in the affluent South East region. The worst local authorities comprise the old industrial areas. These communities lost their main sources of employment, such as the coal, steel and shipping industries, in the rapid restructuring of the 1980s and 1990s when manufacturing jobs were lost at a rate of up to 1,000 per week in industrial centres such as Sheffield,

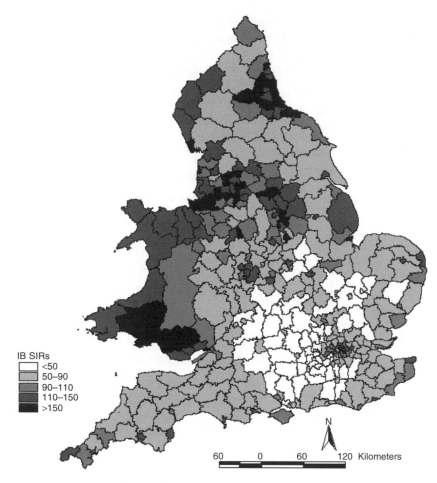

IB SIRs
	<50
	50–90
	90–110
	110–150
	>150

60   0   60   120 Kilometers

100 = National average for England & Wales

Fig. 6.4 Standardised illness ratios of Incapacity Benefit claims by local authority, England and Wales.
Reproduced from Norman and Bambra (2007) with permission from the publishers John Wiley and Sons.

England (Fletcher, 2007). There was not enough in the way of new local employment to replace these large industries, and the service sector jobs that did emerge did not match the skills of the existing workforce. In the 1980s and 1990s, Conservative governments actively encouraged a transition to sickness benefits in these communities as a way of reducing the numbers on unemployment benefits and thereby keeping the politically sensitive unemployment rate artificially low (Adams 1999; Bivand 2002). Further, the higher value of Incapacity Benefit in comparison to unemployment benefit may have acted as

Table 6.2 Local Authorities in England and Wales with the highest and lowest standardised ratios of Incapacity Benefit recipients

Highest		Lowest	
Local Authority	Region	Local Authority	Region
Merthyr Tydfil	Wales	Hart	South-East
Easington	North East	Surrey Heath	South East
Blaenau Gwent	Wales	Wokingham	South East
Neath Port Talbot	Wales	Elmbridge	South East
Rhondda, Cynon, Taff	Wales	South Bucks	South East
Liverpool	North West	Windsor & Maidenhead	South East
Knowsley	North West	Horsham	South East
Caerphilly	Wales	South Oxfordshire	South East
Manchester	North West	Uttlesford	East
Hartlepool	North East	Vale of White Horse	South East

Source: Reproduced from Norman and Bambra (2007) with permission from the publishers John Wiley and Sons.

a financial incentive for individual recipients. It has also been argued that general practitioners in deprived areas may have exacerbated the above trend in recognising that, manual workers in particular would struggle to find employment in the newly de-industrialised areas (Legard *et al.*, 2002; Ritchie *et al.*, 1993).

Beatty and colleagues (2000) have therefore argued that regional differences in employment rates conceal what can be termed 'hidden unemployment'. This concentration of 'hidden unemployment' in the former industrial areas suggests that some regional economies have not fully recovered from the fall-out of de-industrialisation, a conclusion also reached by a number of other researchers (see Turok and Edge, 1999; Webster, 2006; Theodore, 2007). Beatty and colleagues (2007) estimate the 'real' level of unemployment in the UK in 2007 was 2.6 million, compared with 1.6 million in the International Labour Office definition of unemployment and only 0.9 million claiming Jobseeker's Allowance. This is based on a estimate that around 40% of incapacity related benefit recipients could reasonably be expected to have been in work in a genuinely fully employed economy, corresponding to 560,000 men and 450,000 women. However, it is important to point out that the concept of 'hidden unemployment' does not assume any fraudulent claims of sickness and ill health. Incapacity Benefit receipt requires medical assessment and as individual level evidence from recent cohort studies shows, medically certified sickness absence clearly reflects actual morbidity and mortality (Marmot *et al.*, 1995,

Kivimäki *et al.*, 2003c, Vahtera *et al.*, 2004). Population level studies have also found higher associations between Incapacity Benefit claims in England and Wales and morbidity (r=0.98 p<0.01, 2001 census limiting long term illness; r=0.97 p<0.01, 2001 census not good health) and mortality (r=0.80 p<0.01, 2001 Vital Statistics) than unemployment (r=0.72 p<0.01, 2001 census) (Bambra and Norman, 2006; Norman and Bambra, 2007).

Beatty and colleagues (2000) therefore also refer to the term 'hidden sickness'. 'Hidden sickness' refers to those in employment suffering from some form of ill health or disability. Although many such people would be sufficiently sick to be eligible for benefits, they are at the same time able to perform some or all of the duties required in their job, in some cases with modifications agreed with their employer to accommodate their incapacity (such as working part-time or avoiding heavy lifting). Beatty and colleagues argue that in a tight local labour market at full employment, many people with some form of incapacity who are able to do some types or amounts of work are therefore likely to be in employment. In a slack local labour market experiencing high levels of unemployment, many such people will instead claim incapacity related benefits. Consequently, people with ill health remain towards the end of the 'jobs queue' (Berthoud, 2008). The dual concepts of hidden unemployment and hidden sickness together predict that in tight labour markets there will be little hidden unemployment and a lot of hidden sickness, while in slack labour markets there will be little hidden sickness and a lot of hidden unemployment (Beatty *et al.*, 2000). This is in keeping with the 'reserve army of labour' thesis which is examined in Section 6.2.4.

6.2.2 **Cultures of worklessness**

The complex economic, social and geographical connections between health related worklessness and unemployment have fuelled the view that health related welfare claims represent a form of 'welfare scrounging' and act as a disincentive to work (Bambra and Norman, 2006). Such views are not limited to the UK (Organisation for Economic Cooperation and Development, 2003), nor are they particularly new; American Social Security Disability Insurance, for example, was subject to similar debate and was subsequently reformed under the Reagan administration in the early 1980s (Stone, 1986). In the UK, politicians and the media often talk about a 'dependency culture', 'habits of worklessness', or 'cultures of worklessness', particularly in relation to areas of high incapacity benefit receipt. This is despite evidence that a substantial proportion of those in receipt of benefits want to return to work and would do so if they were given appropriate support (Beatty and Fothergill, 2005; Joyce *et al.*, 2010a; Smith *et al.*, 2010). There is little evidence of a lower work ethic amongst workless people (Gallie, 2004). Workless individuals face multiple barriers to employment, such as a lack of relevant job skills and experience as well as problems accessing the work environment (often relating to transport and carer costs), and stigma surrounding ill health and work ability from employers (Danziger et al., 2002). Indeed, poor health and disability make it difficult for some individuals to secure jobs in a competitive labour market in which employers demand flexibility (Houston and Lindsay, 2010). Living in areas of high worklessness can also entail stigma, with whole communities stereotyped as feckless and work shy (Fletcher, 2007). These barriers mean that helping individuals move from 'welfare and into work' may not easily be addressed by single, linear interventions (Gardiner, 1997; Bambra et al., 2005b; Ritchie et al., 2005). This is particularly likely to be the case where changes in local economies have restricted employment options.

A particularly emotive notion, 'worklessness' has negative connotations, with 'cultures of worklessness' implying idleness and fault on the part of the workless individual and their communities, thus implying that such people and places are to blame for their own worklessness and poverty. Grover and Piggott (2007: 735) remark that there is a moralising discourse through which the receipt of incapacity benefit is constructed as being indicative of a 'dependency culture' of sick and disabled people who are encouraged into idleness by the structure of the benefits that they receive. Grover comments that the public, policy and political discourses surrounding worklessness construct 'workless people as those who 'won't work', rather than those people for whom there are few jobs to apply for, who face barriers to work, including various and multiple forms of discrimination' (2007: 536). 'Worklessness' is thus a term that combines together those unable to work through age, illness or disability, alongside those allegedly unwilling to work through lack of aspiration or cultural influences (Welshman, 2006). This echoes the 'undeserving' and 'deserving' poor, implying that the workless are 'undeserving' if they do not at least seek paid employment, regardless of the quality and calibre of that employment. On the other hand, the 'deserving' poor are those who are actively seeking work and who are keen to make a contribution to society in this way (as discussed in Section 6.1.2).

The creation of a 'culture of worklessness' and the association of this with the attitudes and behaviour of marginalised groups owes much to the 'culture of poverty' debates that emerged in the US in the late 1960s in which cultural patterns (family structure, interpersonal relations, value systems, sense of community and spending patterns) were seen as inter-generationally transmitted to reinforce a recurring cycle of poverty (Fletcher, 2007). This idea was taken up in the UK in the 1970s by Keith Joseph with his promotion of the idea of a 'cycle of deprivation' (Fletcher, 2007). In the 1980s, other US theorists such as Charles Murray (1990) used ideas of inter-generational cultures to claim that they could identify an 'underclass'; a culturally distinct and deprived minority that included both the delinquent and the welfare dependent. Illegitimacy, violent crime and non-participation in the labour market were deemed to be key indicators and socially acceptable norms of this 'underclass' (Fletcher, 2007). The creation and existence of the 'underclass' was the fault of an overly generous welfare system, not employers, the macro-economic environment or the wider system of economic inequality. These views have been counteracted by those such as Byrne (2005) who talk about the long term social exclusion of the poor and of deprived communities as a result of government action (or, more usually inaction).

This 'culture of worklessness' approach suggests that worklessness and benefit receipt can only be understood in terms of the 'faulty' attitudes and behaviours of deprived families and communities: *'In some areas a culture of worklessness or poverty of aspirations has developed, locking people into cycles of worklessness'* (HM Treasury and Department for Work and Pensions, 2003: 46). This enlarges the victim blaming discourse around ill health, poverty and welfare receipt from one which focuses on the individual to one that stigmatises entire (working class) communities and ways of life. Such attitudes have a long history in the UK and other European countries, dating back to early twentieth century views of the morally defective nature of slum dwellers (Fletcher, 2007). They have also underpinned entire policy interventions, such as the Working Neighbourhoods programmes in the UK (Fletcher, 2007). Policy debates about Incapacity Benefit and worklessness are thus shaped as much by ideological and political factors as by broader economic trends.

6.2.3 The medicalisation of sickness and sickness absence

'Medicalisation' first came to prominence in the 1970s and it is a term used to describe how medicine extends its power by colonising areas of social life. Conrad (1992) defines medicalisation as:

'The process by which non-medical problems become treated and defined as medical problems usually in terms of illnesses or disorders'.

Conrad (1992: 209)

Conrad traces the roots of the medicalisation thesis to Parsons' influential description of the 'sick role' in which sickness is identified as a social role which has rights and responsibilities (Parsons, 1951[1991]). In terms of rights, a sick person is temporarily exempt from 'normal' social roles (such as paid work) and the more severe the sickness, the greater the exemption. Sickness also entails an absence of blame and the sick person is not held responsible for their condition. Subsequently, the sick person has a right to treatment and support. However, the exemption from normal responsibilities is temporary and conditional upon trying to leave the state of sickness and regain health—to 'get well'. The sick person therefore also has an obligation to seek professional medical help and to cooperate in the recovery process.

Parsons considers the sick role to be a social threat as 'the sick' are relieved of their usual duties within capitalist production (i.e. to work, or to care for the family). Sickness can be used to evade social responsibility. Medical professionals are central to the process of assigning and legitimising the social status accorded to illness. They act as 'gatekeepers' against illness as social deviance and they provide a form of social regulation. The medicalisation thesis developed alongside the anti-psychiatry movement whose exponents, such as Szasz (1964) Laing (1967) and Cooper (1968), criticised medical professionals for acting as agents of social control. The medicalisation thesis thus '*draws attention to the fact that medicine operates as a powerful institution of social control*' (Nettleton, 1995: 27). Freidson (1970) was one of the first researchers to attempt to theorise how medicine established and maintains its social power. He argued that state patronage established orthodox medicine in a dominant position. This cemented a particular form of occupational control over patients and other practitioners within the health sector. However in order to retain this position, medicine has to engage in a continuing political struggle to retain its dominance, in both the healthcare division of labour and its control over the direction of the profession and its work.

Extension of medical power to spheres of life previously beyond it (childbirth is a prominent example), is also a crucial way in which medicine maintains and extends its dominance. Medicine is thus part of a wider bureaucratisation of social life in advanced capitalist economies which disempowers individuals in favour of experts and professionals (Zola, 1972). Medicalisation is a process which strips away the resources and abilities of individuals and communities to cope with their own problems by replacing them with a hegemony of disabling professionals (Illich, 1976 [1995]). Sickness absence and health related welfare benefits are a strong example of the process of medicalisation as doctors are a central part of the administrative and legal sides of the welfare system. They are responsible for assessing the entitlement and legitimacy of all applications for sickness and disability benefits (Finkelstein, 1980). Medicine therefore acts as a gatekeeper to accessing health related welfare benefits. For example, absence from the workplace due to sickness either on a temporary or on a long-term basis is usually regarded as legitimate. However, this legitimacy is dependent upon validation by a medical practitioner who also has the ability to revalidate the legitimacy of such claims or to withdraw their validation.

This gatekeeper role, whilst clearly disempowering for individual workers, has also recently been criticised by government and by employers as effectively disempowering them in their ability to prevent sickness absence and enhance return to work (Organisation for Economic Cooperation and Development, 2009). As discussed in Section 6.2.1, falls in unemployment benefit receipt have to a greater or lesser extent been matched by increases in health related benefit receipt. This has led to the view, as expressed by a high level OECD report (2009), that a predominantly labour market issue has become a medical one:

> 'The purpose of publicly-funded disability benefits [has shifted], from providing a safety net for persons who are unable to secure employment because their ability to compete for work is weakened (*i.e.* a labour market issue), to compensation for permanent loss of functioning due to injury or sickness (*i.e.* a medical issue)'.
>
> Organisation for Economic Cooperation and Development (2009: 18)

This application of the medicalisation thesis contends that the use of medical criteria to assess whether someone is fit for work results in significant numbers of people with partial work capacity being medically deemed incapacitated for work, often on a permanent basis:

> 'Whereby their formal obligation to seek employment ceases and, in most benefit systems, they are also indirectly compelled to remain inactive and assert they are incapable of work in order to continue to receive payments'.
>
> Organisation for Economic Cooperation and Development, (2009: 18)

The medicalisation of worklessness has thus allowed the medical model of disability and sickness, whereby people with a health condition or disability are 'incapacitated' and incapable of participating in the workforce, to dominate this area of labour market policy. It is argued that medicalisation has thus facilitated the entrenchment of a 'benefit culture' (Section 6.2.2) and acted to undermine attempts to reform health related welfare benefits (Organisation for Economic Cooperation and Development, 2009).

Policymakers across advanced market economies have attempted to undermine the historical dominance of the medical model with regard to health related welfare. In the UK, for example, the 'sick note' which was traditionally used to certify sickness absence operated on a zero-sum basis: an individual was either too sick to work or well enough to work. This was replaced, after much government effort, in 2010 with a 'fit note' which is intended to assess fitness for work, as opposed to sickness. The fit note adds the option of being partially fit for work if certain issues are taken into account including a phased return to work, altered hours, amended duties and workplace adaptations. The intention of the fit note is to reduce the number of people on short-term sickness absence who then lose their employment and become long-term benefit recipients. The fit note is also intended to address concerns that general practitioners were too close to their patients and too keen to sign people off—'on the sick' (particularly in areas or times of high unemployment) (Organisation for Economic Cooperation and Development, 2009). Similar reforms have occurred in Australia and Denmark. In Australia, those who are out-of-work due to ill health are subject to a 'job capacity assessment' that determines their work ability. Since 1998, Denmark has operated a scheme of subsidised jobs ('flexjobs'), this offers a permanent wage subsidy to employers of 50% to 65% of the total salary for the employment of people with a permanent reduction in work ability due to illness or disability. The scheme also includes reduced working hours, adapted working conditions, or restricted job demands. Employment in flexjobs has increased dramatically since the introduction of the scheme: from 6,700 in 1999 to 40,600 in 2006 (Whitehead *et al.*, 2009). These changes have to be understood in relation to the wider shifts in welfare policy for those with a health condition or disability from a passive (incapacity) model to a more active (work capability), and ultimately, towards a workfare model (Section 6.1.1).

6.2.4 Sickness, disability, and the reserve army of labour

The 'reserve army of labour' thesis was developed by Marx who describes it as a holding pool, a reservoir of labour which can be accessed by capital at very short notice. It is cheap, highly convenient and also economically efficient as workers are not being retained and paid for by employers during periods of low market demand. The existence of a reserve army also regulates the wages of those in employment as it undermines their wage bargaining capacity:

> 'Taking them as a whole, the general movements of wages are exclusively regulated by the expansion and contraction of the industrial reserve army' *and* 'the industrial reserve army, during the periods of stagnation and average prosperity, weighs down the active army of workers; during periods of over-production and feverish activity, it puts a curb on their pretensions'.

Marx (1867 [1976]: 790 & 792)

Marx argues that the reserve army of labour—or the surplus population—always has three forms: the *floating*, the *latent* and the *stagnant*. The *floating* part refers to the temporarily unemployed, the *latent* part consists of that segment of the population not yet fully integrated into capitalist production—for example, parts of the rural population in the nineteeth century—and the *stagnant* part which consists of marginalised people with extremely irregular employment who dwell in the sphere of pauperism. Applying Marx's analysis to the post-war period, Ginsburg argues that a central function of the welfare state is the production and maintenance of the industrial 'reserve army of labour' which depresses the market price of labour. The state, by providing social security and other welfare services for the 'surplus population', ensures the daily and generational reproduction of labour and collectivises the costs (Gough, 1979; Ginsburg, 1992).

In the 1970s, the reserve army of labour thesis was applied by feminist and anti-racist writers to explain the role of women, ethnic minority and immigrant workers within the labour market and the welfare state. These newer applications of the 'reserve army of labour' thesis also influenced writers from the disability rights movement such as Finkelstein (1980) or Oliver (1990) who then applied the idea to the labour market relationships of people with a disability. There is certainly evidence from the US to show that disabled people experience proportionally larger gains in employment during economic booms, and suffer proportionally greater losses during times of contraction than those without a disability (Yelin and Katz, 1994: 36) with disability benefit claims also rising (Russell, 2002). There are further issues. In Marx's original typology of the 'reserve army of labour', disabled people and those with ill health were placed in the group least likely to become employed: the 'stagnant' reserve army of labour. The passive welfarism of the immediate post-war period incorporated this view (see Section 6.1.1). However, the welfare reforms of the 1990s, the activation agenda and the emergence of workfare in some countries in relation to health related worklessness, have placed more people with a health problem or disability into the 'active' (floating) pool of the reserve army of labour. Enlarging the available pool of labour in this way benefits capital as having more people competing for work keeps wages down (Russell, 2002). Beatty and colleagues' (2000) theories of hidden unemployment and hidden sickness are also relevant in this regard (see Section 6.2.1).

The 'reserve army of labour' thesis has been subjected to a number of criticisms. In relation to health related worklessness, as Grover and Piggott (2005) have argued, it is not the case that all disabled or chronically ill people are part of the 'reserve army of labour' as at least a third of those of working age are in some form of employment. Consequently the idea that all of the long-term sick and disabled, or all women or all ethnic minority and immigrant workers, constitute a 'reserve army of labour' is problematic, and 'membership' is highly stratified by socio-economic class, and local labour market conditions, with low skill levels a clear characteristic of membership of any 'reserve army of labour'. It can also be argued that in some particularly deprived areas, structural unemployment levels and long-term health related benefit receipt are so high and so intransigent that such groups are far removed from the labour market and thus no longer constitute a 'reserve army of labour' so much as a dislocated and socially excluded 'underclass' (see Section 6.2.2). Another perspective is that the high levels of part-time work amongst women, immigrants and those with a disability or chronic illness, suggest that whilst they may not constitute a 'reserve army of labour' in a zero-sum (unemployed-employed) sense, they are under-employed and can thus be fully employed in times of labour market expansion and then under-employed once more in times of contraction.

6.3 Socio-economic inequalities in health related worklessness

Ill health increases the likelihood of long-term worklessness. For example, a study of health related worklessness in the UK using national household survey data found that the employment rates of people with limiting long-term illness (LLTI) or disability were 45.9% compared to 82.4% of those without an illness or disability (Pope and Bambra, 2005). This varies by gender with women with an LLTI having a lower employment rate than men with an LLTI: in the UK, 58.9% of men with an LLTI were employed in 2005 compared to 49.9% of women. Differences in employment rates with respect to health and gender are also present in other advanced market democracies. For example, in 2005, the employment rates of men with a LLTI in Canada were 62.7% compared to 86.4% for those without, in Norway 70.6% to 93.2% and in Sweden 62.6% to 93.3% (Whitehead et al., 2009). The employment rates of women with a LLTI in 2005 were even lower: in Canada they were 53.6% for those with LLTI compared to 74.7% for those without, in Norway 64.3% to 88.6% and in Sweden 64.9% to 88.4% (Whitehead et al., 2009). However, health related worklessness is also unevenly socio-economically distributed. A comprehensive comparative study by Whitehead and colleagues (2009) found that there were significant educational inequalities in the employment rates of people with LLTI (Table 6.3). In the UK, the study found that, in 2005, employment rates of men with a low education and a LLTI were 65.6% less than healthy men with a low education, 58.7% less than highly educated men with LLTI and 68.1% lower than healthy, highly educated men. These patterns were even starker for UK women: those with a low education and LLTI had employment rates of 71.2% less than healthy women with a low education, 72.6% less than highly educated women with LLTI and 79.4% lower than healthy, highly educated women. Internationally, these patterns were repeated to a greater or lesser extent (Whitehead et al., 2009) with the employment gaps between healthy highly educated men and low educated men with LLTI ranging from 30.9% in Norway to 68.1% in the UK, and between healthy highly educated women and low educated women with LLTI ranging from 57.7% in Sweden to 79.4% in the UK.

Table 6.3 Differences in the employment rates of working age people (aged 25–59) with and without limiting long-term illness (LLTI) by educational status in four countries (1980s compared to 2000s)

Rate Differences (%) by educational and health status		UK[a]		Canada[b]		Norway[c]		Sweden[d]	
		1980s	2000s	1980s	2000s	1980s	2000s	1980s	2000s
Men	Low education LLTI v Low education healthy	−51.6	−65.6	−38.1	−47.1	−18.9	−25.2	−21.7	−47.2
	Low education LLTI v High education LLTI	−48.5	−58.7	−28.25	−48.5	−17.4	−27.1	−16.5	−38.7
	Low education LLTI v High education healthy	−58.0	−68.1	−43.6	−57.5	−17.7	−30.9	−21.3	−49.2
Women	Low education LLTI v Low education healthy	−54.0	−71.2	−50.2	−47.7	−18.6	−52.6	−25.5	−47.4
	Low education LLTI v High education LLTI	−51.7	−72.6	−64.9	−62.6	−26.1	−53.4	−32.3	−48.7
	Low education LLTI v High education healthy	−65.0	−79.4	−72.4	−69.4	−29.1	−60.5	−33.9	−57.7

[a] Data from Labour Force Survey 1984–1986 and 2004–2006.

[b] Data from Census 1986 and 2001.

[c] Data from Survey of Living Conditions 1980–1983 and 2002–2005.

[d] Data from Survey of Living Conditions 1982–1984 and 2003–2005.

Source: Author calculations of rate differences using data presented in Tables 5.5 to 5.9 in Whitehead *et al.* (2009).

The Whitehead and colleagues (2009) study also found that the employment situation for low educated people with LLTI had significantly worsened since the 1980s in all the countries studied. In the early 1980s, the employment rates of low educated healthy men in the UK were 82.2% compared to 94.6% for highly educated healthy men, a gap of 13.1%. By the mid-2000s this situation had improved with the gap closing to 7.2% (Whitehead *et al.*, 2009). Over the same period, the employment gap between healthy high and low educated women in the UK increased slightly from 23.9% to 28.5%. However, for low educated men and women with LLTI, the employment gap between them and the rest of the working age population, the healthy and unhealthy, increased massively. In the early 1980s, the gap between men with a low education and LLTI compared to healthy low educated men was 51.6%, by the mid 2000s this had increased to 65.6%. The gap with highly educated men with LLTI increased from 48.5% to 58.7% and the gap with healthy highly educated men increased from 58.0% to 68.1%. For low educated women in the UK with LLTI, the labour market was even more unfavourable with their employment rates falling from 26.6% in the early 1980s to 18.1% in the mid-2000s. This represents an employment gap in the mid-2000s of 71.2% between them and healthy low educated women, compared to 54.0% in the 1980s. The employment gap between low educated women with an LLTI and highly educated women with an LLTI increased from 51.7% to 72.6% and the gap between low educated women with an LLTI and healthy highly educated women rose from 65.0% to 79.4% in the same period. These findings were similar in the other countries studied by Whitehead and colleagues (2009), although the magnitudes of educational inequalities in employment varied. Structural worklessness is of increasing importance to socio-economic inequalities in health.

6.4 **Welfare state regimes and health related worklessness**

The employment rates of people with an illness or disability vary by welfare state regime. This is demonstrated in Table 6.4. Health related worklessness is lowest in the Scandinavian welfare states, where the worklessness rates of people with a LLTI is 30.3% in Iceland, 33.1% in Sweden, 41.6% in Finland and Denmark, and 42.4% in Norway with a welfare state regime average of 37.8% (van der Wel *et al.*, 2010). Health related worklessness is highest in the Anglo-Saxon countries of the UK and Ireland where 49.9% and 64.3% respectively of people with LLTI are workless. The Bismarckian (Luxembourg 40.6%, Austria 42.2%, France 45.8%, Belgium 59.0%, Netherlands 50.8%) and Southern (Cyprus 41.9%, Italy 51.3%, Portugal 48.2%, Spain 58.3%, Greece 62.2%)

Table 6.4 Rates of worklessness in the working age population (aged 25–59) in Western Europe by health status and welfare state regime

Welfare State Regime	Worklessness rate in healthy working age population (%)	Worklessness rate in working age population with limiting long-term illness (%)
Scandinavian	8.0	37.8
Bismarckian	18.1	47.7
Southern	21.4	52.4
Anglo-Saxon	17.7	57.1

Source: Un-weighted welfare state regime averages calculated by the author using data from the European Union Survey of Income and Living Conditions as presented by van der Wel *et al.* (2010).

welfare states hold intermediate positions with average health related worklessness rates of 47.7% and 52.4% respectively. There are also significant cross-national differences in terms of the magnitude of socio-economic inequalities in the employment consequences of ill health. This is evident in Whitehead and colleagues' (2009) research which found that educational inequalities in worklessness were higher in the UK (and to a lesser extent in Canada) than in the Scandinavian countries (as demonstrated in Table 6.3). This issue has also been explored by van der Wel and colleagues (2010) in a comparative study of inequalities in the employment consequences of sickness by welfare state regime. In a multi-level analysis of 25 countries using data from the European Union Survey of Income and Living Conditions, van der Wel and colleagues compared labour force participation by educational status and health. They found that in all countries, people with health problems have lower employment rates than those who are healthy and that worklessness rates are particularly high amongst people who have both a health problem and a low education. However, the study found that the employment rates of those with a health problem and a low education are higher amongst those welfare states—the Social Democratic ones—that invest in active labour market policies, have higher levels of income equality and provide more generous welfare benefits (van der Wel *et al.*, 2010).

These differences by welfare state regime in health related worklessness and inequalities in worklessness may also be linked to the different ways in which sickness absence (both short-term and long-term) is treated in different welfare states. This issue has long been of importance in comparative social policy. The level of sickness absence decommodification was one of the central aspects of Esping-Andersen's *Three Worlds of Welfare* typology (1990) in which welfare state regimes were first conceptualised (see Chapter 2). The Social Democratic welfare states had the highest level of decommodification, particularly in terms of replacement rates, and the Liberal welfare states had the lowest (Esping-Andersen, 1990; Bambra, 2006b). In 2003, the OECD published a more comprehensive taxonomy of welfare states which clustered them in terms of two key aspects of their disability and sickness absence policies: compensation (including benefit replacement rates, eligibility requirements, length of disability, population coverage) and integration (focusing on vocational rehabilitation and employment measures such as work incentives or employer obligations) (Organisation for Economic Cooperation and Development, 2003). This produced a five-fold taxonomy of disability policy clusters: Anglo-American (Canada, US, UK); Scandinavian (Norway, Sweden, Denmark); Germanic (Austria and Germany); Romanic (France, Italy, Portugal, Poland, Spain, Belgium); and a mixed cluster (Netherlands, Australia, Switzerland). The Anglo-American model is characterised by strict medical requirements, relatively low replacement rates, substantial employer responsibilities, weak vocational rehabilitation programmes, and significant return to work incentives (Organisation for Economic Cooperation and Development, 2003. 129). The Scandinavian model is characterised by full population coverage, generous benefit levels, strict medical assessment, a strong focus on employment subsidies and on extensive vocational rehabilitation. The Germanic model offers only labour force coverage; medium benefit levels, work incapacity limited to own occupation, and has a strong rehabilitation focus. The Romanic model has a weak rehabilitation programme, work incapacity limited to own occupation, a strong focus on employment subsidies, and strict medical criteria. Countries in the 'mixed' model have full population coverage (means-testing in Australia), significant employer responsibilities, substantial focus on sheltered employment and varying benefit levels (Organisation for Economic Cooperation and Development, 2003: 130). In terms of the compensation or integration dichotomy, most countries still offer a mix of both of these approaches with Denmark closest to a fully integrationist approach (Organisation for Economic Cooperation and Development, 2003: 129).

6.5 **Conclusion**

In this chapter, I have examined health related worklessness from both a public health and a social policy perspective. With regard to social policy, I have overviewed the historical relationship between health related worklessness and the social security system, with a particular focus on the UK. I have argued that there have been three clear phases in welfare state development with regard to the treatment of people with a disability or health condition, and that recent reforms in the UK and across other advanced market democracies which have introduced workfare, have radically restructured the relationship between the state, society and people with ill health or a disability. I have also examined some of the key debates around health related worklessness including whether it is an employment or a health issue, as well as discussions about how high levels of structural health related worklessness have been attributed to 'cultures of worklessness'. I have also examined the medicalisation of sickness absence and the extent to which health related worklessness creates a 'reserve army of labour'. Socio-economic inequalities in health related worklessness have also been examined as well as variation by welfare state. Here I have shown that whilst there are inequalities in the employment consequences of long-term ill health and disability across all advanced welfare states, they are most pronounced in the Liberal welfare states, and smallest in the Social Democratic ones. This shows that the political, economic and social context has important implications in terms of the employment consequences of ill health and that there are policy mechanisms available to enhance the employment of those with ill health as well as to reduce inequalities in health related worklessness. These are explored in more detail in the next chapter.

6.6 **Further reading**

Stone, D. A. (1986). *The Disabled State*, Basingstoke: Macmillan.

Organisation for Economic Cooperation and Development (2003). *Transforming disability into ability: policies to promote work and income security for disabled people.* Paris: Organisation for Economic Cooperation and Development.

Williams, G. H. (2010). 'Understanding Incapacity'. In: G. Scambler and S. Scambler (eds.), *New Directions in the Sociology of Chronic and Disabling Conditions: Assaults on the Lifeworld.* London, Palgrave.

Chapter 7

Work, health, and welfare interventions

More than a quarter of the European workforce report that work negatively affects their health (European Working Conditions Observatory, 2010) and there are considerable socio-economic class inequalities in this work related ill health (Mazzuco and Suhrcke, 2010). The preceding chapters have shown that work and worklessness are the most important determinants of health and health inequalities and that the effects of work and worklessness on health and health inequalities are to a large extent mediated by welfare state regime. The latter shows that things can be done to change these health effects. Workplace interventions which eradicate or reduce exposure to known hazards in the workplace (both physical and psychosocial) or include health concerns in the planning of production, as well as those welfare interventions which improve the health of the workless may improve population health, and given the uneven social distribution of work related ill health, decrease health inequalities (Hogstedt and Lundberg, 2002). In this chapter, evidence on the effectiveness of interventions which are intended to change the experience of work and worklessness are examined with respect to providing examples of how to create healthier work, healthier experiences of worklessness, and a healthy return to work, even within the constraints of unequal capitalist societies. Strategies to tackle health inequalities are also examined.

7.1 Improving the physical work environment

This section provides some examples of the measures undertaken to reduce the risk to health of the physical work environment (as outlined in Chapter 3) in terms of health and safety regulation and prevention measures.

7.1.1 Health and safety legislation

In the welfare states of advanced capitalist economies, political pressure from workers, public health reformers, trade unions and to a lesser extent, Social Democratic governments (for example the introduction of the Health and Safety at Work Act by the UK Labour government in 1975 which set up the

Health and Safety Executive) have meant that since the 1950s, much has been done to regulate exposure to traditional workplace hazards via health and safety legislation, as well as primary prevention techniques. The European Union has also initiated a number of health and safety directives (Box 7.1). Campaigns often originated around specific conditions, for example the miners' campaign around black lung disease in the US (Berman, 1983). However, whilst regulations exist, for them to be effective they need to be implemented and enforced (Siegrist *et al.*, 2009). There is longstanding evidence that they are often not well enforced. For example, the 1970 Occupational Safety and Health Act in the US included extensive powers for the government's Occupational Safety and Health Administration to inspect workplaces, make citations for violations, and even close down workplaces. Workers could also call in inspectors and show them violations. However, examining data for the first five years after the Act, Berman (1983) found that the Act resulted in little improvement in working conditions as only a small proportion of workplaces were inspected and these were disproportionately the larger worksites with more than 500 employees. Further, the penalties given to employers for violation of the regulations were usually minor (Berman, 1983). Similar experiences were reported in relation to the UK's 1975 legislation (Doyal and Pennell, 1979). More current data also suggests that low fines are common with, for example, the 1,245 prosecutions by the UK Health and Safety Executive in 2008–2009 resulting in an average fine of just £20,000 (20% below the median UK wage of £25,000). The importance to improving health and safety of inspections to enforce legislation is illustrated in a US study by Nelson and colleagues (1997) who examined the effects on injury rates of health and safety legislation in the construction industry. They found that injury rates decreased in those firms where a health and safety inspection took place in comparison to those firms, subject to the same health and safety legislation, which were not inspected. Similarly, a pan-European study by Menendez and colleagues (2009) found that trade union representation in the assessment and control process results in better compliance by employers and a subsequent reduction in injuries and occupational health problems.

7.1.2 Exposure reduction

In terms of chemical hazards, prevention strategies to reduce silica exposure include the substitution of silica containing materials with a less hazardous material or modification of the process or equipment used (National Institute for Occupational Safety and Health, 2002). In cases where this is not possible, primary prevention can also take the form of dust control, for example with the mandatory use of protective respiratory equipment (Rees and Murray, 2007).

Box 7.1 Examples of European Union health and safety legislation

The European Union Council Directive 89/391/EEC of 1989 on the introduction of measures to encourage improvements in the safety and health of workers at work stipulates that every workplace should have a good health and safety management system which protects everyone. It sets out the general principles guiding further EU and member state policies. Under the directive, employers' duties to their workers include:

- Identifying potential hazards and carrying out a risk assessment and, based on the risk assessment, putting in place arrangements for ensuring health and safety at work.

- Providing the necessary organisation, including making specific supervision arrangements, and ensuring that supervisors have the competence and time to carry out their duties.

- Identifying any special measures required for vulnerable individuals such as prohibiting them from using dangerous equipment.

- Providing information on the possible risks that people face in their jobs, and the prevention measures adopted.

- Providing adequate training, instruction and information at recruitment, and following any change of job or changes in the workplace.

- Consulting with workers and their representatives on health and safety matters.

In addition, European Union Council Directive 98/24/EC of 1998 contained specific measures to protect workers against the health and safety risks of chemical agents including:

- Binding occupational exposure limit values.

- Binding biological limit values and health surveillance measures.

- Prohibition for specific agents.

- Risk assessments by employers.

- Action to prevention risk.

- Information and training.

Source: Full text of the legislation is available from: http://eur-lex.europa.eu

In some instances, the use of wet methods can also help to minimise exposure. Control at the individual level also includes risk communication about the hazard and ways to minimise exposure as well as undertaking routine surveillance. Preventative strategies to reduce morbidity and mortality associated with cumulative exposure to coal dust include the use of protective masks, minimising dust levels and ensuring adequate ventilation where possible. Commentators have also suggested that, as smoking worsens the symptoms of silicosis and pneumoconiosis by interfering with lung function, smoking cessation counselling should be delivered to workers with pulmonary signs and symptoms (Ross and Murray, 2004). Legislation has also been passed in many countries, including the EU directive 98/24/EC, limiting levels of acceptable or 'safe' exposure to chemical hazards. However, as described in Chapter 3, 'safe doses' of toxic substances have varied over time and by country with no allowance for variation in individual tolerances (Doyal and Pennell, 1979). The needs of an efficient and profitable production process usually take precedence over public health concerns, with the levels set so that they only minimally interfere with productivity. For example, the 1970 Occupational Safety and Health Act in the US limited the level of airborne lead, but what was allowable under the Act was still considered to be hazardous by many occupational health physicians (Landrigan, 1990).

Health damaging noise exposure is preventable. Regulations have been introduced in a number of countries to limit exposure to noise. Consequently, in the UK, the Control of Noise at Work Regulations 2005 state that hearing protection and hearing protection zones must be made available by employers when noise levels reach 85 decibels (based on average daily or weekly exposure) (Health and Safety Executive, 2005a). Further, the UK regulations require employers to undertake surveillance for putative risks to workers' health (as well as providing information and training) when noise levels reach 80 decibels. The regulations also specify that exposure levels should not exceed 87 decibels even when hearing protection is in place (Health and Safety Executive, 2005a). Interventions to reduce noise exposure include the use of hearing protection including ear plugs or ear muffs (Health and Safety Executive, 2010c). Protections like this are effective if adhered to by employers and workers. For example, a study of 374 workers at an American automobile plant found that the use of hearing protection reduced both systolic and diastolic blood pressure in workers exposed to noises of 85 dBA or over (Lusk *et al.*, 2002). Systolic blood pressure was 3.7 mm Hg lower amongst workers who wore hearing protection and diastolic blood pressure was 2.9 mm Hg. In the longer term, interventions which change job patterns, using equipment with lower noise exposure, changing processes or limiting the duration of exposure per work task to reduce workers' exposure to excess noise levels, can all reduce the development of health problems associated with work related noise (Health and Safety Executive, 2010c).

In terms of vibration, the UK Control of Vibration at Work Regulations 2005 specifies that the daily exposure limit for hand-arm vibration is set at 5 m/s^2 A(8) but importantly the exposure action value (that is the value at which the employer must take reasonable action to limit exposure) is 2.5 m/s^2 A(8) (Health and Safety Executive, 2005b). Prevention and control strategies include identifying alternative work methods; replacing old equipment with vibration reducing tools; improving work stations to reduce the load on hands and wrists; and minimising exposure by adopting work schedules that limit the time a worker spends using vibration creating tools or equipment. Similarly, in terms of whole body vibration, the UK Control of Vibration at Work Regulations 2005 limits the daily exposure for whole body vibration to 1.15 m/s^2 and the daily exposure action value is 0.5 m/s^2 (Health and Safety Executive, 2005b). European Union regulations specify the role of employers in identifying and evaluating possible risks, communicating possible risks to workers, combating risks by for example replacing machines with high risk of exposure to vibration with updated more ergonomic models (Health and Safety Executive, 2010d). In addition, preventive policies are advocated including: using ergonomically designed equipment; minimising the duration and magnitude of exposures; adhering to a regular schedule of rest breaks; and providing training and information for workers on the risks of whole body vibration and ways of minimising exposure (Health and Safety Executive, 2010d).

7.1.3 Ergonomic strategies

In relation to the ergonomic prevention of work related musculoskeletal disorders, Kuorinka (1998) describes the need for a multi-pronged preventive strategy which is both flexible and participatory in nature. The UK Health and Safety Executive (2004) stipulate that employers should make all possible attempts to minimise the need for hazardous manual handling while also assessing and reducing the risk of injury from unavoidable manual handling. The UK Health and Safety Executive (2010e) also encourages employers to consider a number of strategies to reduce exposure to repetitive tasks, including limiting repetitive and intensive tasks to short durations; allowing for regular breaks rather than one mid-shift break; rotating workers between tasks to reduce monotony; making the pace of work manageable; and designing work stations and/or equipment appropriately for the required tasks. A systematic review of 26 studies examined the effects on musculoskeletal disorders of reducing the amount of manual physical lifting undertaken by employees (especially industrial workers and health care workers) (van der Molen *et al.*, 2005). The review focused on two types of intervention: ergonomic interventions especially the introduction of mechanical lifting devices and lifting aids, and educational interventions such as training and information on how to reduce physical work demands. The review concluded that the ergonomic interventions were generally successful in terms of reducing physical work demands and that this usually resulted in a decrease in musculoskeletal complaints – particularly with respect to lower back pain. In terms of the education interventions, training workers to perform their work tasks in ways that reduced physical loads, as well as involving them in discussions of workloads, were also beneficial in terms of reducing physical workloads and improved musculoskeletal symptoms, but usually only when ergonomic interventions were also present.

There is more of a debate about the effectiveness of prevention interventions in terms of the health effects of repetitive work. For example, a systematic review of 24 studies of ergonomic, exercise and job rotation interventions to prevent carpal tunnel syndrome (a form of repetitive strain injury—RSI) amongst clerical workers, concluded that none of the included studies conclusively demonstrated that the interventions (e.g. redesigned computer keyboards and workstations) were effective (Lincoln *et al.*, 2000). In contrast, there is research in industrial settings which suggests that tool redesign can be effective in reducing the onset – or at least the severity—of RSI. For example, Yassi (1997) describes a study of automobile workers which found that using ergonomically designed tools, assembly fixtures to eliminate pinched grips, and job rotation within the assembly line reduced operations for RSI by 50%. Similarly, a review of 14 studies by Kilborn across different industrial settings found that job redesigns were the most effective prevention strategy (Kilborn, 1988).

7.1.4 Shift work interventions

Various different interventions have been suggested to address the negative effects of shift work (Harrington, 2001). These include interventions at the individual level: exposure to bright light or napping; training; countermeasures against sleep problems and problems with appetite and digestion; counselling and educational interventions (e.g. to help workers to cope with shift work); regular medical surveillance and pharmaceutical interventions (e.g. melatonin administration); and selection strategies to remove the most vulnerable (Health and Safety Executive, 2006b; Monk and Folkard, 1992; Wedderburn and Rankin, 2001). At the organizational level, interventions include decreased shift length (especially on night shift); redesign of shift work schedules (according to ergonomic criteria or to increase flexibility); improvements in working conditions (reducing noise or improving unfavourable working environments); and legislation that limits working hours or exposure to shift work (e.g. the European Union's Working Time Directive and its subsequent revisions) (Harrington, 2001).

A systematic review of the 26 studies on the health and well-being effects of changing the organisation of shift work showed that three types of intervention (switching from slow to fast rotation; changing from backward to forward rotation; and self-scheduling of shifts) can improve the health of employees, their work-life balance, or both (Table 7.1) (Bambra *et al.*, 2008a). Studies which reported on a change from a slow to a fast rotation of shifts (a change from six or seven consecutive shifts of the same type e.g. seven consecutive morning shifts, to a maximum of three or four) found consistent positive outcomes in relation to sleep, fatigue and to work-life balance. Changing from

Table 7.1 Systematic reviews of work environment interventions

Citation	Intervention(s)	Summary of results
Bambra *et al.* (2007b)	Task structure work reorganisation: task variety, team working, autonomous groups.	Task structure interventions did not generally alter levels of employee control. However, where job control decreased (and psychosocial demands increased), self-reported mental (and sometimes physical) health appeared to get worse.
Egan *et al.* (2007)	Organisational level work reorganisation: participatory committees, control over hours of work.	Participatory committee interventions which increased employee control had a consistent and positive impact on self-reported health.
Bambra *et al.* (2008a)	Changes to the organization of shift work schedules	Switching from slow to fast shift rotation; changing from backward to forward shift rotation; and the self-scheduling of shifts were found to benefit health and work-life balance.
Bambra *et al.* (2008b)	Changing from an 8hr, 5 day week to a Compressed Working Week (CWW) of a 12hr/10hr, 4 day week.	Health effects were inconclusive, although there was seldom a detrimental effect. Work-life balance was often improved.
Joyce *et al.* (2010b)	Flexible work interventions including self-scheduling, overtime, gradual/partial retirement, involuntary part-time work and fixed-term contracts.	Interventions (such as self-scheduling or partial retirement) which offered flexibility favouring the employee and over which the employee had more control tended to have beneficial effects on health and wellbeing.

Source: Adapted and reproduced from Bambra *et al.*, (2010c) with permission from BMJ publishing.

a backward (night, afternoon, morning) to a forward shift rotation (morning, afternoon, night), also improved health, particularly in terms of sleep. Self-scheduling (worker control over shifts, start times, or rest days) was also associated with positive outcomes in relation to health, and work-life balance. Another popular organisational level intervention is changing the hours of shift work by introducing a Compressed Working Week which increases the hours worked per day, whilst decreasing the days worked. The compressed working week, therefore, represents a radical break from the eight-hour working day length traditionally favoured by workers and trade unions (McOrmond, 2004) and it is therefore vital that a cap still remains on the total number of hours worked per week (e.g. a maximum of 48 hours under the European Union Working Time Directive) (McOrmond, 2004). A systematic review of 40 studies (Table 7.1) of the health and work-life balance effects of changing from five eight-hour days to a Compressed Working Week of four twelve-hour days, found that health, particularly mental health, and work-life balance improved (Bambra *et al.*, 2008b).

7.2 **Improving the psychosocial work environment**

The strong epidemiological relationship between key elements of the psychosocial work environment and health (as outlined in Chapter 4) has resulted in academic and policy discussions about how it can be improved in order to enhance public health and potentially reduce health inequalities. Karasek categorised workplace psychosocial interventions by distinguishing organisational level interventions aimed at changing the psychosocial environment, from individual level interventions aimed at changing the way individuals behave in or cope with that environment. He argued that organisational interventions were preferable as preventative measures because they addressed the structural causes of unhealthy working environments (Karasek, 1992). There are two types of organisational interventions, micro and macro (Bambra *et al.*, 2009b). Micro-organisational changes to the work environment focus on the nature of work tasks, whereas macro-organisational changes are designed to increase employees' opportunities to make decisions or participate in workplace decision-making processes. The health improvement potential of such interventions is of increasing relevance to policymakers as, for example, in 1994 the European Union issued a directive to increase participation at work. In addition, high profile reports by the Department of Health and Human Services in the US (2007), the English Department of Health (Marmot, 2010), as well as the World Health Organisation (WHO, 2008) have all highlighted the potential health benefits of changing the psychosocial work environment. Sweden and Norway have implemented extensive regulation of the psychosocial

> ## Box 7.2 Key psychosocial aspects of the 1991 Swedish Work Environment Act
>
> The 1991 Swedish Work Environment Act amended legislation from the 1970s. In terms of the psychosocial work environment, it specified that:
>
> - There should be opportunities for employees to participate in designing their own work situation.
> - Work organisation and job content should be designed in ways that reduce exposure to unhealthy physical and mental loads.
> - Pay systems and work schedules that increase the risk of ill health should be avoided (e.g. piece work).
> - Strictly controlled work should be restricted.
> - All jobs should include task variety, social contact, and cooperation.
> - Employers should provide opportunities for personal development and autonomy.
>
> Source: As described in Landsbergis, 2009: 195.

work environment (Box 7.2) in order to prevent occupational ill health (Schnall *et al.*, 2009; Landsbergis, 2009).

7.2.1 Micro-organisational changes to the psychosocial work environment

Karasek (1992) suggested that micro-organisational changes to work tasks can take three forms:

  (i) Job enrichment and enlargement (task variety),

 (ii) Collective coping and decision-making (team working), and

(iii) The use of autonomous production groups (autonomous groups).

Task variety interventions increase the skills used by workers by increasing the variety of work tasks which are required as part of their jobs. Team working interventions give workers more collective responsibility and decision-making power. However, workers are still individualised, responsibility is not shared and supervisory structures remain in place. This intervention type is also designed to enhance collective coping and provide support within the workplace. Autonomous group interventions are specific to mass production environments where they are often used to reduce the prevalence of traditional production line characteristics (such as individualised, repetitive tasks) by increasing skill variety and collective involvement. They combine aspects of job enrichment and team working as well as increased worker participation within the work team.

Karasek hypothesised that task restructuring interventions would improve levels of job control and social support although, in line with the characteristics of more active jobs, demands may also be high. Given the literature on the psychosocial work environment and health as outlined in Chapter 4, it can further be hypothesised that interventions which improve the psychosocial work environment in this way would also have a beneficial effect on health, while, conversely, interventions that result in higher demands and lower control would have an adverse effect on health outcomes. A systematic review examined this hypothesis by synthesising the available evidence on the health effects of changes to the psychosocial work environment brought about by the reorganisation of work task structures (see Table 7.1) (Bambra *et al.*, 2007b). The review also explored whether those health effects differed by socio-economic class.

The review synthesised a total of nineteen studies: eight examined task variety interventions, seven evaluated team working and six looked at autonomous production groups (two of the studies examined interventions which entailed both changes to task variety and increased team working). It found that those interventions that improved the psychosocial work environment by increasing task variety either had no effect or a limited positive effect on health. The team working interventions tended to improve the psychosocial work environment in most studies, although not for all workers, but the health effects were less apparent. The autonomous work groups, contrary to the stated aims of such interventions, caused deterioration in the psychosocial work environment, and, as would be predicted from the demand-control-support model, the resulting health effects were correspondingly adverse, though in some cases they were negligible. It is important to note that some interventions did not greatly alter the psychosocial work environment at all, and so could not be expected to have a measurable effect on health. This may have been due to poor implementation of the interventions or, in some cases, because of concurrent negative changes occurring in the macro work environment. It may also be simply because some of the interventions were not substantial enough to alter the psychosocial work environment in a meaningful way.

This review concluded that changes in the levels of job control appeared to be a more important factor for health than changes in levels of social support. Interventions which altered levels of control tended to report significant changes in self-reported mental and physical health: decreased levels of control almost invariably resulted in adverse health outcomes and, albeit to a lesser extent, increased levels of control resulted in improved health outcomes. When the interventions increased demand and decreased control, this negatively affected health, and increases to workplace support had minimal mediating effects.

7.2.2 **Macro-organisational changes to the psychosocial work environment**

Following Karasek (1992), macro-organisational changes are those designed to increase employees' opportunities to make decisions about their work environment and/or participate in wider workplace decision-making processes. Examples of these interventions would include workers councils (as are common in Germany), or problem-solving committees of workers or their representatives (Landsbergis, 2009). These are considered to operate at a macro level because managerial structures and workplace hierarchies may need to change in order to accommodate an increase in employee participation and control.

In 2007, Egan and colleagues systematically reviewed the health effects of organizational level interventions designed to increase employee participation or control (see Table 7.1). The systematic review identified a total of 18 studies, six of which examined the health effects of 'participatory' or 'problem-solving' committees of employee representatives (the other 12 were of participatory interventions implemented in combination with individual level interventions, ergonomic improvements, or organisational downsizing). These were usually established to identify ways of tackling workplace stressors, although one had wider powers in areas such as budgeting and personnel. These studies generally found that if the committees were effective in increasing levels of employee control, then they had beneficial health effects. For example, one controlled prospective cohort study (Bond and Bunce, 2001) examined the effects of a workers' steering committee of volunteer employee representatives, moderated by an external consultant in a UK central government office. It found that after one year, mean scores for 'sense of control' increased in the intervention group, in contrast to a decrease in the control group. Mean mental ill health scores also improved in the intervention group relative to the control group, whose scores increased. The intervention group also experienced a decrease in routinely recorded sickness absence.

The review concluded that interventions that improved workplace control and/or workplace support tended to improve employee health. Health improvements did not occur when either control or support worsened. Interventions that reduced demands also improved health, but sometimes health improved even when the intervention appeared to increase demands. The importance of control at work was also the conclusion of a Cochrane systematic review of flexible working which found that employee control over working hours had some positive health effects (see Table 7.1) (Joyce *et al.*, 2010b).

7.3 Mitigating the ill health effects of unemployment

Chapter 5 outlined the ill health effects of unemployment. In terms of interventions, there are two broad issues: welfare payments for the unemployed, and interventions to aid return to work.

7.3.1 Social benefits and welfare rights

Epidemiological research has shown that welfare rights, as well as the level of out-of-work benefits paid to the unemployed can be important factors in whether unemployment leads to an increased population risk of ill health. For example, a 2001 study compared means-tested and non-means-tested unemployment benefits. It found that amongst the unemployed, those in receipt of non-means-tested benefits had better self-perceived health than those in receipt of means-tested benefits (Rodriguez, 2001). The study used household panel data from 8,726 adult respondents in Britain (1991–1993), 11,086 in Germany (1991–1993), and 11,668 in the US (1985–1987). In each country, the study compared the perceived health of unemployed people in receipt of different benefits with those in full-time employment. After adjusting for baseline health, employment history, socio-economic and demographic characteristics, the likelihood of reporting poor health was significantly higher amongst the means-tested group but there were no significant differences between the entitlement and employed groups. In Britain, people on means-tested benefits were 59% more likely to report poor health than those in employment (adjusted OR = 1.59, 95% CI 1.08 to 2.35), in Germany they were 123% more likely (adjusted OR = 2.23, 95% CI 1.14 to 4.35), and 141% in the US (adjusted OR = 2.41, 95% CI 1.43 to 4.06). The study concluded that whilst entitlement benefits were sufficient to ameliorate the negative health effects of unemployment, means-tested benefits were not. This is probably a result of the combination of both material and psychosocial factors: means-tested benefits are usually lower in value than entitlement benefits, and they also attract stigma.

The 'minimum income for healthy living' (MIHL) is potentially a way of ensuring that welfare benefits are of a sufficient level to maintain health and wellbeing, and that there is a right to a certain standard of living. Based on the link between income and health, Morris and colleagues (2000) have illustrated how, in relation to older people and young men, health can be improved and inequalities in health reduced via the public provision of a minimum income to meet basic and social needs relating to nutrition, physical activity, housing, psychosocial interactions, transport, medical care and hygiene. The MIHL would include funding to enable:

> 'Consumption of a healthy diet, for example five portions of fruit and vegetables a day, two portions of fish a week; expenses related to exercise costs, for example, the cost of trainers, bicycles and swimming in a local leisure centre; as well as costs related to social integration and support networks (e.g. telephone rental, television)'.

> Marmot (2010: 121)

In their first analysis, Morris and colleagues (2000) calculated the MIHL for healthy young British men aged 18–30. The minimum costs were assessed to be £131.86 per week (UK, 1999 prices). This compared with a net income from the national minimum wage of £105.84 at 18–21 years and £121.12 at 22+ years for a thirty-eight hour working week. State welfare benefits were considerably less. More recent analysis has shown that the MIHL for an older single person would be around £144.20 per week (UK, 2008 prices) (Morris, 2009). This was higher than the poverty line (60% of median income—£115 per week), and more than the minimum pension credit (£124.05 per week). As the Marmot Review of Health Inequalities in England states:

> 'A minimum income for healthy living will improve the standard of living for those on low incomes. It would ensure that all would receive an appropriate income for their stage in the life course, and would reduce overall levels of poverty as well as child poverty'.

> Marmot (2010: 121)

The MIHL provides a model for determining the welfare safety net required to counteract poverty, improve living standards and increase the life chances for those most at risk (Morris and Deeming, 2004). The 2010 Marmot Review recommended implementation of the MIHL (Marmot, 2010), and it is also supported as a policy to tackle health inequalities by the World Health Organisation (Bambra et al., 2009a, 2010b).

7.3.2 Active labour market policies

In addition to the payment of out-of-work welfare benefits, governments fund a number of programmes to reduce levels of unemployment. This is referred to as Active Labour Market Policy (ALMP). ALMP can be defined as work, training or other programmes designed to help the unemployed move back into employment and/or secure higher earnings (Robinson, 1998). In the UK, ALMP is quite often referred to using the term 'welfare to work'. It is contrasted to 'traditional' labour market policy—the passive payment of unemployment and other related benefits (Robinson, 1998). ALMP has become increasingly popular across both the European Union and the wider countries of the Organisation for Economic Cooperation and Development (OECD). Three types of ALMP can be identified (Robinson, 2000):

(1) Measures to enhance successful job search.

(2) Measures to raise the skills of job seekers e.g. training courses.

(3) Measures to directly subsidise employment opportunities for target groups e.g. public works programmes and recruitment/wage subsidies to private employers.

Target groups vary by country and across time. For example, in the late 1990s in the UK it was the long-term unemployed and young people who were the main focus of ALMP, in the US it was single parents; and in Sweden and the Netherlands, the focus was on disabled people (Robinson, 1998: 87). However, more recently in the UK the focus has shifted towards people with a chronic illness or disability (see Chapter 6). There are three aims behind ALMP (Robinson, 1998):

◆ To increase demand for labour from target groups.

◆ To improve the effective supply of labour by enhancing participants' chances of obtaining a regular job via job search, training and work experience programmes.

◆ To check the eligibility of participants to receive benefits.

Workfare is a more restrictive form of ALMP (see Chapters 2 and 6). Perhaps unsurprisingly, there have been various calls (Smith, 1993; Acheson 1998; World Health Organisation Commission on the Social Determinants of Health, 2008) for research on the health effects of ALMP policies. However, there is a shortage of evidence on the effects of ALMP on health and well-being, and what exists is rather conflicting. In a review of the evidence base prepared for the Strategic Review of Health Inequalities in England Post 2010 (Marmot Review), Coutts (2009) concludes that the weight of evidence suggests that participation within ALMPs, specifically government training programmes, can have a positive effect on the well-being (psychological health) of the participants compared to those who remain unemployed and economically inactive (Coutts, 2009: 3). Further, he argues that these health improvements occur as a result of psychosocial (not material) mechanisms such as increases in social contact, social support, and feelings of control and self-worth. He cites evidence from a number of studies which recorded an improvement amongst ALMP participants in terms of psychological well-being, depression, anxiety, self-esteem, and emotional functioning.

In contrast, Dorling (2009) argues that the health and well-being effects of ALMP are less positive. He cites a UK study which compared the experiences of 46 young people who were unemployed, or on a youth training scheme

(early form of ALMP) or employed as apprentices, and which found significant differences in terms of depression, with the employed being less depressed
than the other three groups (Branthwaite and Garcia, 1985). Depression levels
amongst the ALMP group were not significantly different from the unemployed. Further, more recent evidence from a series of qualitative studies of
unemployed men and women in the North of England shows that the 'empow-
erment' and 'feelings of control' which ALMP may engender can be short
lived, especially if there are no jobs at the end of the training period (Joyce
et al., 2010a; Smith *et al.*, 2010). The quantitative evidence summarised by
Coutts (2009) also highlights the short-term nature of the health gains associated with ALMP, with the longest recorded benefits lasting just four months,
and most disappearing immediately after participation ends. The importance
to health and well-being of participating in what were perceived by the programme participants as 'better' or 'worse' ALMP activities is also demonstrated
by a Swedish study by Westerlund and colleagues (2004) which found that
during the 'better' programme activities there was a temporary reduction in
stress levels, whilst involvement in the 'worse' activities led to a temporary
increase. Whether involvement in ALMP is voluntary or compulsory is also
likely to mediate the health impacts. The health and wellbeing effects of ALMP
therefore really depend on the type and quality of ALMP offered, as well as the
wider welfare state and labour market context.

7.4 Enhancing the health and employment of the chronically ill

Most welfare state countries have adopted active labour market policies
for people who are disabled or chronically ill (as previously discussed in
Chapter 6). Policy strategies are directed at either the supply-side—enhancing
the ability of individuals with a disability or chronic illness to be employed, or
the demand-side—increasing the desirability to employers of recruiting and
retaining this particular group of workers (Bambra, 2006c).

Supply-side strategies are concerned with increasing the availability and
work readiness of individuals with a disability or chronic illness. They are
designed to overcome some of the employment barriers which people with a
disability or chronic illness face, particularly in terms of lack of skills or work
experience, and financial uncertainty about the transition into paid employment (Gardiner, 1997). Supply-side interventions typically include:

◆ *Education, training and work placement schemes* which aim to increase
  employment rates by providing vocational skills, work experience and
  exposure to employers, or recognised qualifications.

- *Vocational advice and support services* which are designed to help movement into employment by enhancing job search skills, matching individuals to jobs, arranging access to training and education schemes, offering information about in-work benefits, and providing other forms of individualised vocational advice and support.

- *Vocational rehabilitation* is a long established form of return to work policy in many developed countries. Rehabilitation (both medical and vocational) is particularly used to help people who develop a disability or chronic illness whilst in work to retain their employment (Bloch and Prins, 2001).

- *In-work benefits* aim to increase employment by overcoming fears about taking low paid jobs, the loss of future benefit entitlement if they become out-of-work again, the additional costs of employment such as transport costs, or the financial difficulties that the initial loss of benefits could create.

Demand-side interventions focus on increasing the demand for disabled or chronically ill workers. They tend to focus on reducing the costs or risks to employers of employing them or placing requirements on employers in their recruitment and retention (Bambra *et al.*, 2005b; Bambra, 2006c). They are attempts to combat the other type of employment barriers faced by people with a disability: employer uncertainty and the physical difficulties of workplaces (Gardiner, 1997). There are four common demand-side policies:

- *Financial incentives for employers* aim to encourage recruitment by offering wage subsidies to cover the initial costs of employment or to compensate for any reduced productivity associated with employing someone with a disability or chronic illness.

- *Mandatory employment quotas* are still operated in some countries such as Poland, Luxembourg and Spain (Organisation for Economic Cooperation and Development, 2009). These require that 2 to 5% of the workforce of a company must be disabled or chronically ill (the UK operated a similar scheme of 3% from 1944 to 1995).

- *Employment rights legislation* such as the UK's Disability Discrimination Act, or the Americans with Disabilities Act, or the comparable legislation operating in Sweden, the Netherlands or Australia, is increasingly being used instead of employment quotas. Since 2006, all EU member states are obliged to have such legislation (Organisation for Economic Cooperation and Development, 2009).

- *Accessibility interventions* are designed to facilitate employment by reducing physical workplace barriers, for instance by providing specialist ergonomic equipment, for people with a disability or chronic illness.

Various evidence reviews have examined the effectiveness of welfare to work interventions on employment rates in the UK (Bambra *et al.*, 2005b; Bambra, 2006c; Clayton *et al.*, 2011). With regard to supply-side interventions, the review evidence suggests that vocational advice and employment and training interventions have positive impacts on employment rates ranging from 11% to 50% depending on the characteristics of participants, such as 'job-readiness' or type of illness, as well as the local labour market context (Bambra *et al.*, 2005b). However, the vast majority of evaluations are uncontrolled and it is therefore impossible to determine if the improved employment chances are due to the effectiveness of the welfare to work interventions themselves or to external factors such as a general upturn in UK employment rates. There is little evidence that in-work benefits were effective in increasing employment (Bambra, 2006c).

In terms of demand side interventions, the UK evidence base suggests that such interventions have a very limited impact on the employment of people with a disability or chronic illness. For example, financial interventions designed to incentivise employers were ineffective because they did not adequately off set the perceived risks and costs of employing a disabled person (Bambra, 2006c). The employment rights approach was similarly found to be ineffective in increasing the employment rates of people with a disability or chronic illness. The UK evidence suggests that the legislation had no effect on employers' recruitment decisions (with the majority of employers unaware of its employment provisions) (Roberts *et al.*, 2004) and that the employment gap between those with and without a health condition or disability actually increased after the introduction of the Disability Discrimination Act (Pope and Bambra, 2005). A further study found that after the legislation socio-economic inequalities in the consequences of ill health increased with no significant effect on the employment rates of professional workers in classes 1 and 2 (−2.7%, 95% CI −8.7% to 2.99%) but a large significant decrease of 10.7% (95% CI −6.16% to −15.24%) in the employment of less skilled workers (social classes IV and V) with a health condition or disability (Bambra and Pope, 2007). Of the demand-side interventions, only accessibility interventions appear to have a more positive employment impact (Hillage *et al.*, 1998; Beinart *et al.*, 1996).

Beyond the UK, evaluations have similarly found little evidence of the effectiveness of vocational rehabilitation interventions. For example, evaluations of the wide scale US 'Ticket to Work' scheme (a voucher based system which entitles disabled people to purchase rehabilitation services from a variety of private and voluntary sector providers who are financially rewarded only for positive employment outcomes) revealed limited uptake and minimal employment outcomes for participants (Thornton *et al.*, 2004). An international evidence synthesis also found limited evidence on successful return to work outcomes (Waddell *et al.*, 2008). Employment quotas have been found to have only limited success with a third of employers ignoring them (possibly because the sanctions that exist to penalise non-compliance are limited, amounting to around 1% of company payroll) resulting in only 60% of quota places being filled (Organisation for Economic Cooperation and Development, 2003: 210). Similarly, whilst the US has one of the most extensive disability employment rights acts in the world (1990 Americans with Disabilities Act), the research evidence suggests that it has had minimal influence on increasing the employment of disabled people (DeLeire, 2000; Russell, 2002). Finally, an international systematic review of the employment effects of restricting entitlements to welfare benefits for people with ill health or a disability in the UK, Canada, Denmark, Sweden and Norway concluded that:

> 'There is insufficient evidence, and what there is [is] equivocal, to indicate whether changes in benefit eligibility requirements . . . will have an impact on the employment of people with disabilities and chronic illness in well developed welfare states'.

> Barr *et al.* (2010)

A possible factor behind the rather limited success of these ALMPs for this particular group of workless people is that they focus almost exclusively on employment. There is little attention to the health needs of this population, who, after all, are workless in the first place as a result of ill health. Recognising the importance of sickness as a barrier to employment would result in more innovative 'health first' approaches. Whilst such medical and psychosocial rehabilitation has been a common feature of interventions in the Nordic countries, more recently it is beginning to be applied in the UK. For example, recent international evidence based guidance produced by England's National Institute for Health and Clinical Excellence (National Institute for Health and Clinical Excellence, 2009b) has recommended a 'health first' case management approach to improving the health and employment of people with a chronic illness (Box 7.3). The National Institute for Health and Clinical Excellence guidance on managing long-term sickness absence and incapacity for work recommends that integrated programmes which combine traditional vocational training approaches, financial support, and health management on an ongoing case management basis should be commissioned to help Incapacity Benefit recipients enter or return to work. The UK National Institute for Health and Clinical Excellence considers these integrated approaches to be the most effective ways of enhancing the employment of people who are workless due to ill health (Gabbay *et al.*, 2011). This approach is being piloted in the North East of England (County Durham), an area with high levels of health related worklessness (Bambra, 2010b).

Box 7.3 National Institute for Health and Clinical Excellence recommendation on return to work interventions for Incapacity Benefit recipients

Who is the target population?
People with health problems who are unemployed and claiming Incapacity Benefit or Employment Support Allowance.

Who should take action?
Department for Work and Pensions and other bodies or organisations which may commission services for those who are unemployed and claiming Incapacity Benefit or Employment Support Allowance.

What action should they take?
Commission an integrated programme to help claimants enter or return to work (paid or unpaid). The programme should include a combination of interventions such as:

- An interview with a trained adviser to discuss the help they need to return to work.

- Vocational training, including that offered by *New Deal for Disabled People* (for example, help producing a curriculum vitae, interview training and help to find a job or a work placement).

- A *condition management* component run by local health providers to help people manage their health condition.

- Financial measures to motivate them to return to work (such as return-to-work credit).

- Support before and after returning to work (this may include one or more of the following: mentoring, a job coach, occupational health support or financial advice).

Source: National Institute for Health and Clinical Excellence (2009b) and Gabbay *et al.*, (2011).

7.5 **Tackling health inequalities**

Conventionally, approaches to addressing health inequalities fall into three broad but interlinked categories (Graham and Kelly, 2004):

(1) Focusing on improving the position of the most disadvantaged groups.

(2) Reducing the gap between the best and worst off.

(3) Reducing the entire social gradient in health.

More recently, a fourth hybrid approach called 'proportionate universalism' has emerged (Marmot, 2010). Work and worklessness interventions to tackling health inequalities tend to reflect these different approaches and the recommendations of the World Health Organisation on how the workplace and social protection for the workless can decrease health inequalities are detailed in Box 7. 4.

Box 7.4 World Health Organisation Commission on the Social Determinants of Health recommendations on reducing health inequalities via employment, work and social protection interventions

Fair employment and decent work

Employment and working conditions have powerful effects on health equity. When these are good, they can provide financial security, social status, personal development, social relations and self-esteem, and protection from physical and psychosocial illness. The Commission calls for:

- Full and fair employment and decent work, to be a central goal of national and international social and economic policymaking.
- Economic and social policies that ensure secure work for men and women with a living wage that takes into account the real and current cost of healthy living.
- All workers to be protected through international core labour standards and policies; and
- improved working conditions for all workers.

Social protection throughout life

Everyone needs social protection throughout their lives, as young children, in working life, and in old age. People also need protection in case of specific shocks, such as illness, disability, and loss of income or work. Four out of five people worldwide lack the back-up of basic social security coverage. Extending social protection to all people, within countries and globally, will be a major step towards achieving health equity within a generation. The Commission calls for:

- Establishing and strengthening universal comprehensive social protection policies.
- Ensuring social protection systems include those who are in precarious work, including informal work and household or care work.

Source: World Health Organisation Commission on the Social Determinants of Health (2008).

7.5.1 **Focusing on disadvantaged groups**

This approach focuses on improving the health of the most disadvantaged groups by concentrating on absolute levels of health by improving social conditions, reducing risk factors and increasing life opportunities (Graham and Kelly, 2004). The advantages of this approach are threefold:

 (i) It directs attention to marginalised groups.

 (ii) Monitoring and evaluation of the effectiveness of interventions is relatively straightforward by employing case control designs or making comparisons with the general population.

 (iii) It enables synergy with other policies such as social inclusion and community regeneration (Graham and Kelly, 2004).

Area based initiatives are often employed to enable measurement of disadvantage using household (e.g. Job Seekers Allowance claimants) or individual (e.g. teenage mothers) indicators. There are, however, disadvantages associated with this type of approach, not least the problems associated with equating the language of inequality to the language of disadvantage. The consequence of which, as Graham and Kelly (2004) describe, is a shift in the focus of reducing inequalities from the whole population to a smaller proportion of people and the potential for a widening health gap when compared with the general population. In terms of work and worklessness interventions, area based ALMPs are underpinned by this approach.

7.5.2 **Reducing the gap**

This approach entails strategies which focus on reducing the gap between the best and worst off, by implementing interventions targeted towards those people with the greatest burden of disadvantage in terms of risk factors, social exclusion or being hard to reach (Graham and Kelly, 2004). Driven by the realisation that improvements in health have been paralleled by a widening of disparities between the best and worst off in the population, interventions under this category would necessitate 'raising the health of the poorest, fastest' (Graham and Kelly, 2004: 8). In the UK, programmes like Health Action Zones and Sure Start have tended to adopt this strategy, the benefits of which include the capacity to set targets to facilitate monitoring and evaluation (Graham and Kelly, 2004). There are, however, a number of constraints associated with this type of approach. As with improving the health of the most disadvantaged, this strategy would again target only a small section of the population and perhaps more importantly, this type of approach tends to engender a focus on lifestyle factors as the cause of inequalities and ignores wider societal influences. There is concern, also that this approach fails to appreciate social differentials and the effects of disadvantage on health for those just outside the most deprived group (ibid.). Workplace health checks, in which members of staff are screened for such problems as diabetes or cardiovascular disease, are often targeted at those with the greatest burden of disease or highest risk factor profile.

7.5.3 Reducing the social gradient

This strategy considers the whole social gradient and seeks to focus not only on people in the most deprived groups within society but also on those who, although not at the bottom of the social hierarchy, nonetheless suffer disadvantage in relation to health outcomes. In other words this strategy:

> 'Locates the causes of health inequality, not in the disadvantaged circumstances and health damaging behaviours of the poorest groups, but in the systematic differences in life chances, living standards and lifestyles associated with people's unequal position in the socio-economic hierarchy'.

Graham and Kelly (2004: 10)

The benefits of this type of approach are to refocus attention to the largest proportion of the population sitting between the two extremes of the hierarchy, thereby achieving maximum health gains for the majority. It is common for workplace interventions to take this more universal approach with, for example, health and safety legislation applying across the whole workforce.

7.5.4 Proportionate universalism

A more recent approach, this strategy advocates the combination of the first and last approaches with the intention of improving the health of all, but the health of the poorest the most. This underpins the recommendations to tackle embedded patterns of health inequality made by the recent Marmot Review of health inequalities in England and Wales (Marmot, 2010): *Fair Society, Healthy Lives*. It proposes the use of interventions which are universally targeted *'but with a scale and intensity that is proportionate to the level of disadvantage'*—proportionate universalism (Marmot, 2010: 15). This is similar to developments in other areas of social policy particularly in the UK, where what is called *progressive* universalism has, for example, resulted in means-tested supplements to the universal flat rate state pensions for those in most financial need. The 'minimum income for healthy living' could be viewed as a proportionate universalism intervention.

7.6 Conclusion

In this chapter I have provided examples of policies and interventions in the workplace and the welfare system which may reduce the negative effects of the work environment and of worklessness on health. I have shown that in terms of the physical work environment the most important issue in advanced market democracies is the more stringent enforcement of existing health and safety legislation. There is still too much focus on the individual worker, who must adapt to or cope with the hazardous working conditions, rather than the employer being required to redesign the production process (Doyal and Pennell, 1979). In the psychosocial work environment, the evidence presented here supports the health benefits of workplace interventions which increase worker control, give them a voice in workplace decision-making, and break down the isolation, disempowerment and alienation felt by workers—especially those in lower skilled posts or on the periphery of the labour market. However, whilst enhancing the control of individual workers is potentially a way of decreasing alienation, the effects of any reforms would be limited unless the means of production were also more socialised. Larger health benefits would therefore require more radical solutions, such as the creation of workers' cooperatives (Landsbergis, 2009). In terms of worklessness, a right to welfare state support and a minimum income level are vital in terms of ensuring that people who experience unemployment are not driven into poverty and social isolation. It is also therefore an important way of reducing the ill health effects of unemployment. The type of return to work intervention may also be important in this regard. In terms of ill health related worklessness, a 'health first' approach should be taken towards those who are workless due to a chronic health condition. Employability focused 'welfare to work' interventions have only had limited effects on actually increasing employment, and they may actually be damaging to the well-being of participants.

Given the uneven social distribution of unhealthy work environments and of unemployment and ill health related worklessness, it would be expected that any interventions would also reduce the social gradient in occupational health. However, the evidence base is fairly inconclusive on this point. This could be because there is a lack of evidence on the effects of interventions on health inequalities, or, more likely because the interventions are small scale and piecemeal. Their health effects are thus likely to be limited unless they are implemented on a wide scale and are accompanied by changes in the levels of material rewards and social status given to different types of work, and different levels of worker. The results of ecological and welfare state studies show strongly that a greater degree of equality, not just in the workplace but across all areas of society in terms of power and resource redistribution, is what is most required in terms of significantly improving population health and reducing health inequalities (Wilkinson and Pickett, 2009). Work and production may be the basis for all means of public and private welfare (Hogstedt and

Lundberg, 2002) but changes to the workplace or the experience of worklessness will not on their own produce large health improvements for all or reduce health inequalities. This requires far more radical political changes in terms of how the wider political economy is structured and the role of work and workers within it.

7.7 **Further reading**

Karasek, R. (1992). Stress prevention through work reorganisation: a summary of 19 case studies, *Conditions of Work Digest*, 11:23–42.

Landsbergis, P.A. (2009). 'Interventions to Reduce Job Stress and Improve Work Organization and Worker Health, In: P.L. Schnall, M. Dobson, and E. Rosskam (eds.) *Unhealthy Work: Causes, Consequences, Cures*. New York, Baywood.

Morris, J.N., Donkin, A.J, Wonderling, D. *et al.* (2000). A minimum income for healthy living. *Journal of Epidemiology and Community Health*, 54: 885–889.

Chapter 8

Conclusion[1]

Political economy approaches have a long, if often subdued, history in the study of public health and health inequalities. Engels was arguably the first to analyse public health in this way in his study of the conditions of the working class in Manchester (Engels, 1844 [2009]). More recent examples include the work of Doyal and Pennell (1979), Coburn (2004) and the large body of work developed over a number of years by Navarro and colleagues (such as Navarro et al., 2003). This political economy research has shown the importance of political and economic systems for population health and health inequalities.

In this book, I have applied such approaches to the study of work and worklessness. I have shown how work and worklessness impact on population health. I have also emphasised the role of public policy interventions in mediating the relationships between work, worklessness and health. Above all however, I have argued that work and the socio-economic class polarities it creates play a fundamental role in creating inequalities in the distribution of morbidity and mortality, via uneven exposure to physical hazards and psychosocial risks in the workplace, as well as via inequalities in exclusion from the labour market and the absence of paid work. Further, in this book I have shown that the relationships between work, worklessness and health inequalities are influenced by the broader political and economic context in the form of welfare state regimes. I have argued that work and worklessness are not the discrete activities of individuals but are essential parts of the way in which the totality of society is politically, socially and economically organised.

In this concluding chapter, I summarise the evidence on health inequalities presented in the previous chapters, and I then develop a model of the political economy of health inequalities to show how different types of public policy interventions can mitigate health inequalities. I apply the model to the case of work and worklessness. I conclude by arguing that politics matter in the aetiology of health inequalities.

---

[1] Material in this chapter is reproduced from Bambra (2011) with permission from BMJ Publishing Group.

8.1 **Work and health inequalities**

8.1.1 **Physical work environment and health inequalities**

Chapter 3 has shown that workers in low occupation jobs are more exposed to adverse physical working conditions. European Working Conditions Survey data show that professionals have at least 50% less exposure to the major physical hazards (exposure to dangerous chemicals, noise, vibrations, repetitive work, shift work, and heavy lifting) than the bottom occupational groups (European Working Conditions Observatory, 2005). Industries with a high percentage of workers in lower socio-economic classes (such as construction or manufacturing) are also those at elevated risk of occupational injuries and accidents, restricted posture, repetitive movements and heavy lifting (Siegrist *et al.*, 2009). Often workers' exposures to such risks are multiple. The health problems associated with the adverse aspects of the physical work environment are more prevalent amongst manual than non-manual workers. For example, industrial injury rates in the UK exhibit significant occupational inequalities with professional occupations having a fatal injury rate of 0.2 per 100,000 compared to a rate of 1.9 per 100,000 for the lowest grade occupations (Health and Safety Executive, 2010b). Similarly, the all reported injury rate for professionals was 188.6 per 100,000, as opposed to 1,725.1 per 100,000 for the lowest grade workers (Health and Safety Executive, 2010b). Lower grade workers are also more likely to develop ill health after exposure to hazards. For example, in the case of lead exposure, poor nutritional conditions such as irregular food intake, high fat intake and deficiencies in calcium and iron, augment the physiological effects of lead uptake (Mahaffey, 1995).

8.1.2 **Psychosocial work environment and health inequalities**

Chapter 4 showed that the distribution of adverse psychosocial working conditions is also socially patterned, with jobs at the lower end of the socio-economic class scale more likely to entail a higher exposure to adverse conditions than those towards the higher end. European Working Conditions Survey data (2005) show that in terms of social support at work, there are few differences by occupation, with the lowest and the highest occupational groups reporting broadly similar levels of social support. However, in terms of job demands (repetition, tight deadlines, machine paced, monotonous) and control at work (control over tasks or speed of tasks, consulted about changes), there are stark differences by occupational status between the highest and lowest occupations. For example, in terms of demands at work, monotonous work was around 50% higher amongst the lowest occupational groups. Similarly, workers in the two highest occupational groups were almost twice as likely to report that they were consulted about changes to the organisation of work as those in the two lowest occupational groups (European Working Conditions Observatory, 2005). The Whitehall studies have demonstrated that occupational class differences in the psychosocial work environment are important in terms of explaining the social gradient in health, with adjustment for adverse psychosocial working conditions reducing the inequality in coronary heart disease between the top and bottom occupational grades by 64% in men and 51% in women (Marmot *et al.*, 1997b). Differences in psychosocial working conditions are also linked to inequalities in the distribution and development of musculoskeletal disease (Gillen *et al.*, 2007). Similarly, socio-economic inequalities in psychological disorders are also strongly associated with inequalities in exposures to harmful psychosocial work environments (Stansfield *et al.*, 2003).

8.2 **Worklessness and health inequalities**

8.2.1 **Unemployment, health, and health inequalities**

Chapter 5 showed how economic recessions influence health and health inequalities and that one of the main ways was by increasing the number of people without work. Unemployment is associated with poverty and social exclusion, and it tends to be concentrated in lower socio-economic classes: Employment rates are consistently higher amongst more educated groups (Arber, 1987). For example, according to English census data, in 2001 in London, 90.1% of men and 81.5% of women with a university degree were employed compared to just 69.2% of men and 51.8% of women with no qualifications (Bambra and Popham, 2010). Ill health related job loss also has a social gradient, with adverse employment consequences more likely for those in lower socio-economic classes (Bartley and Owen, 1996). The importance of unemployment to health inequalities was demonstrated in a recent English study which found that for both men and women, not being in paid employment accounted for up to 81% of the inequalities in the prevalence of self-rated poor health between the most affluent and the least affluent socio-economic classes in the English working age population (Bambra and Popham, 2010). As an example, 5.6% of men living in owner occupied housing had not good general health compared to 19.1% of men in social rented housing, an age-adjusted difference of 13% points. After further adjustment for employment status this difference reduced to 2.5% points, a reduction of 81%. Adjusting for employment status reduced the prevalence of poor self-reported health in all socio-economic classes, thereby substantially reducing the social gradient.

8.2.2 Inequalities in health related worklessness

In Chapter 6, the concept of health related worklessness was examined. Ill health increases the likelihood of long-term worklessness. For example, a study of health related worklessness in the UK using national household survey data found that the employment rates of people with a chronic illness or disability were 45.9% compared to 82.4% of those without an illness or disability (Bambra and Pope, 2007). However, the worklessness associated with ill health (health related worklessness) is also significantly unevenly socio-economically and spatially distributed. A comprehensive comparative study found that there were significant educational inequalities in the employment rates of people with a limiting long-term illness with the employment gaps between healthy highly educated men and women and low educated men and women with ill health ranging from 30.9% in Norway to 68.1% in the UK for men and from 57.7% in Sweden to 79.4% in the UK for women (Whitehead *et al.*, 2009). Similarly, the geographical distribution of health related worklessness is also skewed with the levels highest in the deprived de-industrialised areas (e.g. the North East of England, the West of Scotland and South Wales) and smallest in the more affluent, mainly semi-rural non-deprived commuter and 'stockbroker' belt areas (e.g. in the South East region of England) (Norman and Bambra, 2007).

8.3 Public policy and the political economy of health

8.3.1 Work, worklessness, and welfare state regimes

Chapter 2 examined welfare state regimes and the health effects of different political and economic arrangements within welfare state capitalism. The remaining chapters applied this framework to the work environment, unemployment and health related worklessness. This suggested important variations by welfare state regime. In terms of the work environment, whilst there is little evidence of variation across advanced welfare states in terms of the influence of the physical work environment (although the Liberal welfare states are the least regulatory) on health outcomes (Rosskam, 2009), studies have shown important variation in the psychosocial work environment, work related stress and the health effects of adverse psychosocial working conditions (Salavecz, 2010). For example, the relationship between job insecurity and poor health is less in those countries with more extensive social security systems which improve the ability of individuals to cope with stressful events (Bartley and Blane, 1997). Similarly, recent epidemiological work has shown that relationships between stressful psychosocial work environments and health differ by welfare state regime with a lower prevalence of work related stress in Social Democratic countries which have more comprehensive welfare states and where the psychosocial work environment is more regulated (Siegrist *et al.*, 2009; Dragano *et al.*, 2010; Sekine *et al.*, 2009). These studies have also found that the effects on health and health inequalities of adverse psychosocial work environments are lessened in these countries (Dragano *et al.*, 2010; Sekine *et al.*, 2009).

Social protection (particularly wage replacement rates) during unemployment varies by welfare state regime. A recent study examined the extent to which relative health inequalities between unemployed and employed people varied across European welfare state regimes (Bambra and Eikemo, 2009). We found that in all countries, the relative health of the unemployed was consistently worse than that of those in work, and that these relative inequalities were largest for both men and women in the Liberal welfare states where benefit levels were lowest and where means-testing was more common. Similarly, with respect to health related worklessness, recent studies have shown that the employment rates of people with an illness vary by welfare state regime (Whitehead *et al.*, 2009; van der Wel *et al.*, 2010). Health related worklessness is lowest in the Social Democratic welfare states, where the worklessness rates of people with a chronic illness is less than 40% and it is highest in the Liberal countries where it is over 50% (van der Wel *et al.*, 2010). Socio-economic inequalities in the employment consequences of ill health are also higher in the Liberal welfare states than in the Social Democratic ones (Whitehead *et al.*, 2009; van der Wel *et al.*, 2010).

8.3.2 **A model of the political economy of health inequalities**

The effects of work and worklessness on health and health inequalities are therefore mediated by political, economic and social organisations—by welfare state regime. Drawing on this, Figure 8.1 sets out a conceptual framework for understanding how socio-economic class inequalities in health are a result of interactions between the political and economic systems, the (welfare) state, the social security system, the labour market and the organisation of work. In this framework, political power relations and the economic system set the landscape and the structural parameters within which the social determinants of health operate (Bambra *et al.*, 2005a). Politics is given prominence in the model both as an overarching macro actor which has the ability to shape and reshape all the determinants (including the economic system), and also as an important factor working across the macro, meso and micro levels, contextualising the various intervention points (A–C). The (welfare) state is given a quasi-independent role in which it mediates the effects of the economic system, the organisation of work and the labour market on

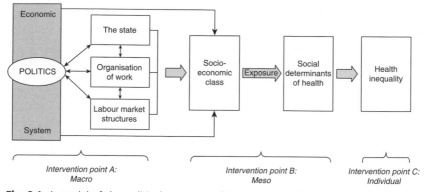

Fig. 8.1 A model of the political economy of health inequalities.
Source: Reproduced from Bambra (2011) with permission from BMJ Publishing Group.

the extent of socio-economic class inequality and exposure to the social determinants of health.

The intervention points (A–C) can be understood in the following ways: Intervention point A includes macro-level changes to the political and economic context (the economy, the state, the organisation of work, the social security system or the labour market); point B refers to meso-level environmental changes to the social determinants (such as housing or the work environment); and interventions at point C focus on the individual and 'treating' the structural effects of inequality. A and B can thus be considered as primary and secondary prevention intervention points, whilst point C is effectively the treatment point. Interventions at point A are expected to be the most beneficial in terms of reducing health inequalities and those at point C the least. Interventions at points A and B treat the causes, whilst interventions at point C treat the symptoms.

8.3.3 **Work, health, and welfare policy Interventions**

This model can be applied to the specific work, health and welfare policy interventions that were examined in Chapter 7. The Minimum Income for Healthy Living proposed by Morris and colleagues (2000) is an example of a macro primary prevention policy intervention. The Minimum Income for Healthy Living is a way of ensuring that social security benefits and wages are of a sufficient level to maintain health and well-being (a living wage), and that there is a right to a certain standard of living for all citizens (a citizen's income) regardless of their employment status. Based on the link between income and health, Morris and colleagues (2000) have illustrated how health can be improved and inequalities in health reduced via the public provision of a minimum income to meet basic and social needs relating to nutrition, physical activity, housing, psychosocial interactions, transport, medical care and hygiene. The 2010 Marmot Review recommended implementation of the Minimum Income for Healthy Living, and it is also supported as a policy to tackle health inequalities by the World Health Organisation. Less specific examples would include improving job security, making wages more equitable and increasing income equality (either at source as is the case in Japan or via the tax system as is the case in Sweden), or reducing the unemployment rate (via public employment for example).

Changes to the physical and psychosocial work environments can be considered as secondary prevention measures. Health and safety legislation to reduce exposure to the adverse aspects of the physical work environment, such as the 1975 Health and Safety at Work Act in the UK or the 1970 Occupational Safety and Health Act in the US, are examples of secondary prevention. However, whilst regulations exist, for them to be effective they need to be well implemented and enforced (Berman, 1983; Siegrist, 2009). In terms of the psychosocial work environment, systematic review evidence suggests that organisational changes which increase workers' control and participation improve occupational health (Joyce et al., 2010b; Egan et al., 2007; Bambra et al., 2007b). In 1994 the European Union issued a directive to increase participation at work and countries such as Sweden and Norway have implemented extensive regulation of the psychosocial work environment in order to prevent occupational ill health (Landsbergis, 2009).

In terms of 'treatment' interventions, most measures to improve the health of the workless or enhance the employment of the chronically ill would come under this category as they are dealing with existing inequality and ill health. For example, many interventions intended to increase the employment rates of people with a disability or chronic illness are supply-side focused and thus target the individual (in terms of skills, job searching, interview skills—employability) rather than trying to increase demand from employers or alter the structural barriers which people may face in terms of, say, workplace design or working hours (Bambra, 2006c). Other examples of individual focused interventions to reduce health inequalities would include workplace strategies to help workers cope better with workplace stress or with the desynchronisation of shift work (Whitehead, 2007; Bambra et al., 2008a, 2008b).

8.4 **Conclusion**

In this final chapter I have summarised the epidemiological research presented elsewhere in the book to show the importance of work and worklessness to the development of health inequalities. I have shown that the health effects of work and worklessness vary by welfare state regime and that therefore *politics matter:* how society is economically and socially organised is vital in terms of influencing the social determinants of health and health inequalities. I have set out a model of the political economy of health inequalities and I have applied this to the case of work, worklessness and health. This political economy analysis has led me to conclude that, even within the constraints of unequal capitalist societies, policies underpinned by the political principles of equality, participation and fairness—Social Democracy—can improve population health and reduce (if not eliminate) health inequalities.

8.5 **Further reading**

Navarro, V. (2009). What we mean by the social determinants of health. *International Journal of Health Services*, 39, 423–441.

Wilkinson, R. and Pickett, K. (2009). *The spirit level: Why more equal societies almost always do better.* London: Penguin.

Whitehead, M. (2007). A typology of actions to tackle social inequalities in health. *Journal of Epidemiology and Community Health*, 61, 473–78.

References

Abrahamson, P. (1999). The welfare modelling business. *Social Policy & Administration*, **33**, 394–415.

Acheson, D. (1998). *Independent inquiry into inequalities in health*. London: TSO.

Adams, E. (1999). *Invalidity Benefit in Glasgow: Comparative study*. Glasgow: Institute of Social and Economic Research.

Adewusi, S.A., Rakheja, S., and Marcotte, P. (2010). Vibration transmissibility characteristics of the human hand-arm system under different postures, hand forces and excitation levels. *Journal of Sound and Vibration*, **329**, 2953–2971.

Ahonen, E.Q., Benavides, F.G. and Benach, J. (2007). Immigrant populations work and health—a systematic literature review. *Scandinavian Journal of Work, Environment & Health*, **33**, 96–104

Aittomaki, A., Lahelma, E., Rahkonen, O., Leino-Arjas, P. and Martikainen, P. (2007). The contribution of musculoskeletal disorders and physical workload to socioeconomic inequalities in health. *European Journal of Public Health*, **17**, 145–150.

Akerstadt, T. (1990). Psychological and psychophysiological effects of shift work. *Scandinavian Journal of Work, Environment & Health*, **16**, 67–73.

Alberti, K.G.M.M., Zimmet, P. and Shaw, J. for the IDF Epidemiology Task Force Consensus Group. (2005). The metabolic syndrome—a new worldwide definition. *Lancet*, **366**, 1059–1062.

Albertsen, K., Rafnsdottir, G.L., Grimsmo, A., Tomasson, K. and Kauppinen, K. (2008). Workhours and worklife balance. *Scandinavian Journal of Work, Environment & Health*, **5**, 14–21.

Alcock, P., Beatty, C., Fothergill, S., Macmillan, R. and Yeandle, S. (2003). *Work to Welfare: How men become detached from the labour market*. Cambridge: Cambridge University Press.

Alterman, T., Shekelle, R.B., Vernon, S,W, and Burau, K.D. (1994). Decision Latitude, Psychologic Demand, Job Strain, and Coronary Heart Disease in the Western Electric Study. *American Journal of Epidemiology*, **139**, 620–627.

Althusser, L. (1971). *Lenin and philosophy and other essays*. London: Monthly Review Press.

Amick, B. and Kasl, S. (2000). Work stress, in C. MacDonald (ed.) *Epidemiology of work-related diseases* (second edition), London: BMJ Books.

Arber, S. (1987). Social class, non-employment, and chronic illness: continuing the inequalities in health debate. *BMJ*, **294**, 1069–1073.

Artazcoz, L., Benach, J., Borrell, C. and Cortès, I. (2005). Social inequalities in the impact of flexible employment on different domains of psychosocial health. *Journal of Epidemiology and Community Health*, **59**, 761–767.

Aspalter, C. (2006). The East Asian welfare model. *International Journal of Social Welfare,* **15**, 290–301.

Åström, C., Rehn, B., Lundström, R., Nilsson, T., Burström, L. and Sundelin, G. (2006). Hand-arm vibration syndrome (HAVS) and musculoskeletal symptoms in the neck and the upper limbs in professional drivers of terrain vehicles—A cross sectional study. *Applied Ergonomics,* **37**, 793–799.

Aust, B. and Ducki, A. (2004). Comprehensive health promotion interventions at the workplace: experiences with health circles in Germany. *Journal of Occupational Health Psychology,* **9**, 258–270.

Aust, B., Peter, R. and Siegrist, J. (1997). Stress management in bus drivers: A pilot study based on the model of effort-reward imbalance. *International Journal of Stress Management,* **4**, 297–305.

Avendano, M., Jürges, H. and Mackenbach, J.P. (2009). Educational level and changes in health across Europe: longitudinal results from SHARE. *Journal of European Social Policy,* **19**, 301–316.

Bahro, R. (1984). *From red to green.* London: Verso.

Bambra, C. (2004). The worlds of welfare: Illusory and gender-blind? *Social Policy and Society,* **3**, 201–212.

Bambra, C. (2005). Cash versus services: 'worlds of welfare' and the decommodification of cash benefits and health care services. *Journal of Social Policy,* **34**, 195–213.

Bambra, C. (2006a). Health status and the worlds of welfare. *Social Policy and Society,* **5**, 53–62.

Bambra, C. (2006b). Decommodification and the worlds of welfare revisited. *Journal of European Social Policy,* **16**, 73–80.

Bambra, C. (2006c). The influence of government programmes and pilots on the employment of disabled workers, in K. Needels and B. Schmitz (ed.) *Economic and Social Costs and Benefits to Employers for Retaining, Recruiting and Employing Disabled People and/or People with Health Conditions or an Injury: A review of the evidence.* London: Department for Work and Pensions Research Report no 400. Available at: http://www.dwp.gov.uk/asd/asd5/rrs2006.asp#economic.

Bambra, C. (2007a). Going Beyond the Three Worlds: Regime Theory and Public Health Research. *Journal of Epidemiology and Community Health,* **61**, 1098–1102.

Bambra, C. (2007b). 'Sifting the wheat from the chaff': A two-dimensional discriminant analysis of welfare state regime theory'. *Social Policy and Administration,* **41**, 1–28.

Bambra, C. (2008). Incapacity Benefit reform and the politics of ill health. *British Medical Journal,* **337**, 517.

Bambra, C. (2009). Welfare state regimes and the political economy of health. *Humanity and Society,* **33**, 99–117.

Bambra, C. (2010a). Yesterday once more? An analysis of unemployment and health in the 21st century. *Journal of Epidemiology and Community Health,* **64**, 213–215.

Bambra, C. (2010b). Doctors are key to healthcare reform. *British Medical Journal,* **341**, 941.

Bambra, C. (2011a). Work, worklessness and the political economy of health inequalities. *Journal of Epidemiology and Community Health* doi: 10.1136/jech.2009.102103.

Bambra, C. (2011b). 'Social inequalities in health: Interrogating the Nordic welfare state puzzle'. In: J. Kvist, J. Fritzell, B. Hvinden and O. Kangas (eds.) *Changing Equality: The Nordic Welfare Model in the 21st Century.* Bristol, Policy Press.

Bambra, C. and Eikemo, T. (2009). Welfare state regimes, unemployment and health: A comparative study of the relationship between unemployment and self-reported health in 23 European countries. *Journal of Epidemiology and Community Health,* **63**, 92–98.

Bambra, C. and Norman, P. (2006). What is the association between medically certified long term sickness absence, and morbidity and mortality? *Health and Place,* **12**, 728–733.

Bambra, C. and Pope, D. (2007). What are the effects of anti-discriminatory legislation on socio-economic inequalities in the employment consequences of ill health and disability? *Journal of Epidemiology and Community Health,* **61**, 421–426.

Bambra, C. and Popham, F. (2010). Worklessness and regional differences in educational inequalities in health: Evidence from the 2001 Census. *Health and Place,* **16**, 1014–1021.

Bambra, C. and Smith, K. (2010). No longer deserving? Sickness benefit reform and the politics of (ill) health. *Critical Public Health,* **20**, 71–84.

Bambra, C., Fox, D. and Scott-Samuel, A. (2005a). Towards a politics of health. *Health Promotion International.* **20**, 187–193.

Bambra, C., Whitehead, M. and Hamilton, V. (2005b). Does 'welfare to work' work? A systematic review of the effectiveness of the UK's welfare to work programmes for people with a chronic illness or disability. *Social Science and Medicine,* **60**, 1905–1918.

Bambra, C., Fox, D. and Scott-Samuel, A. (2007a). A politics of health glossary. *Journal of Epidemiology and Community Health,* **61**, 571–574.

Bambra, C., Egan, M., Thomas, S., Pettigrew, M., Whitehead, M. (2007b). The psychosocial and health effects of workplace reorganisation 2: A systematic review of task restructuring interventions. *Journal of Epidemiology and Community Health,* **61**, 1028–37.

Bambra, C., Whitehead, M., Sowden, A., Akers, J. and Petticrew, M. (2008a). Shifting schedules: the health effects of reorganising shift work. *American Journal of Preventive Medicine,* **34**, 427–434.

Bambra, C., Whitehead, M., Sowden, A., Akers, J. and Petticrew, M. (2008b). A hard day's night? The effects of Compressed Work Week interventions on the health and wellbeing of shift workers: a systematic review. *Journal of Epidemiology and Community Health,* **62**, 764–777.

Bambra, C., Joyce, K. and Maryon-Davies, A. (eds.) (2009a). *Priority health conditions– Task Group 8 Report to the Strategic Review of Health Inequalities in England post-2010 (Marmot Review).* Available at: http://www.ucl.ac.uk/gheg/marmotreview/Documents.

Bambra, C., Gibson, M., Sowden, A., Wright K., Whitehead, M. and Petticrew, M. (2009b). Working for health? Evidence from systematic reviews on the health effects of changes to the psychosocial work environment. *Preventive Medicine,* **48**, 454–461.

Bambra, C., Netuveli, G. and Eikemo, T. (2010a). Welfare state regime life courses: The development of Western European welfare state regimes and age related patterns of educational inequalities in self-reported health. *International Journal of Health Services,* **40**, 399–420.

Bambra, C., Joyce, K., Bellis, M., Greatley, A., Greengross, S., Hughes, S. *et al.* (2010b). Reducing health inequalities in priority public health conditions: Developing an evidence based strategy? *Journal of Public Health,* **32**, 496–505.

Bambra, C. Gibson, M., Sowden, A., Wright, K., Whitehead, M. and Petticrew, M. (2010c). 'Tackling the wider social determinants of health and health inequalities: evidence from systematic reviews', *Journal of Epidemiology and Community Health,* **64**: 284–291.

Barbrook, R. (2006). *The Class of the New*. London: OpenMute.

Barham, C. and Begum, N. (2005). *Sickness absence from work in the UK. Labour market trends*. London: Office for National Statistics.

Barnes, C. (1991). *Disabled people in Britain and discrimination: a case for anti-discrimination legislation*. London: Hurst Calgary.

Barnes, C. (2002). Disability, policy and politics. *Policy and Politics*, **30**, 311–318.

Barnes, C. and Mercer, G. (1997). *Doing disability research*. Leeds: Disability Press.

Barnes, C. and Mercer, G. (2003) (eds.). *Implementing the social model: theory and practice*. Leeds: Disability Press.

Barnes, C. and Mercer, G. (2004) (eds.). *Disability policy and practice: applying the social model*. Leeds: Disability Press.

Barr, B., Clayton, S., Whitehead, M., Thielen, K., Burström, B., Nylén, L. *et al.* (2010). To what extent have relaxed eligibility requirements and increased generosity of disability benefits acted as disincentives for employment? A systematic review of evidence from countries with well-developed welfare systems. *Journal of Epidemiology and Community Health*, doi:10.1136/jech.2010.111401.

Bartley, M. (2004). *Health Inequality: An Introduction to Theories, Concepts and Methods*. Cambridge: Polity Press.

Bartley, M. and Blane, D. (1997). Health and the lifecourse: Why safety nets matter. *British Medical Journal*, **314**, 1194–1196.

Bartley, M. and Lewis, I. (2002). Accumulated labour market disadvantage and limiting long-term illness: data from the 1971–1991 ONS longitudinal study. *International Journal of Epidemiology*, **31**, 336–341.

Bartley, M. and Owen C. (1996). Relation between socioeconomic status, employment, and health during economic change, 1973–93. *British Medical Journal*, **313**, 445–449.

Bartley, M., Ferrie, J. and Montgomery, S. (2006). Health and labour market disadvantage: unemployment, non-employment, and job insecurity. In: M. Marmot and R.G. Wilkinson (ed.) *Social determinants of health*; pp.78–96, Oxford: Oxford University Press.

Batuman, V., Landy, E., Maesaka, J.K. and Wedeen, R.P. (1983). Contribution of lead to hypertension with renal impairment. *The New England Journal of Medicine*, **309**, 17–21.

Beatson, M. (1995). *Labour market flexibility*. London: Department of Employment.

Beatty, C. and Fothergill, S. (2002). Hidden unemployment among men: a case study. *Regional Studies*, **36**, 811–823.

Beatty, C. and Fothergill, S. (2005). The diversion from 'unemployment' to 'sickness' across British regions and districts. *Regional Studies*, **39**, 837–854.

Beatty, C., Fothergill, S. and Lawless, P. (1997). Geographical variation in the labour-market adjustment process: the UK coalfields 1981–91. *Environment and Planning A*, **29**, 2041–2060.

Beatty, C., Fothergill, S. and Macmillan, R. (2000). A theory of employment, unemployment and sickness. *Regional Studies*, **34**, 617–630.

Beatty, C., Fothergill, S. and Powell, R. (2007). Twenty years on: has the economy of the UK coalfields recovered? *Environment and Planning A*, **39**, 1654–1675.

Beatty, C., Fothergill, S., Houston, D., Powell, R. and Sissons, P. (2010). *Women on Incapacity Benefits*. University of Sheffield: Centre for Regional and Economic Social Research.

Beck, U, (1999). *The New Statesman Essay—Goodbye to all that wage slavery.* The New Statesman, 5 March 1999. Available at: http://www.newstatesman. com/199903050020.

Beckfield, J. and Krieger, N. (2009). Epi + demos + cracy: Linking Political Systems and Priorities to the Magnitude of Health Inequities—Evidence, Gaps, and a Research Agenda. *Epidemiologic Reviews,* **31**, 152–177.

Beinart, S., Smith, P. and Sproston, K. (1996). *The Access to work programme—a survey of recipients, employers, employment service managers and staff.* London: Social and Community Planning Research.

Belkic, K.L., Landsbergis, P.A., Schnall, P.L. and Baker, D. (2004). Is job strain a major source of cardiovascular disease risk? *Scandinavian Journal of Work, Environment & Health,* **30**, 85–128.

Bell, D. (1974). *The coming of post-industrial society: a venture in social forecasting.* London: Heinemann Educational.

Bellavia, G.M. and Frone, M.R. (2005). *Work-Family Conflict.* In: J. Barling, E.K. Kelloway and M.R. Frone (eds.) *Handbook of Work Stress.* Thousand Oaks: Sage.

Benach, J., Amable, M., Muntaner, C. and Benavides, F.G. (2002). The consequences of flexible work for health: are we looking at the right place? *Journal of Epidemiology and Community Health,* **56**, 405–406.

Benach, J. and Muntaner, C. (2007). Precarious employment and health: Developing a research agenda. *Journal of Epidemiology and Community Health,* **61**, 276–277.

Benach, J., Muntaner, C. and Santana, V. (chairs) (2007). Employment conditions and health inequalities. Final Report to the WHO Commission on Social Determinants of Health. Geneva, WHO.

Benach, J., Muntaner, C., Solar, O., Santana, V. and Quinlan, M. (2010). Introduction to the WHO Commission on Social Determinants of Health Employment Conditions Network (EMCONET) study, with a glossary on employment relations. *International Journal of Health Services,* **40**, 195–207.

Benavides, F.G., Benach, J., Diez-Roux, A.V. and Roman, C. (2000). How do types of employment relate to health indicators? Findings from the Second European Survey on Working Conditions. *Journal of Epidemiology and Community Health,* **54**, 494–501.

Beresford, S.A., Thompson, B., Feng, Z., Christianson, A., McLerran, D. and Patrick, D. (2001). Seattle 5 a day worksite program to increase fruit and vegetable consumption. *Preventative Medicine,* **32**, 230–238.

Berman, D. (1983). Why work kills: a brief history of occupational safety and health in the US. In: V. Navarro and D. Berman (ed.) *Health and Work under Capitalism: an international perspective;* pp. 168–192, New York: Baywood.

Berthoud, R. (2008). Disability employment penalties in Britain. *Work Employment and Society,* **22**, 129–148.

Beynon, H. and McMylor, P. (1985). Decisive power: The new Tory state against the miners, in H. Beynon (ed.) *Digging Deeper: Issues in the miner's strike.* London: Verso.

Bivand, P. (2002). *Economic inactivity and social exclusion.* Centre for Economic and Social Inclusion. Available at: http://www.uuy.org.uk/projects/wb/w132/html/inactivity.html.

Black, C. (2008). *Dame Carol Black's Review of the health of the working age population—Working for a healthier tomorrow.* London: The Stationery Office.

Black, D., Morris, J.N., Smith, C. and Townsend, P. (1980). *Inequalities in health: The Black Report.* London: Pelican.

Blair, T. (2002). Full text of speech on welfare reform. Available at: http://www.guardian.co.uk/society/2002/jun/10/socialexclusion.politics1 (accessed 6 July 2011).

Blakely, T., Tobias, M. and Atkinson, J. (2008). Inequalities in mortality during and after restructuring of the New Zealand economy: repeated cohort studies. *British Medical Journal,* **336**, 371–375.

Blane, D. (2006). The life course, the social gradient, and health. In: M. Marmot and R.G. Wilkinson (ed.) *Social Determinants of Health,* pp.54–77, Oxford: Oxford University Press.

Bloch, F. and Prins, R. (ed.) (2001). *Who returns to work and why?* London: Transaction.

Blondal, S. and Pearson, M. (1995). Unemployment and other non-employment benefits. *Oxford Review of Economic Policy,* **11**, 136–169.

Bøggild, H. (2000). *Shift work and heart disease: Epidemiological and risk factor aspects.* PhD Thesis. Aalborg, Aalborg Regional Hospital: Centre for Working Time Research.

Bonde, J.P., Mikkelsen, S., Andersen, J.H., Fallentin, N., Bælum, J., Svendsen, S.W. *et al.* (2005). Understanding work-related musculoskeletal pain: does repetitive work cause stress symptoms? *Occupational and Environmental Medicine,* **62**, 41–48.

Bond, F.W., and Bunce, D. (2001). Job control mediates change in a work reorganization intervention for stress reduction. *Journal of Occupational Health Psychology,* **6**, 290–302.

Bondi, L. (2005). Working the Spaces of Neoliberal Subjectivity: Psychotherapeutic Technologies, Professionalisation and Counselling. *Antipode,* **37**, 497–514.

Bongers, P.M., de Winter, C.R., Kompier, M.A.J. and Hildebrandt, V.H. (1993). Psychosocial factors at work and musculoskeletal disease. *Scandinavian Journal of Work, Environment & Health,* **19**, 297–312.

Bonoli, G. (1997). Classifying welfare states: A two-dimension approach. *Journal of Social Policy,* **26**, 351–372.

Borrell, C., Espelt, A., Rodrıguez-Sanz, M., Navarro, V. and Kunst, A. (2007). Explaining variations between political traditions in the magnitude of socio-economic inequalities in self-perceived health. *Tackling Health Inequalities in Europe: Eurothine,* Rotterdam: Erasmus Medical Centre. pp. 213–229.

Bosma, H., Marmot, M.G., Hemingway, H., Nicholson, A.C., Brunner, E. and Stansfeld, S.A. (1997). Low job control and risk of coronary heart disease in Whitehall II (prospective cohort) study. *British Medical Journal,* **314**, 558–565.

Bosma, H., Peter, R., Siegrist, J. and Marmot, M. (1998). Two alternative job stress models and the risk of coronary heart disease. *American Journal of Public Health,* **88**, 68–74.

Bourbonnais, R., Brisson, C., Vinet, A., Vezina, M., Abdous, B. and Gaudet, M. (2006). Effectiveness of a participative intervention on psychosocial work factors to prevent mental health problems in a hospital setting. *Occupational and Environmental Medicine,* **63**, 335–342.

Bovenzi, M., Franzinelli, A., Scattoni, L. and Vannuccini, L. (1994). Hand-arm vibration syndrome among travertine workers: a follow up study. *Occupational and Environmental Medicine,* **51**, 361–365.

Brandth, B. and Kvande, E. (2001). Flexible Work and Flexible Fathers. *Work, Employment & Society*, **15**, 251–267.

Branthwaite, A. and Garcia, S. (1985). Depression in the young unemployed and those on Youth Opportunities Schemes. *British Journal of Medical Psychology*, **58**, 67–74.

Braverman, H. (1974). *Labour and monopoly capital: the degradation of work in the twentieth century*. New York; London: Monthly Review Press.

Brenner, M.H. (1971). Economic changes and heart disease mortality. *American Journal of Public Health*, **61**, 606–611.

Brenner, M.H. (1987a). Relation of economic change to Swedish Health and Social Wellbeing, 1950–1980. *Social Science & Medicine*, **25**, 183–195.

Brenner, M.H. (1987b). Economic Change, Alcohol Consumption and Heart Disease Mortality in Nine Industrialized Countries. *Social Science & Medicine*, **25**, 119–131.

Brenner, M.H. (2005). Economic growth is the basis of mortality rate decline in the 20th century—experience of the United States 1901–2000. *International Journal of Epidemiology*, **34**, 1214–1221.

Brenner, M.H. and Mooney, A. (1982). Economic change and sex-specific cardiovascular mortality in Britain 1955–1976. *Social Science & Medicine*, **16**, 431–442.

Breslow, L. (1955). Industrial aspects of bronchogenic neoplasm. *Dis Chest*, **28**, 121 30

Britton, A. and Shipley, M.J. (2010). Bored to death? *International Journal of Epidemiology*, **39**, 370–371.

Broom, D.H., D'Souza, R.M., Strazdins, L., Butterworth, P., Parslow, R. and Rodgers, B. (2006). The lesser evil: Bad jobs or unemployment? A survey of mid-aged Australians. *Social Science & Medicine*, **63**, 575–586.

Brown, J., Hanlon, P., Turok, I., Webster, D., Arnott, J. and Macdonald, E.B. (2009). Mental health as a reason for claiming incapacity benefit- a comparison of national and local trends. *Journal of Public Health*, **31**, 74–80.

Brown, J., Smith, J., Webster, D., Arnott, J., Turok, I., Macdonald, E. *et al.* (2010). *Changes in incapacity benefit receipt in UK cities 2000–2008*. University of Glasgow: Scottish Observatory for Work and Health

Brunner, E.J. (1997). Socioeconomic determinants of health: Stress and the biology of inequality *British Medical Journal*, **314**, 1472–1476.

Brunner, E.J., Marmot, M.G., Nanchahal, K., Shipley, M.J., Stansfeld, S.A., Juneja, M *et al.* (1997). Social inequality in coronary risk: central obesity and the metabolic syndrome. Evidence from the WII study. *Diabetologia*, **40**, 1341–1349.

Brunner, E.J., Chandola, T. and Marmot, M.G. (2007). Prospective Effect of Job Strain on General and Central Obesity in the Whitehall II Study. *American Journal of Epidemiology*, **165**, 828–837.

Bryan, B., Dadzie, S. and Scafe, S. (1985). *The Heart of the Race: Black Women's Lives in Britain*. London: Virago.

Bryson, L., Warner-Smith, P., Brown, P. and Fray, L. (2007). Managing the work–life roller-coaster: Private stress or public health issue? *Social Science & Medicine*, **65**, 1142–1153.

Bulmer, M. and Rees, A.M. (ed.) (1996). *Citizenship today: the contemporary relevance of T.H. Marshall*. London: UCL Press.

Bunn, A.R. (1979). Ischemic Heart Disease Mortality and the Business Cycle in Australia. *American Journal of Public Health*, **69**, 772–781.

Burdorf, A. and Sorock, G. (1997). Positive and negative evidence of risk factors for back disorders. *Scandinavian Journal of Work, Environment & Health*, **23**, 243–256.

Burghes, L. (1987). *Made in the USA: A Review of Workfare*. London: Unemployment Unit.

Burstrom, B. and Fredlund, P. (2001). Self-rated health: Is it as good a predictor of subsequent mortality among adults in lower as well as in higher social classes? *Journal of Epidemiology and Community Health*, **55**, 836–840.

Butland, B., Jebb, S., Kopelman, P., McPherson, K., Thomas, S., Mardell, J. *et al.* (2007). *Tackling obesities: Future choices—Project Report*. London: Government Office for Science.

Byrne, D.S. (2002). Industrial culture in a post-industrial world: the case of the North East of England. *City*, **6**, 279–289.

Byrne, D.S. (2005). *Social Exclusion*. Milton Keynes: Open University.

Byrne, U. (2005). Work-life balance. *Business Information Review*, **22**, 53–59.

Campbell, B. (1984). *Wigan Pier Revisited*. London: Virago.

Campbell, M. (2000). Reconnecting the long term unemployed to labour market opportunity: the case for a 'local active labour market policy', *Regional Studies*, **34**, 655–668.

Canfield, R.L., Henderson, C.R., Cory-Slechta, D.A., Cox, C., Juski, T.A. and Lanphear, B.P. (2003). Intellectual Impairment in Children with Blood Lead concentrations below 10 μg per Deciliter. *The New England Journal of Medicine*, **348**, 1517–1526.

Carta, P., Aru, G., Barbieri, M.T., Avataneo, G. and Casula, D. (1996). Dust exposure, respiratory symptoms, and longitudinal decline of lung function in young coal miners. *Occupational and Environmental Medicine*, **53**, 312–319.

Castles, F.G. and Mitchell, D. (1993). Worlds of welfare and families of nations. In: F.G. Castles (ed.) *Families of Nations: Patterns of Public Policy in Western Democracies*, Aldershot: Dartmouth.

Cavelaars, A., Kunst, A., Geurts, J., Crialesi, R., Grotvedt, L., Helmert, U. *et al.* (2000). Educational differences in smoking: international comparison. *British Medical Journal*, **320**, 1102–1107.

Centers for Disease Control and Prevention. (2003). Surveillance for Elevated Blood Lead Levels—United States, 1997—2001. *Morbidity and Mortality Weekly Report*, **52**, 1–21.

Centre for Social Justice. (2009). *Dynamic benefits: towards welfare that works*. London: Centre for Social Justice.

Cerami, A. and Vanhuysse, P. (ed.) (2009). Post-Communist Welfare Pathways. *Theorizing Social Policy Transformations in Central and Eastern Europe*. Basingstoke: Palgrave Macmillan.

Chandola, T., Brunner, E. and Marmot, M. (2006). Chronic stress at work and the metabolic syndrome: prospective study. *BMJ*, **332**, 521–524.

Chandola, T., Britton, A., Brunner, E., Hemingway, H., Malik, M., Kumari, M. *et al.* (2008). Work stress and coronary heart disease: what are the mechanisms? *European Heart Journal*, **29**, 640–648.

Chetter, I.C., Kent, P.J. and Kester, R.C. (1998). The hand arm vibration syndrome: a review. *Cardiovascular Surgery*, **6**, 1–9.

Chu, C., Driscoll, T. and Dwyer, S. (1997). The health-promoting workplace: an integrative perspective. *Australian and New Zealand Journal of Public Health*, **21**, 377–385.

Chu, C., Breucker, G., Harris, N., Stitzel, A., Gan, X., Gu, X. *et al*. (2000). Health-promoting workplaces—international settings development. *Health Promotion International,* 15, 155–167.

Chung, H. and Muntaner, C. (2006). Political and welfare state determinants of infant and child health indicators: an analysis of wealthy countries. *Social Science & Medicine,* 63, 829–842.

Chung, H. and Muntaner, C. (2007). Welfare State Matters: A Typological Multilevel Analysis Of Wealthy Countries. *Health Policy,* 80, 328–339.

Clayton, S., Bambra, C., Gosling, R., Povall, S. Misso, K. and Whitehead, M. (2011). Assembling the evidence jigsaw: insights from a systematic review of UK studies of return to work initiatives for disabled and chronically ill people. *BMC Public Health* 11, 170.

Coburn, D. (1979). Job alienation and wellbeing. *International Journal of Health Services,* 9, 41–59.

Coburn, D. (2004). Beyond the Income Inequality Hypothesis: Class, Neo-Liberalism, and Health Inequalities. *Social Science & Medicine,* 58, 41–56.

Concha-Barrientos, M , Nelson, D.I., Driscoll, T., Steenland, N.K., Punnett, L., Fingerhut, N.A *et al.* (2004). Selected Occupational Risk Factors. In: M. Ezzati, A.D. Lopez, A. Rodgers, and C.J.L. Murray (ed.) *Comparative quantification of health risks: global and regional burden of diseases attributable to selected major risk factors,* Geneva: World Health Organisation. Available at: http://www.who.int/healthinfo/global_burden_disease/cra/en/ (accessed 6 July 2011).

Conley, D. and Springer, K. (2001). Welfare state and infant mortality. *American Journal of Sociology,* 107, 768–807.

Conrad, P. (1992). Medicalization and Social Control. *Annual Review of Sociology,* 18, 209–232.

Coombes, M. and Raybould, S. (2004). Finding work in 2001: Urban-rural contrasts across England in employment rates and local job availability. *Area,* 36, 202–222.

Cooper, D. (1968). *The Dialectics of Liberation.* Penguin,

Corden, A. and Sainsbury, R. (2001). *Incapacity Benefits and Work Incentives.* Department of Social Security Research Report No. 141. Leeds: CDS.

Corden, A. and Nice, K. (2006). *Incapacity Benefit Reforms Pilot: Findings from the second cohort in a longitudinal panel of clients.* Department for Work and Pensions Research Report, No. 345. Leeds: CDS.

Coutts, A. (2009). Active Labour Market Programmes (ALMPs) and health: an evidence-base Review prepared for the Strategic Review of Health Inequalities in England Post 2010 (Marmot Review). Oxford: University of Oxford. Available at: http://www.marmotreview.org/AssetLibrary/pdfs/full%20tg%20reports/economic%20active%20labour%20market%20full%20report.pdf (accessed 6 July 2011).

Crinson, I. and Yuill, C. (2008). What can alienation theory contribute to an understanding of social inequalities in health. *International Journal of Health Services,* 38, 455–470.

Crisp, R. (2008). Motivation, morals and justice: discourses of worklessness in the welfare reform green paper. *People, Place and Policy Online,* 2/3, 172–185.

Croissant, A. (2004). Changing Welfare Regimes in East and Southeast Asia: Crisis, Change and Challenge. *Social Policy and Administration,* 38, 504–524.

Dahl, E. and Elstad, J.I. (2001). Recent changes in social structure and health inequalities in Norway. *Scandinavian Journal of Public Health*, **55**, 7–17.

Dahl, E., Fritzell, J., Lahelma, E., Martikainen, P., Kunst, A.E. and Mackenbach, J.P. (2006). Welfare state regimes and health inequalities. In: J. Siegrist and M. Marmot (eds.) *Social inequalities in health*, pp. 193–222, Oxford: Oxford University Press.

Dahlen-Gisselmann, M. and Hemstrom, O. (2008). The contribution of maternal working conditions to socio-economic inequalities in birth outcome. *Social Science & Medicine*, **66**, 1297–1309.

Dahlgren, G. and Whitehead, M. (1991). *Policies and strategies to promote social equity in health.* Stockholm: Institute for Futures Studies.

Dahlgren, G., Nordgren, P. and Whitehead, M. (1996). *Health impact assessment of the EU Common Agricultural Policy.* Swedish National Institute of Public Health.

Danieli, A. and Wheeler, P. (2006). Employment policy and disabled people: old wine in new glasses? *Disability & Society*, **21**, 485–98.

Danson, M. (2005). Old industrial areas and employability. *Urban Studies*, **42**, 285–300.

Danziger, S., Corcoran, S., Danziger, C., Heflin, A., Kalil, J., Rosen, K., *et al.* (2002). *Barriers to the employment of welfare recipients.* Population Studies Center, University of Michigan.

Dean, H. and Taylor-Gooby, P. (1992). *Dependency culture: The explosion of a myth.* London: Harvester Wheatsheaf.

Dearlove, J. and Saunders, P. (1991). *Introduction to British Politics.* Cambridge: Blackwell.

Dehejia, R. and Lleras-Muney, A. (2004). Booms, Busts, and Babies Health. *The Quarterly Journal of Economics*, 1091–1130.

De Lange, A.H., Taris, T.W., Kompier, M.A.J., Houtman, I.L.D. and Bongers, P.M. (2003). The very best of the Millennium: Longitudinal research and the Demand-Control-(Support) Model. *Journal of Occupational Health Psychology*, **8**, 282–305.

DeLeire, T. (2000). The wage and employment effects of the Americans with Disabilities Act. *The Journal of Human Resources*, **35**, 693–715.

Department of Health and Human Services (USA). (2007). *The Changing Organization of Work and the Safety and Health of Working People: Knowledge Gaps and Research Directions.* National Occupational Research Agenda Report. Publication No. 2002–116.

Department for Work and Pensions. (DWP) (2006). *A New Deal for Welfare: empowering people to work.* London: TSO.

Department for Work and Pensions. (DWP) (2008). *No One Written Off: Reforming Welfare to Reward Responsibility.* London: TSO.

Department for Work and Pensions. (DWP) (2009). *Building Britain's Recovery: Achieving Full Employment.* London: TSO.

Department for Work and Pensions. (DWP) (2010a). *Benefit rates.* Available at: http://www.direct.gov.uk/en/MoneyTaxAndBenefits/BenefitsTaxCreditsAndOtherSupport/Employedorlookingforwork/DG_10018757 (accessed 6 July 2011).

Department for Work and Pensions. (DWP) (2010b). *White paper on welfare reform.* London: DWP.

Department for Work and Pensions. (DWP) (2010c). *Building Bridges to Work–helping the long term unemployed back to work.* London, TSO.

Dex, S. and Bond, S. (2005). Measuring work-life balance and its covariates. *Work, Employment & Society,* **19**, 627–637.

Diderichsen, F. (2002). Impact of income maintenance policies. In: J. Mackenbach and M. Bakker (eds.) *Reducing inequalities in health: a European perspective,* pp. 53–66, London: Routledge.

Di Viggiani, N. (1997). *A basis for health promotion.* London: South Bank University.

Ditch, J. (1991). The undeserving poor: Unemployed people, then and now. In: M. Loney, R. Bocock, J. Clarke, A.D. Cochrane, P.A.M. Graham, M.J. Wilson (eds.) *The State or the Market: Politics and Welfare in Contemporary Britain,* SAGE.

Dobson, M. and Schnall, P. (2009). From stress to distress: the impact of work on mental health. In: P. Schnall, M. Dobson, E. Rosskam (eds.) *Unhealthy Work: Causes, Consequences, Cures,* New York: Baywood.

Doll, R. (1955). Mortality from lung cancer in asbestos workers. *British Journal of Industrial Medicine,* **12**, 81–86.

Dominelli, L. (1991). *Women across Continents.* Hemel Hempstead: Harvester Wheatsheaf.

Doran, T., Drever, F. and Whitehead, M. (2004). Is there a north-south divide in social class inequalities in health in Great Britain? Cross sectional study using data from the 2001 census. *British Medical Journal,* **328**, 1043–1045.

Dorling, D. (2009). Unemployment and health: Health benefits vary according to the method of reducing unemployment. *British Medical Journal,* **338**, 1087.

Doyal, L. and Pennell, I. (1979). *The Political Economy of Health.* London: Pluto Press.

Dragano, N., Siegrist, J. and Wahrendorf, M. (2010). Welfare regimes, labour policies and workers' health: A comparative study with 9917 older employees from 12 European countries. *Journal of Epidemiology and Community Health* doi:10.1136/jech.2009.098541.

Driscoll, T. and Hanson, M. (1997). Work-related injuries in trade apprentices. *Australian and New Zealand Journal of Public Health,* **21**, 767–772.

Dugdill, L., Brettle, A., Hulme, C., McCluskey, S, and Long, A.F. (2007). *A review of effectiveness of workplace health promotion interventions on physical activity and what works in motivating and changing employees' health behaviour.* London: National Institute for Health and Clinical Excellence.

Duguid, J.B. and Lambert, M.W. (1964). The pathogenesis of coal miner's pneumoconiosis. *The Journal of Pathology and Bacteriology,* **88**, 389–403.

Eales, M.J. (1989). Shame among unemployed men, *Social Science & Medicine,* **28**, 783–789.

Easterlow, D. and Smith, S.J. (2003). Health and employment: towards a New Deal. *Policy and Politics,* **31**, 511–33.

Economou, A., Nikolaou, A. and Theodossiou, I. (2008). Are recessions harmful to health after all? Evidence from the European Union. *Journal of Economic Studies,* **35**, 368–384.

Egan, M., Bambra, C., Thomas, S., Petticrew, M., Whitehead, M. and Thomson, H. (2007). The psychosocial and health effects of workplace reorganisation 1: a systematic review of organisational-level interventions that aim to increase employee control. *Journal of Epidemiology and Community Health,* **61**, 945–954.

Egan, M., Bambra, C., Petticrew, M. and Whitehead, M. (2009). Reviewing evidence on complex social interventions: appraising implementation in systematic reviews of the health effects of organisational level workplace interventions. *Journal of Epidemiology and Community Health,* **63,** 4–11.

Ehrlich, G.E. (2003). *Low Back Pain. Bulletin of the World Health Organisation,* 81, 671–676.

Eikemo, T.A. and Bambra, C. (2008). The Welfare State: A Glossary For Public Health. *Journal of Epidemiology and Community Health,* **62,** 3–6.

Eikemo, T., Bambra, C., Joyce, K. and Dahl, E. (2008a). Welfare state regimes and income related health inequalities: a comparison of 23 European countries. *European Journal of Public Health,* **18,** 593–599.

Eikemo, T.A., Bambra, C., Judge, K. and Ringdal, K. (2008b). Welfare State Regimes and Differences in Self-Perceived Health in Europe: A Multi-Level Analysis. *Social Science & Medicine,* **66,** 2281–2295.

Eikemo, T.A., Huisman, M., Bambra, C. and Kunst, A. (2008c). Health inequalities according to educational level under different welfare regimes: a comparison of 23 European countries. *Sociology of Health and Illness,* **30,** 565–582.

Eikemo, T., Skalicka, V. and Avendano, M. (2009). Variations in relative health inequalities: are they a mathematical artefact? *International Journal of Health Equity,* **8,** 32.

Elovainio, M., Kivimäki, M. and Vahtera, J. (2002). Organizational justice: Evidence of a new psychosocial predictor of health. *American Journal of Public Health,* **92,** 105–108.

Elovainio, M., Kivimäki, M., Puttonen, S., Lindholm, H., Pohjonen, T. and Sinervo, T. (2006a). Organizational injustice and impaired cardiovascular regulation among female employees. *Occupational Environmental Medicine,* **63,** 141–144.

Elovainio, M., Leino-Arjas, P., Vahtera, J. and Kivimäki, M. (2006b). Justice at work and cardiovascular mortality: a prospective cohort study. *Journal of Psychosomatic Research,* **61,** 271–274.

Elovainio, M., Ferrie, J.E., Singh-Manoux, A., Gimeno, D., De Vogli, R., Shipley, M. *et al.* (2010). Organisational justice and markers of inflammation: the Whitehall II study. *Occupational and Environmental Medicine,* **67,** 78–83.

Engbers, L.H., van Poppel, M.N.M., Chin A., Paw, M.J.M., van Mechelen, Wl. (2005). Worksite health promotion programs with environmental changes: a systematic review. *American Journal of Preventative Medicine,* **29,** 61–70.

Engels, F. (1844 [2009]) *Conditions of the Working Class in England.* London, Penguin.

Engels, F. (1877 [1969]). *Anti-Duhring.* London, Lawrence and Wishart.

Erdem, E. and Glyn, A. (2001). Job deficits in UK regions. *Oxford Bulletin of Economics and Statistics,* **63,** 737–752.

Espelt, A., Borrell, C., Rodríguez-Sanz, M., Muntaner, C., Pasarín, M., Benach, J. *et al.* (2008). Inequalities in health by social class dimensions in European countries of different political traditions. *International Journal of Epidemiology,* **37,** 1095–1105.

Esping-Andersen, G. (1985). *Politics against Markets: The Social Democratic Road to Power.* London, Macmillan.

Esping-Andersen, G. (1987). Citizenship and Socialism: Decommodification and Solidarity in the Welfare State In: G. Esping-Andersen and L. Rainwater (eds.) *Stagnation and Renewal in Social Policy: The Rise and Fall of Policy Regimes,* London, Sharpe.

Esping-Andersen, G. (1990). *The Three Worlds of Welfare Capitalism.* London: Polity.

Esping-Andersen, G. (1996). After the Golden Age? Welfare State Dilemmas in a Global Economy. In: G. Esping-Anderson (eds.) *The Welfare State in Transition: National Adaptations in Global Economies*, pp. 1–31, London: Sage.

Esping-Andersen, G. (1999). *Social Foundations of Post-Industrial Economies*. Oxford: Oxford University Press.

European Agency for Safety and Health at Work. (2006). *European Risk Observatory Report Occupational Safety and Health in figures*. Brussels: Institute for Occupational Safety and Health.

European Agency for Safety and Health at Work. (2000). *Research on work-related low back disorders*. Luxembourg: Office for Official Publications of the European Communities.

European Foundation for the Improvement of Living and Working Conditions. (2004) *Part-time work in Europe 2004*. Available at: http://www.eurofound.europa.eu/ewco/reports/TN0403TR01/TN0403TR01_2.htm (accessed 6 July 2011).

European Foundation for the Improvement of Living and Working Conditions. (2000). *BEST European Studies on time: Shift work and health*. Dublin: European Foundation.

European Foundation for the Improvement of Living and Working Conditions. (2009). *ERM case studies: employment impact of relocation of multinational companies across the EU*. Dublin: European Foundation.

European Union Online. (1994) *EU Council Directive 94/45/EC*. European Union: Brussels.

European Working Conditions Observatory. (2005). *European Working Conditions Survey 2005*. Available at: http://www.eurofound.europa.eu/ewco/surveys/index.htm (accessed 6 July 2011).

European Working Conditions Observatory. (2010). *European Working Conditions Survey 2010*. Available at: http://www.eurofound.europa.eu/ewco/surveys/index.htm (accessed 6 July 2011).

Eurostat. (2000). *Social Protection in the EU Member States*. Luxembourg, EU.

Fawcett, J., Blakely, T. and Kunst, A. (2005). Are mortality differences and trends by education any better or worse in New Zealand? A comparison study with Norway, Denmark and Finland, 1980–1990s. *European Journal of Epidemiology*, 20, 683–691.

Fereday, J. and Oster, C. (2010). Managing a work life balance: the experiences of midwives working in a group practice setting. *Midwifery*, 26, 311–318.

Ferrera, M. (1996). The southern model of welfare in social Europe. *Journal of European Social Policy*, 6, 17–37.

Ferrie, J.E., Martikainen, P., Shipley, M.J., Marmot, M.G., Stansfeld, S.A. and Davey Smith, G. (2001). Employment status and health after privatisation in white collar civil servants: prospective cohort study. *BMJ*, 322, 647–651.

Ferrie, J.E., Shipley, M.J., Stansfeld, S.A. and Marmot, M.G. (2002). Effects of chronic job insecurity and change in job security on self-reported health, minor psychiatric morbidity, physiological measures, and health-related behaviours in British civil servants: the Whitehall II study. *Journal of Epidemiology and Community Health*, 56, 450–454.

Ferrie, J.E., Head, J., Shipley, M.J., Vahtera, J., Marmot, M.G. and Kivimäki, M. (2006). Injustice at work and incidence of psychiatric morbidity: the Whitehall II study. *Occupational Environmental Medicine*, 63, 443–450.

Fieldhouse, E. and Hollywood, E. (1999). Life after mining: hidden unemployment and changing patterns of economic activity amongst miners in England and Wales 1981–1991. *Work, Employment & Society*, **13**, 483–502.

Finkelstein, V. (1980). *Attitudes and Disabled People. World Rehabilitation Monograph* No5. New York.

Fletcher, D. (2007). A culture of worklessness? Historical insights from the Manor and Park areas of Sheffield. *Policy and Politics*, **35**, 65–85.

Floyd, M. and Curtis, J. (2000). An examination of changes in disability and employment policy in the UK. *European Journal of Social Security*, **2**, 303–322.

Foresight Mental Capital and Wellbeing Project. (2008). Final Project report–Executive summary. London: The Government Office for Science.

Fothergill, S. (2001). The true scale of the regional problem in the UK. *Regional Studies*, **35**, 241.

Fothergill, S. (2010). Welfare to work: time for a rethink? *People, Place and Policy Online*. **4/1**, 3–5.

Fothergill, S. and Wilson, I. (2007). A Million off Incapacity Benefit: how achievable is Labour's target? *Cambridge Journal of Economics*, **31**(5), 1007–1024.

Frank, A. (2000). Injuries related to shift work. *American Journal of Preventative Medicine*, **18**, 33–6.

Fredriksson, K., Bildt, C., Hägg, G. and Kilbom, Å. (2001). The impact on musculoskeletal disorders of changing physical and psychosocial work environment conditions in the automobile industry. *International Journal of Industrial Ergonomics*, **28**, 31–45.

Freidson, E. (1970). *Profession of medicine: a study of the sociology of applied knowledge*. New York: Dodd, Mead.

Freud, D. (2007). *Reducing Dependency, Increasing Opportunity: Options for the Future of Welfare to Work. An Independent Report to the Department for Work and Pensions*. Leeds: Corporate Document Services.

Fritzell, J. and Lundberg, O. (2005). Fighting inequalities in health and income: one important road to welfare and social development. In: O. Kangas and J. Palme (eds.) *Social Policy and Economic Development in the Nordic Countries*, Basingstoke: Palgrave Macmillan.

Frohlich, K. and Potvin, L. (2008). The inequality paradox: the population approach and vulnerable population. *American Journal of Public Health*, **98**, 216–221.

Frone, M.R., Russell, M. and Cooper, M.L. (1997). Relation of work-family conflict to health outcomes: A four-year longitudinal study of employed parents. *Journal of Occupational and Organizational Psychology*, **70**, 325–335.

Fryer, D.M. (1986). Employment, deprivation and personal agency during unemployment: a critical discussion of Jahoda's explanation of the psychological effects of unemployment. *Social Behavior*, **3**, 23.

Fu, H. and Boffetta, P. (1995). Cancer and occupational exposure to inorganic lead compounds: a meta-analysis of published data. *Occupational and Environmental Medicine*, **52**, 73–81.

Fuchs, V.R. (1979). Economics, Health and Post-industrial society. *The Milbank Memorial Fund Quarterly. Health and Society*, **57**(2), 153–182.

Fulcher, J. and Scott, J. (2003). *The state, social policy and welfare, in Sociology*. Oxford: Oxford University Press.

Furlong, A. and Cartmel, F. (2004). *Vulnerable young men in fragile labour markets: Employment, unemployment and the search for long-term security.* Joseph Rowntree Foundation: York.

Futatsuka, M., Maeda, S., Inaoka, T., Nagano, M., Shono, M. and Miyakita, T. (1998). Whole-Body Vibration and Health Effects in the Agricultural Machinery Drivers. *Industrial Health,* **36,** 127–132.

Gabbay, M., Taylor, L., Sheppard, L., Hillage, J., Bambra, C., Ford, F. *et al.* (2011). NICE's Guidance on long term sickness and incapacity. *British Journal of General Practice,* **61:** e118–124.

Gallie, D. (2004). *Resisting marginalisation: Unemployment experience and social policy in the European Union.* Oxford: Oxford University Press.

Gamble, A. (2009). *The spectre at the feast: capitalist crisis and the politics of recession.* Basingstoke: Palgrave.

Gardella, C. (2001). Lead Exposure in Pregnancy: A Review of the Literature and Argument for Routine Prenatal Screening. *Obsterical and Gynecological Survey,* **56,** 231–238.

Gardiner, K. (1997). *Bridges from benefit to work.* York: Joseph Rowntree Foundation.

Gerdtham, U. and Johannesson, M. (2005). Business cycles and mortality: results from Swedish microdata. *Social Science & Medicine,* **60,** 205–218.

Gerdtham, U. and Ruhm, C. (2006). Deaths rise in good economic times: Evidence from the OECD. *Economics and Human Biology,* **4,** 298–316.

Gillen, M., Yen, I.H., Trupin, L., Swig, L., Rugulies, R., Mullen, K. *et al.* (2007). The association of socioeconomic status and psychosocial and physical workplace factors with musculoskeletal injury in hospital workers. *American Journal of Industrial Medicine,* **50,** 245–260.

Ginsburg, N. (1979). *Class, Capital and Social Policy.* London: Macmillan.

Ginsburg, N. (1992). *Divisions of Welfare: A Critical Introduction to Comparative Social Policy.* London: Sage.

Glasgow, R., Terborg, J., Stryker, L., Boles, S. and Hollis, J.F. (1997). Take heart 2: replication of a worksite health promotion trial. *Journal of Behavioural Medicine,* **20,** 143–159.

Gleeson, B. (1991). *Notes Towards a Materialist History of Disability.* University of Bristol: Geography Dept Occasional Paper.

Godin, I. and Kittel, F. (2003). Can we disentangle life course processes of accumulation, critical period and social mobility? An analysis of disadvantaged socio-economic positions and myocardial infarction in the Stockholm Heart Epidemiology Program (SHEEP). *Social Science & Medicine,* **58,** 1543–1553.

Godin, I., Kittel, F., Coppieters, Y. and Siegrist, J. (2005). A prospective study of cumulative job stress in relation to mental health. *BMC Public Health,* **5,** 67.

Goldstone, C. and Meager, N. (2002). *Barriers to employment for disabled people.* London: Department for Work and Pensions.

Gough, I. (1979). *The Political Economy of the Welfare State.* London: Macmillan.

Gouldner, A.W. (1960). The norm of reciprocity: a preliminary statement. *American Sociological Review,* **25,** 161–178.

Gorz, A. (1980). *Ecology as politics.* Boston: South End Press.

Gorz, A. (1982). *Farewell to the working class: an essay on post-industrial socialism.* London: Pluto.

Graham, H. and Kelly, M.P. (2004). Health inequalities: concepts, frameworks and policy. London: Health Development Agency.

Graham, J.D., Chang, B.H. and Evans, J.S. (1992). Poorer is Riskier. *Risk Analysis,* **12**, 333–337.

Grandey, A.A. and Cropanzano, R. (1999). The conservation of resources model applied to work-family conflict and strain. *Journal of Vocational Behavior,* **54**, 350–370.

Gravelle, H., Hutchinson, G. and Stern, J. (1981). Mortality and unemployment: a critique of Brenner's time series analysis. *The Lancet,* **318**, 675–679.

Greenhaus, J.H., Collins, K.M. and Shaw, J.D. (2003). The relation between work–family balance and quality of life. *Journal of Vocational Behavior,* **63**, 510–531.

Grice, M.M., Feda, D., McGovern, P., Alexander B.A., McCaffrey, D. and Ukestad, L. (2007). Giving Birth and Returning to Work: The Impact of Work–Family Conflict on Women's Health After Childbirth. *Annals of Epidemiology,* **17**, 791–798.

Grint, K. (2005). *The sociology of work: an introduction.* Cambridge: Polity.

Grover, C. (2007). The Freud Report on the Future of Welfare to Work: some critical reflections. *Critical Social Policy,* **27**, 534–545.

Grover, C. and Piggott, L. (2005). Disabled people, the reserve army of labour and welfare reform. *Disability & Society,* **20**, 705–717.

Grover, C. and Piggott, L. (2007). Social security, employment and Incapacity Benefit: A critical reflection of *A new deal for welfare. Disability & Society,* **22**, 733–746.

Grover, C. and Piggott, L. (2010). From Incapacity Benefit to Employment and Support Allowance: social sorting, sickness and impairment, and social security. *Policy Studies,* **31**, 265–282.

Grzywacz, J.G., Arcury, T.A. Marın, A., Carrillo, L., Burke, B., Coates, M.L. *et al.* (2007). Work–Family Conflict: Experiences and Health Implications Among Immigrant Latinos. *Journal of Applied Psychology,* **92**, 1119–1130.

Habermas, J. (1976). *Legitimation Crisis.* London: Heineman.

Hadden, W., Muntaner, C., Benach, J., Gimeno, D. and Benavides, F.G. (2007). A glossary for the social epidemiology of work organization: Part 3. Terms from the sociology of labour markets. *Journal of Epidemiology and Community Health,* **61**, 6–8.

Hagquist, C., Silburn, S.R., Zurbrick, S.R., Lindberg, G. and Ringbäck, W.G. (2000). Suicide and mental health problems among Swedish youth in the wake of the 1990s recession. *International Journal of Social Welfare,* **9**, 211–219.

Hall, S. and Jacques, M. (1983). *The Politics of Thatcherism.* London: Lawrence & Wishart.

Hamberg-van Reenen, H.H., Ariëns, G.A.M., Blatter, B.M., van Mechelen, W. and Bongers, P.M. (2007). A systematic review of the relation between physical capacity and future low back and neck/shoulder pain. *Pain,* **130**, 93–107.

Han, S., Pfizenmaier, D.H., Garcia, E., Eguez, M.L., Ling, M., Kemp, F.W. *et al.* (2000). Effects of Lead Exposure before Pregnancy and Dietary Calcium during Pregnancy on Fetal Development and Lead Accumulation. *Environmental Health Perspectives,* **108**, 527–531.

Hannerz, H., Albertsen, K., Nielsen, M.L., Tuchsen, F. and Burr, H. (2004). Occupational factors and 5-year weight change among men in a Danish national cohort. *Health Psychology,* **23**, 283–288.

Hanson, L.L.M., Theorell, T., Oxenstierna, G., Hyde, M. and Westerlund, H. (2008). Demand, control and social climate as predictors of emotional exhaustion symptoms in working Swedish men and women. *Scandinavian Journal of Public Health,* **36**, 737–743.

Harrington, J. (2001). Health effects of shift work and extended hours of work. *Occupational and Environmental Medicine,* **58**, 60–72.

Harrington, J., Gill, F., Aw, T. and Gardiner, K. (1998). *Occupational Health* (4th edition). London: Blackwell.

Hartvigsen, J., Lings, S., Leboeuf-Yde, C., and Bakketeig, L. (2004). Psychosocial factors at work in relation to low back pain and consequences of low back pain; a systematic, critical review of prospective cohort studies. *Occupational and Environmental Medicine,* **61**, e2.

Harvey, D. (2000). *Spaces of Hope,* Edinburgh: Edinburgh University Press.

Hay, C. (1995). Structure and Agency: Holding the Whip Hand. In: D. Marsh and G. Stoker (eds.) *Theory and Methods in Political Science;* pp.189–208, London: Macmillan.

Hay, C. (1996). *Re-Stating Social and Political Change.* Milton Keynes: Open University Press.

Head, J., Kivimäki, M., Siegrist, J., Ferrie, J.E., Vahtera, J., Shipley, M.J. *et al.* (2007). Effort-reward imbalance and relational injustice at work predict sickness absence: the Whitehall II study. *Journal Psychosomatic Research,* **63**, 433–440.

Head, J., Martikainen, P., Kumari, M., Kupor, H. and Marmot, M. (2002). *Work Environment, Alcohol Consumption and Ill-Health: The Whitehall II Study.* Suffolk: HSE Books.

Health and Safety Executive. (2002). *Control of lead at work regulations.* Available at: http://www.hse.gov.uk/pubns/priced/l132.pdf (accessed 6 July 2011).

Health and Safety Executive. (2004). *Getting to grips with manual handling.* Available at: http://www.hse.gov.uk/pubns/indg143.pdf (accessed 6 July 2011).

Health and Safety Executive. (2005a). *The Control of Noise at Work Regulations 2005.* Available at: http://www.opsi.gov.uk/si/si2005/20051643.htm (accessed 6 July 2011).

Health and Safety Executive. (2005b). *The Control of Vibration at Work Regulations 2005.* Available at: http://www.opsi.gov.uk/si/si2005/20051093.htm (accessed 6 July 2011).

Health and Safety Executive. (2006a). *Shift work and fatigue.* Available from: http://www.hse.gov.uk/humanfactors/shiftwork/index.htm (accessed 6 July 2011).

Health and Safety Executive. (2006b). *Managing shift work: health and safety guidance.* London: Health and Safety Executive Books.

Health and Safety Executive. (2009) *Disease Statistics.* Available at: http://www.hse.gov.uk/statistics/causdis/index.htm (accessed 6 July 2011).

Health and Safety Executive. (2010a). *Pneumoconiosis and Silicosis.* Available at: http://www.hse.gov.uk/statistics/causdis/pneumoconiosis/(accessed 6 July 2011).

Health and Safety Executive. (2010b). *Injury Statistics.* Available at: http://www.hse.gov.uk/statistics/(accessed 6 July 2011).

Health and Safety Executive. (2010c). *Noise at work.* Available at: http://www.hse.gov.uk/noise/keyfacts.htm (accessed 6 July 2011).

Health and Safety Executive. (2010d). *Vibration at Work.* Available at: http://www.hse.gov.uk/vibration/(accessed 6 July 2011).

Health and Safety Executive. (2010e). *Reducing the risk of upper limb disorders (ULDs) in the workplace.* Available at: http://www.hse.gov.uk/msd/uld/whatareulds.htm (accessed 6 July 2011).

Hemmingway, H. and Marmot, M. (1999). Psychosocial factors in the aetiology and prognosis of coronary heart disease: systematic review of prospective cohort studies. *British Medical Journal,* **318**, 1460–1467.

Henning Bjorn, N., Pico Geerdsen, L. and Jensen, P. (2004). *The threat of compulsory participation in active labour market programmes for the unemployed: systematic review protocol.* The Campbell Library, 2004.

Her Majesty's Stationery Office [HMSO]. (1995). *Disability Discrimination Act.*

Hill, E.J., Grzywacz, J.G., Allen, S., Blanchard, V.L., Matz-Costa, C., Shulkin, S. *et al. (2008). Defining and conceptualizing workplace flexibility. *Community, Work, & Family,* **11**, 149–163.

Hillage, J., Williams, M. and Pollard, E. (1998). *Evaluation of access to work.* Brighton: Institute for Employment Studies.

Hine, R.C. and Wright, P.W. (1998). Trade with low wage economies, employment and productivity in UK manufacturing. *The Economic Journal,* **108**, 1500–1510.

HM Treasury. (1998). *Principles into Practice.* London, HMSO.

HM Treasury. (2003). *Employment for All.* London: HMSO.

HM Treasury and Department for Work and Pensions [DWP]. (2003). *Full employment in every region.* London: The Stationery Office.

Hodson, C. (2001). *Psychology and Work.* Hove: Routledge.

Hogstedt, C. and Lundberg, I. (2002). Work-related policies and interventions, in J. Mackenbach and M. Bakker (ed.) *Reducing inequalities in health: a European perspective,* pp. 85–103, London: Routledge.

Hopkins, S. (2006). Economic stability and health status: Evidence from East Asia before and after the 1990s economic crisis. *Health Policy,* **75**, 347–357.

Hoogendoorn W.E., van Poppel, M.N., Bongers, P.M., Koes B.W., and Bouter L.M. (2000). Systematic review of psychosocial factors at work and private life as risk factors for back pain. *Spine,* **25**, 2114–2125.

Horan, A.P. (2002). An effective workplace stress management intervention: Chicken Soup for the Soul at Work Employee Groups. *Work,* **18**, 3–13.

Houston, D. and Lindsay, C. (2010). Fit for work? Health, employability and challenges for the UK welfare reform agenda. *Policy Studies,* **31**, 133–142.

Huijts, T. and Eikemo, T.A. (2009). Causality, selectivity or artefacts? Why socioeconomic inequalities in health are not smallest in the Nordic countries. *European Journal of Public Health,* **19**, 452–453.

Hyyppä, M.T., Erkki, K. and Alanen, E. (1997). Quality of sleep during economic recession in Finland: a longitudinal cohort study. *Social Science & Medicine,* **45**, 731–738.

Illich, I. (1976 [1995]). *Limits to medicine: medical nemesis: the exploration of health.* London: Boyars.

Institute for Environment and Health. (1998). *Recent UK Blood Lead Surveys.* Medical Research Council.

Institute for Environment and Health. (2005). *Shift Work and Breast Cancer: Report of an Expert Meeting 12 November 2004 (Web Report W23), Leicester, UK, MRC Institute for*

Environment and Health. Available at: http://www.silsoe.cranfield.ac.uk/ieh/pdf/w23. pdf (accessed 6 July 2011).

Jahoda, M. (1982). *Employment and Unemployment. A Social Psychological Analysis.* Cambridge: Cambridge University Press.

Jamieson, R. (2011). *Employability and govermentality.* PhD thesis. Durham: Durham University.

Jansen, N.W.H., Kant, I., Kristensen, T.S. and Nijhuis, F.J.N. (2003). Antecedents and consequences of work-family conflict: a prospective cohort study. *Journal of Occupational and Environmental Medicine,* **45**, 479–491.

Jansen, N.W.H., Kant, I.J., van Amelsvoort, L.G.P.M., Kristensen, T.S., Swaen, G.M.H. and Nijhuis, F.J.N. (2006). Work–family conflict as a risk factor for sickness absence. *Occupational and Environmental Medicine,* **63**, 488–494.

Jessop, B. (1990) *State Theory: Putting the Capitalist State in its Place.* Cambridge, Polity.

Jessop, B. (1991). The Welfare State in Transition from Fordism to Post-Fordism. In: B. Jessop, H. Kastendiek, K. Nielsen and O.K. Pedersen (eds.) *The Politics of Flexibility: Restructuring State and Industry in Britain, Germany and Scandinavia,* pp. 82–105, Aldershot: Edward Elgar.

Jessop, B. (1994a). The Transition to Post-Fordism and the Schumpeterian Workfare State In: R. Burrows and B. Loader (eds.) *Towards a Post-Fordist Welfare State?* pp. 13–37, London: Routledge.

Jessop, B. (1994b). Post-Fordism and the State In: A. Amin (ed.) *Post-Fordism: A Reader,* pp. 251–279, Oxford: Blackwell.

Jessop, B. (2010). A cultural political economy of crises. Seminar, Department of Geography, Durham University, March 2010.

Johansson, E., Böckerman, P., Prärättälä, R. and Uutela, A. (2006). Alcohol-related mortality, drinking behavior, and business cycles: Are slumps really dry seasons? *European Journal of Health Economics,* **7**, 215–220.

Johansson, G. (1989). Job demands and stress reactions in repetitive and uneventful monotony at work. *International Journal of Health Services,* **19**, 365–377.

Johansson, G. (2002). Work–life balance: the case of Sweden in the 1990s. *Social Science Information,* **41**, 303–17.

Johnson, J. (2009). The Growing imbalance: class, work and health in an era of increasing inequality. In: P. Schnall, M. Dobson, E. Rosskam (eds.) *Unhealthy Work: Causes, Consequences, Cures,* New York: Baywood.

Johnson, J.V. and Hall, E.M. (1988). Job strain, work place social support, and cardiovascular disease: a cross-sectional study of a random sample of the Swedish working population. *American Journal of Public Health,* **78**, 1336–1342.

Johnson, J.V. and Lipscomb, J. (2006). Long working hours, occupational health and the changing nature of work organization. *American Journal of Industrial Medicine,* **49**, 921–929.

Johnston, J.M., Landsittel, D.P., Nelson, N.A., Gardner, L.I. and Wassell, J.T. (2003). Stressful Psychosocial Work Environment Increases Risk for Back Pain Among Retail Material Handlers. *American Journal of Industrial Medicine,* **43**, 179–187.

Joyce, K. and Bambra, C. (2010). Health inequalities in developed nations. *Social Alternatives,* **2**, 21–27.

Joyce, K.E., Smith, K.E., Sullivan, C. and Bambra, C. (2010a). 'Most of industry's shutting down up here . . .': Employability initiatives to tackle worklessness in areas of low labour demand. *Social Policy and Society*, **9**, 337–353.

Joyce, K., Pabayo, R., Critchley, J.A., and Bambra, C. (2010b). Flexible working conditions and their effects on employee health and well being. *Cochrane Library*, Issue 2, Feb 2010.

Karasek R. (1979). Job demands, job decision latitude and mental strain: implications for job design. *Administrative Science Quarterly*, **24**, 285–308.

Karasek R. (1992). Stress prevention through work reorganisation: a summary of 19 case studies. *Conditions of Work Digest*, **11**, 23–42.

Karasek, R.A. and Theorell, T. (1990). *Healthy Work: Stress, Productivity, and the Reconstruction of Working Life*. New York, NY: Basic Books.

Karim, S.A., Eikemo, T.A. and Bambra, C. (2010). Welfare state regimes and population health: integrating the East Asian welfare states. *Health Policy*, **94**, 45–53.

Kasza, G. (2002). The Illusion of Welfare Regimes. *Journal of Social Policy*, **31**, 271–287.

Katz, J.N. and Simmons, B.P. (2002). Carpal tunnel syndrome. *The New England Journal of Medicine*, **346**, 1807–1812.

Katz, M.B. (1986). *In the Shadow of the Poorhouse: A social history of welfare in America*. New York: Basic Books.

Kawachi, I., Kennedy, B.P., Lochner, K. and Prothrow-Stith, D. (1997). Social Capital, Income Inequality, and Mortality. *American Journal of Public Health*, **87**, 1491–1498.

Kawachi, I., Subramanian, S.V. and Almeida-Filho, N. (2002). A glossary for health inequalities. *Journal of Epidemiology and Community Health*, **56**, 647–652.

Kemp, P. (2006). Comparing trends in disability benefit receipt. In: P. Kemp, A. Sunden and B. Bakker Tauritz, (eds.) *Sick societies? Trends in disability benefits in post-industrial welfare states*, pp.7–22, Geneva: International Social Security Association.

Kemp, P. and Davidson, J. (2008). *Routes onto Incapacity Benefit: Findings from a survey of recent claimants*. DWP Research Report No. 469. Leeds: Corporate Document Services.

Kemp, P. and Davidson, J. (2009). Gender Differences Among New Claimants of Incapacity Benefit. *Journal of Social Policy*, **38**, 589–606.

Kessler, R.C., Turner, J.B. and House, J.S. (1987). Intervening processes in the relationship between unemployment and health. *Psychological Medicine*, **17**, 949–961.

Kilborn, A. (1988). Intervention programmes for work-related neck and upper limb disorders: strategies and evaluation. *Ergonomics*, **31**, 735–747.

Kim, I-H., Muntaner, C., Khang, Y-H., Paek, D. and Cho, S-I. (2006). The relationship between nonstandard working and mental health in a representative sample of the South Korean population. *Social Science & Medicine*, **63**, 566–574.

King, D.A. and Thomas, S.M. (2007). Big Lessons for a Healthy Future. *Nature*, **449**, 791–792.

Kinnunen, U. and Mauno, S. (1998). Antecedents and Outcomes of Work-Family Conflict Among Employed Women and Men in Finland. *Human Relations*, **51**(2), 157–177.

Kivimäki, M., LeinoArjas, P., Luukkonen, R., Riihimäki, H., Vahtera, J. and Kirjonen, J. (2002). Work stress and risk of cardiovascular mortality: prospective cohort study of industrial employees. *British Medical Journal*, **325**, 857–860.

Kivimäki, M., Elovainio, M., Vahtera, J. and Ferrie, J.E. (2003a). Organisational justice and health of employees: prospective cohort study. *Occupational and Environmental Medicine*, **60**, 27–34.

Kivimäki, M., Vahtera, J., Virtanen, M., Elovainio, M., Pentti, J. and Ferrie, J.E. (2003b). Temporary employment and risk of overall and cause specific mortality, *American Journal of Epidemiology*, **158**, 663–668.

Kivimäki, M., Head, J. Ferrie, J., Shipley, M. Vahtera, J. and Marmot, M. (2003c). Sickness absence as a global measure of health: evidence from mortality in the Whitehall II prospective cohort study. *British Medical Journal*, **327**, 364–370.

Kivimaki, M., Ferrie, J.E., Brunner, E., Head, J., Shipley, M.J., Vahtera, J. *et al.* (2005). Justice at work and reduced risk of coronary heart disease among employees: the Whitehall II Study. *Archive of Internal Medicine*, **165**, 2245–2251.

Kjuus, H., Istad, H. and Langard, S. (1981). Emphysema and occupational exposure to industrial pollutants. *Scandinavian Journal of Work, Environment & Health*, **7**, 290–297.

Knight, T., Dickens, S., Mitchell, M. and Woodfield, K. (2005). *Incapacity Benefit Reforms—The Personal Adviser role and practices: Stage Two*, DWP Research Report 278. Leeds: Corporate Document Services.

Kock, S., Andersen, T., Kolstad, H.A., Kofoed-Nielsen, B., Wiesler, F. and Bonde, J.P. (2004). Surveillance of noise exposure in the Danish workplace: a baseline survey. *Occupational and Environmental Medicine*, **61**, 838–843.

Kompier, M. (2006). New systems of work organization and workers' health. *Scandinavian Journal of Work, Environment & Health*, **32**, 421–430.

Kondo, N., Subramanian, S., Kawachi, I., Takeda, Y. and Yamagata, Z. (2008). Economic recession and health inequalities in Japan: analysis with a national sample, 1986–2001. *Journal of Epidemiology and Community Health*, **62**, 869–875.

Korpi, T. (2001). Accumulating disadvantage: longitudinal analyses of unemployment and physical health in representative samples of the Swedish population. *European Sociological Review*, **17**, 255–274.

Korpi, W. (1983). *The Democratic Class Struggle*. London: Routledge.

Korpi, W. and Palme, J. (1998). The paradox of redistribution and the strategy of equality: welfare state institutions, inequality and poverty in the Western countries. *American Sociological Review*, **63**, 662–687.

Kposowa, A. (2001). Unemployment and suicide: a cohort analysis of social factors predicting suicide in the US National Mortality Study. *Psychological Medicine*, **31**, 127–138.

Krieger, N. (2008). Ladders, pyramids and champagne: the iconography of health inequities. *Journal of Epidemiology and Community Health*, **62**, 1098–1104.

Krieger, N., Rehkopf, D.H., Chen, J.T., Waterman, P.D., Marcelli, E. and Kennedy, M. (2008). The fall and rise of US inequities in premature mortality: 1960–2002. *PLoS Medicine*, **5**, 227–241.

Kumar, K. (1978). *Prophecy and Progress: the sociology of industrial and post industrial society*. London: Allen Lane.

Kumar, K. (1995). *From Post-Industrial to Post-Modern Society: New Theories of the Contemporary World*. Blackwell.

Kuper. H. and Marmot, M. (2003). Job strain, job demands, decision latitude, and risk of coronary heart disease within the Whitehall II study. *Journal of Epidemiology and Community Health*, **57**, 147–53.

Kuper, H., Marmot, M. and Hemmingway, H. (2002). Systematic Review of Prospective Cohort Studies of Psychosocial Factors in the Etiology and Prognosis of Coronary Heart Disease. *Seminars in Vascular Medicine*, **2**, 267–314.

Kuorinka, I. (1998). The influence of industrial trends on work-related musculoskeletal disorders (WMSDs). *International Journal of Industrial Ergonomics*, **21**, 5–9.

Lahelma, E., Kivela, K., Roos, E., Tuominen, T., Dahl, E., Diderichsen, F. *et al.* (2002). Analysing changes of health inequalities in the Nordic welfare states. *Social Science & Medicine*, **55**, 609–625.

Lahelma, E., Laaksonen, M. and Aittomaki, A. (2009). Occupational class inequalities in health across employment sectors: the contribution of working conditions. *International Archives of Occupational and Environmental Health*, **82**, 185–190.

Laing, R.D. (1967). *The Politics of Experience*. New York: Ballantine.

Lake, A. and Townshend, T. (2006). Obesogenic environments: Exploring the built and food environments. *Journal of the Royal Society for the Promotion of Health*, **126**, 262–267.

Lalonde, M. (1974). *A new perspective on the health of Canadians*. Ottawa: Ministry of Supply and Services.

Lallukka, T., Lahelma, E., Rahkonen, O., Roos, E., Laaksonen, E., Martikainen, P. *et al.* (2008). Associations of job strain and working overtime with adverse health behaviors and obesity: evidence from the Whitehall II Study, Helsinki Health Study, and the Japanese Civil Servants Study. *Social Science & Medicine*, **66**, 1681–1698.

Lallukka, T., Chandola, T., Hemmingway, H., Marmot, M., Lahelma, E. and Rahkonen, O. (2009). Job strain and symptoms of angina pectoris among British and Finnish middle-aged employees. *Journal of Epidemiology and Community Health*, **63**, 980–985.

Landrigan, P.J. (1990). Lead in the modern workplace. *American Journal of Public Health*, **80**, 907–908.

Landsbergis, P.A. (2009). Interventions to Reduce Job Stress and Improve Work Organization and Worker Health. In: P. Schnall, M. Dobson, and E. Rosskam (eds.) *Unhealthy Work: Causes, Consequences, Cures*, New York: Baywood.

Landsbergis, P.A. (2010). Assessing the Contribution of Working Conditions to Socioeconomic Disparities in Health: A Commentary. *American Journal of Industrial Medicine*, **53**, 95–103.

Landbergis, P.A, Schnall, P. and Dobson, M. (2009). The workplace and cardiovascular disease. In: P. Schnall, M. Dobson, E. Rosskam (eds.) *Unhealthy Work: Causes, Consequences, Cures*, New York: Baywood.

Laney, A. and Attfield, M. (2010). Coal workers' pneumoconiosis and progressive massive fibrosis are increasingly more prevalent among workers in small underground coal mines in the United States. *Occupational and Environmental Medicine*, **67**, 428–431.

Leeni, T. and Berntsson, L.K. (2001). Long-term illness and psychosomatic complaints in children aged 2–17 years in the five Nordic countries: Comparison between 1984 and 1996. *European Journal of Public Health*, **1**, 35–42.

Lefebvre, H. (1984). *Everyday Life in the Modern World*, S. Rabinovitch (trans.) New Brunswick: Transaction Publishers.

Legard, R., Lewis, J., Hiscock, J. and Scott, J. (2002). *Evaluation of the Capability Report: Identifying the work-related capabilities of Incapacity Benefits recipients. DWP Research Report 162.* Leeds: Corporate Document Services.

Leibfroid, S (1992), Towards a European welfare state. In: Z. Ferge and J.E. Kolberg (ed.) *Social policy in a changing Europe,* Frankfurt: Campus-Verlag.

Leka, S., Griffiths, A. and Cox, T. (2003). *Work organization and stress. World Health Organization Protecting Workers' Health Series No. 3.* Nottingham: Institute of Work, Health and Organizations.

Letz, R., Cherniack, M.G., Gerr, F., Hershman, D. and Pace, P. (1992). A cross sectional epidemiological survey of shipyard workers exposed to hand-arm vibration. *British Journal of Industrial Medicine,* **49**, 53–62.

Lewis, G. and Sloggett, A. (1998). Suicide, deprivation and unemployment: record linkage study. *BMJ,* **317**, 1283–1286.

Lewis, J. (1992). Gender and the Development of Welfare regimes. *Journal of European Social Policy,* **2**, 159–173.

Lewis, O. (1968). *The Culture of Poverty.* New York: Random House Inc.

Li, C.Y. and Sung, E.C. (1999). A review of the healthy worker effect in occupational epidemiology. *Occupational Medicine,* **49**, 225–229.

Lidwall, U., Marklund, S. and Voss, M. (2010). Work-family interference and long-term sickness absence: a longitudinal cohort study. *European Journal of Public Health,* **20**, 676–681.

Lin, J.L., Lin-Tan, D.T., Hsu, K.H. and Yu, C.C. (2003). Environmental Lead Exposure and progression of Chronic Renal Diseases in Patients without Diabetes. *The New England Journal of Medicine,* **348**, 277–286.

Lincoln, A., Vernick, J., Ogaitis, S, Smith, G., Mitchell, S. and Agnew, J. (2000). Interventions for the Primary Prevention of Work-Related Carpal Tunnel Syndrome. *American Journal of Preventative Medicine,* **18**, 37–50.

Lindsay, C., McQuaid, R.W. and Dutton, M. (2007). New approaches to employability in the UK: combining 'Human Capital Development' and 'Work First' strategies? *Journal of Social Policy,* **36**, 539–560

Lings, S. and Leboeuf-Yde, C. (2000). Whole-body vibration and low back pain: a systematic, critical review of the epidemiological literature 1992–1999. *International Archives of Occupational and Environmental Health,* **73**, 290–297

Loomis, D. (2010). Time for global occupational health. *Occupational and Environmental Medicine,* **67**, 145.

Loumidis, J., Youngs, R., Lessof, C. and Stafford, B. (2001). *New Deal for Disabled People: National survey of Incapacity Benefits recipients. DWP Research Report 160.* Leeds: Corporate Document Services.

Lundberg, O. and Lahelma, E. (2001). Nordic health inequalities in the European context. In: M. Kautto, J. Fritzell, B. Hvinden, J. Kvist and H. Uusitalo (eds.) *Nordic welfare states in the European context,* pp. 42–65, London: Routledge.

Lundberg, O., Diderichsen, F. and Yngwe, M.A. (2001). Changing health inequalities in a changing society? Sweden in the mid-1980s and mid-1990s. *Scandinavian Journal of Public Health,* **55**, 31–39.

Lundberg, O., Yngwe, M.A., Stjärne, M., Björk, M.L., Fritzell, J. (2007). *The Nordic experience: welfare states and public health (NEWS).* Report for the Commission on Social Determinants of Health. Stockholm, Centre for Health Equity Studies (CHESS).

Lundberg, O., Yngwe, M., Kölegård Stjärne, M., Elstad, J., Ferrarini, T., Kangas, O. *et al.* (2008). The role of welfare state principles and generosity in social policy programmes for public health: an international comparative study. *Lancet*, **372**, 1633–1640.

Lunt, N. and Thornton, P. (1994). Disability and employment: towards an understanding of discourse and policy. *Disability and Society*, **9**, 223–238.

Luoto, R., Poikolainen, K. and Uutela, A. (1998). Unemployment, sociodemographic background and consumption of alcohol before and during the economic recession of the 1990s in Finland. *International Journal of Epidemiology*, **27**, 623–629.

Lusk, S.L., Hagerty, B.M., Gillespie, G. and Caruso, C.C. (2002). Chronic Effects of Workplace Noise on Blood Pressure and Heart Rate. *Archives of Environmental Health: An International Journal*, **57**, 273–281.

Lynch, J.W., Davey Smith, G., Kaplan, G.A. and House, J.S. (2000). Income inequality and mortality: importance to health of individual income, psychosocial environment, or material conditions. *British Medical Journal*, **320**, 1200–1204.

Lynch, K.M. and Smith, W.A. (1935). Pulmonary asbestosis III: Carcinoma of the lung in asbestos-silicosis. *American Journal of Cancer*, **24**, 56–64.

MacDonald, C. (ed.) (2000). *Epidemiology of work-related diseases* (second edition). London: BMJ Books.

MacEachen, E., Polzer, J. and Clarke, J. (2008). 'You are free to set your own hours': Governing worker productivity and health through flexibility and resilience. *Social Science & Medicine*, **66**, 1019–33.

MacKay, R. (1999). Work and nonwork: a more difficult labour market. *Environment and Planning A*. **31**, 487–502.

MacKay, R. and Davies, L. (2007). Unemployment, permanent sickness, and nonwork in the United Kingdom. *Environment and Planning A*, **40**, 464–481.

Macintyre, S. (1997). The Black Report and Beyond: what are the issues? *Social Science & Medicine*, **44**, 723–45.

Mackenbach, J. (2009). Politics is nothing but medicine as a larger scale: reflections on public health's biggest idea. *Journal of Epidemiology and Community Health*, **63**, 181–184.

Mackenbach, J., Kunst, A., Cavelaars, A., Groenhof, F. and Geurts, J. (1997). Socioeconomic inequalities in morbidity and mortality in Western Europe. *Lancet*, **349**, 1655–1659.

Mackenbach, J., Bakker, M., Kunst, A. and Diderichsen, F. (2002). Socio-economic inequalities in health in Europe: an overview. In: J. Mackenbach and M. Bakker (eds.) *Reducing inequalities in health: A European perspective*, pp. 3–24, London: Routledge.

Mackenbach, J.P., Bos, V., Andersen, O., Cardano, M., Costa, G., Harding, S. *et al.* (2003). Widening socioeconomic inequalities in mortality in six Western European countries. *International Journal of Epidemiology*, **32**, 830–837.

Mackenbach, J., Stirbu, I., Roskam, A., Schaap, M., Menvielle, G., Leinsalu, M. *et al.* (2008). Socioeconomic Inequalities in Health in 22 European Countries. *New England Journal of Medicine*, **358**, 2468–2481.

Madsen, S.J., John, C.R. and Miller, D. (2005). Work-Family Conflict and Health: A Study of Workplace, Psychological, and Behavioral Correlates. *Journal of Behavioral and Applied Management*, **6**, 225–247.

Mahaffey, K.R. (1995). Nutrition and Lead: Strategies for Public Health. *Environmental Health Perspectives Supplements*, **103**, 191–196.

Maki, N. (2010). *Mortality among the unemployed differs greatly by the magnitude of workplace downsizing; a register-based follow-up study of Finnish men and women. 13th Biennial Congress of the European Society for Health and Medical Sociology*, 26–28 August 2010 Ghent, Belgium.

Manderbacka, K., Lahelma, E. and Rahkonen, O. (2001). Structural changes and social inequalities in health in Finland, 1986–1994. *Scandinavian Journal of Public Health*, **55**, 41–54.

Maniadakis, N. and Gray, A. (2000). The economic burden of back pain in the UK. *Pain*, **84**, 95–103.

Marmot, M. (2006). Introduction, in M. Marmot and R.G. Wilkinson (ed.) *Social Determinants of Health*, pp. 1–5, Oxford: Oxford University Press.

Marmot, M. (Chair) (2010). *Fair Society, Healthy Lives: the Marmot review*. London: University College.

Marmot, M. and Brunner, E. (2005). Cohort Profile: The Whitehall II study. *International Journal of Epidemiology*, **34**, 251–256.

Marmot, M. and Wilkinson, R.G. (2001). Psychosocial and material pathways in the relation between income and health: a response to Lynch *et al*. *British Medical Journal*, **322**, 1233–1236.

Marmot, M. and Wilkinson, R.G. (2006) (eds). *Social Determinants of Health*. Oxford: Oxford University Press.

Marmot, M., Shipley, M.J. and Rose, G. (1984). Inequalities in death—specific explanations of a general pattern. *Lancet*, **323**, 1003–1006.

Marmot, M., Stansfeld, S., Patel, C., North, F., Head, J., White, I. *et al*. (1991). Health inequalities among British civil servants–the Whitehall II study. *Lancet*, **337**, 1387–1393.

Marmot, M., Feeney, A., Shipley, M., North, F. and Syme, S.L. (1995). Sickness absence as a measure of health status and functioning: from the UK Whitehall II study. *Journal of Epidemiology and Community Health*, **49**, 124–130.

Marmot, M., Ryff, C.D., Bumpass, L.L., Shipley, M. and Marks, N.F. (1997a). Social inequalities in health: Next questions and converging evidence. *Social Science & Medicine*, **44**, 901–910.

Marmot, M., Bosma, H., Hemingway, H., Brunner, E. and Stansfeld, S. (1997b). Contribution of job control and other risk factors to social variations in coronary heart disease. *Lancet*, **350**, 235–240.

Marmot, M., Siegrist, J. and Theorell, T. (2006). Health and the psychosocial work environment, in M. Marmot and R.G. Wilkinson (ed.) *Social Determinants of Health*, pp. 97–130, Oxford: Oxford University Press.

Marreilha Dos Santos, A.P., Andrade, V., Mateus, M.L., Aschner, M. and Batoreu, M.C. (2010). Occupational exposure of miners to manganese and lead—A preliminary study. *Toxicology Letters*, 196 (S1), p.S79.

Marsden, D. and Duff, E. (1975). *Workless: Some unemployed men and their families*. London, Pelican.

Marshall, A. (1989). The sequel of unemployment: The changing role of part-time and temporary work in Western Europe. In: G. Rodgers and J. Rodgers (eds.) *Precarious*

Jobs in Labour Market Regulation: The Growth of Atypical Employment in Western Europe, Geneva: International Institute for Labour Studies.

Marshall, T.H. (1950). *Citizenship and social class, and other essays*. Cambridge. Cambridge University Press.

Marshall, T.H. (1963). *Sociology at the Crossroads*. London: Hutchinson.

Martikainen, P., Bartley, M. and Lahelma, E. (2002). Psychosocial determinants of health in social epidemiology. *International Journal of Epidemiology*, 31, 1091–1093.

Martikainen, P. and Valkonen, T. (1996). Excess mortality of unemployed men and women during a period of rapidly increasing unemployment. *Lancet*, 348, 909–912.

Martikainen, P., Lahelma, E., Marmot, M., Sekine, M., Nishi, N. and Kagamimori, S. (2004). A comparison of socioeconomic differences in physical functioning and perceived health among male and female employees in Britain, Finland and Japan. *Social Science & Medicine*, 54, 1287–1295.

Marx, K. (1963). *Karl Marx: Early writings*. London: C Watts.

Marx, K. ((1844 [1970]). *Philosophical and Economic Manuscripts*. London, Lawrence and Wishart.

Marx, K. ((1867 [1976]). *Capital Volume 1*. London: Penguin.

Massarelli, N. (2009). European Union Labour Force Survey: Annual results 2008. *Eurostat: Data in Focus*, 33.

Mathers, C.D. and Schofield, D.J. (1998). The health consequences of unemployment: the evidence. *The Medical Journal of Australia*, 168, 178–183.

Matthews, S., Hertzman, C., Ostry, A. and Power, C. (1998). Gender, Work Roles and Psychosocial Work Characteristics as Determinants of Health. *Social Science & Medicine*, 46, 1417–1424.

Mazzuco, S. and Suhrcke, M. (2010). Health inequalities in Europe: new insights from European Labour Force Surveys. *Journal of Epidemiology and Community Health*, doi:10.1136/jech.2009.096271.

McCarthy, M. (2006). Transport and health. In: M. Marmot and R. Wilkison (eds.) *The Social Determinants of Health*, Oxford: Oxford University Press.

McCormick, J. (2000). *On the sick: incapacity and inclusion*. Edinburgh, Scottish Council Foundation.

McDonough, P. and Amick, B. (2001). The social context of health selection: a longitudinal study of health and employment. *Social Science & Medicine*, 53, 135–145.

McOrmond, T. (2004). Changes in working trends over the past decade. *Labour Market Trends*, 112, 1–11.

Mead, L.M. (1997). Citizenship and Social Policy: T.H. Marshall and Poverty. *Social Philosophy and Policy*, 14, 197–230.

Menéndez, M., Benach, J. and Vogel, L. (2009). *The impact of safety representatives on occupational health: A European perspective*. ETUI: Health and Safety Department.

Menzel, N.N., Brooks, S.M., Bernard, T.E. and Nelson, A. (2004). The physical workload of nursing personnel: association with musculoskeletal discomfort. *International Journal of Nursing Studies*, 41, 859–867.

Meyer, P.A., Pivetz, T., Digman, T.A., Homa, D.M., Schoonover, J. and Brody, D. (2003). Surveillance for Elevated Blood Lead Levels Among Children—United States, 1997–2001. *Morbidity and Mortality Weekly Reports*, 52, 1–21.

Millstone, E. (1997). *Lead and Public Health*. London: Earthscan Publications Limited.

Mishra, R. (1984). *The Welfare State in Crisis: Social Thought and Social Change*. London: Wheatsheaf.

Mishra, R. (1999). *Globalisation and the Welfare State*. Cheltenham: Edward Elgar.

Mitchell, R. (2005). The decline of death–how do we measure and interpret changes in self reported health across cultures and time? *International Journal of Epidemiology*, **34**, 306–308.

Mitchell, R., McClure, R. and Driscoll, T. (2008). Refining estimates of hospitalised work-related injury in NSW, 2000–01 to 2004–05. *Australian and New Zealand Journal of Occupational Health and Safety*, **24**, 33–42.

Monk, T. and Folkard, S. (1992). *Making shift work tolerable*. London: Taylor and Francis.

Montgomery, S.M., Cook, D.G., Bartley, M. and Wadsworth, M.E. (1999a). Unemployment pre-dates symptoms of depression and anxiety resulting in medical consultation in young men. *International Journal of Epidemiology*, **28**, 95–100.

Montgomery, S.M., Cook, D.G., Bartley, M. and Wadsworth, M.E. (1999b). Unemployment, cigarette smoking, alcohol consumption and body weight in young British men. *European Journal of Public Health*, **8**, 21–27.

Moore, D. (2009). *Bad for business: Good for health?* MSc thesis. Durham: Durham University.

Moran, M. (2007). *The British regulatory state: High modernism and hyper innovation*. Oxford: Oxford University Press.

Moreau, M., Valente, F., Mak, R., Pelfrene, E., de Smet, P., de Backer, G. *et al.* (2004). Occupational stress and incidence of sick leave in the Belgian workforce: the Belstress study. *Journal of Epidemiology and Community Health*, **58**, 507–516.

Morrell, S.L., Taylor, R.J. and Kerr, C.B. (1998). Unemployment and young people's health. *The Medical Journal of Australia*, **168**, 236–240.

Morris, J. and Deeming, C. (2004). Minimum incomes for healthy living: next thrust in UK social policy? *Policy and Politics*, **32**, 441–454.

Morris, J.K., Cook, D.G. and Shaper, A.G (1994). Loss of employment and mortality. *BMJ*, **308**, 1135–1139.

Morris, J.N., Donkin, A.J., Wonderling, D., Wilkinson, P., Dowler, E.A. (2000). A minimum income for healthy living. *Journal of Epidemiology and Community Health*, **54**, 885–889.

Morris, J.N., Wilkinson, P., Dangour, A.D., Deeming, C., Fletcher, A. (2007). Defining a minimum income for healthy living (MIHL): older age, England. *International Journal of Epidemiology*, **36**, 1300–1307.

Morris, J., Wilkinson, P., Dangour, A. and Deeming, C. (2009). *Minimum Incomes for Healthy Living*. Evidence submitted to the Marmot Commission (unpublished research).

Morris, W. (1884 [1979]) 'How we live and how we might live'. In: A. Morton (ed.) *Political Writings of William Morris*. London, Lawrence and Wishart, 148–149.

Moser, K.A., Fox, A.J. and Jones, D.R. (1984). Unemployment and mortality in the OPCS Longitudinal Study. *Lancet*, **324**, 1324–1329.

Moshammer, H. and Neuberger, M. (2004). Lung cancer and dust exposure: results of a prospective cohort study following 3260 workers for 50 years. *Occupational and Environmental Medicine*, **61**, 157–162.

Mozurkewich,E,. Luke, B., Avni, M. and Wolf, F. (2000). Working conditions and adverse pregnancy outcome: a meta-analysis. *Obstetrics and Gynecology*, **95**, 623–35.

Muntaner, C. and Lynch, J. (1999). Income inequality, social cohesion, and class relations: A critique of Wilkinson's neo-Durkheiminan research program. *International Journal of Health Services*, **29**, 59–81.

Murray, C.A. (ed.) (1990). *The emerging British underclass*. London: Institute of Economic Affairs.

Myung, K., Sacker, A., Kelly, Y. and Nazroo, J. (2010). Health selection operating between classes and across employment statuses. *Journal of Epidemiology and Community Health*, doi:10.1136/jech.2009.107995.

Nakamura, K., Shimai, S., Kikuchi, S., Takahashi, H., Tanaka, M., Nakano, S. *et al.* (1998). Increases in body mass index and waist circumference as outcomes of working overtime. *Occupational Medicine*, **48**, 169–173.

National Academy of Sciences. (1993). *Measuring Lead Exposure in Infants, Children, and Other Sensitive Populations*. Washington: National Academy Press.

National Cancer Institute. (2009). *Asbestos Exposure and Cancer Risk*. Available at: http://www.cancer.gov/cancertopics/factsheet/Risk/asbestos (accessed 6 July 2011).

National Institute for Health and Clinical Excellence. (2008). *Public Health Guidance 13: Workplace health promotion: how to encourage employees to be physically active*. London: NICE.

National Institute for Health and Clinical Excellence. (2009a). *Public Health Guidance 22: Promoting mental wellbeing through productive and healthy working conditions: guidance for employers*. London: NICE.

National Institute for Health and Clinical Excellence. (2009b). *Public Health Guidance 19: Managing long-term sickness absence and incapacity for work*. London: NICE.

National Institute for Occupational Safety and Health (NIOSH). (2002). *Centers for Disease Control and Prevention. Health Effects of Occupational Exposure to Respirable Crystalline Silica. DHHS (NIOSH) Publication No. 2002–129*.

Naidoo, J. and Wills, J. (2000). *Health promotion: foundations for practice*. London: Bailliere Tindall.

Navarro, V. (1978). *Class struggle, the state, and medicine: an historical and contemporary analysis of the medical sector in Great Britain*. London: Robertson.

Navarro, V. (1982). The labour process and health: a historical materialist interpretation. *International Journal of Health Services*, **12**, 5–29.

Navarro, V. (2009). What we mean by the social determinants of health. *International Journal of Health Services*, **39**, 423–441.

Navarro, V. and Shi, L. (2001). The political context of social inequalities and health. *International Journal of Health Services Research*, **31**, 1–21.

Navarro, V., Borrell, C., Benach, J. and Muntaner, C. (2003). The Importance of the Political and the Social In Explaining Mortality Differentials Among The Countries Of The OECD, 1950–1998. *International Journal of Health Services Research*, **33**, 419–494.

Navarro, V., Muntaner, C., Borrell, C. and Benach, J. (2006). Politics and Health Outcomes. *Lancet*, **368**, 1033–1037.

Need, A., Steijn, B. and Gesthuizen, M. (2005). Long-term effects of flexible work. In: B. Peper, A. van Doorne-Huiskes, and L. den Dulk (eds.) *Flexible working and organisational change. The integration of work and personal life*, Cheltenham: Edward Elgar.

Nelson, N.A., Kaufman, J., Kalat, J. and Silverstein, B. (1997). Falls in construction: injury rates for OSHA-inspected employers before and after citation for violating the Washington State Fall Protection Standard. *American Journal of Industrial Medicine*, **31**, 296–302.

Netemeyer, R.G., Boles, J.S. and McMurrian, R. (1996). Development and validation of work-family conflict and family-work conflict scales. *Journal of Applied Psychology*, **81**, 400–410.

Netterstrøm, B. and Suadicani, P. (1993). Self-Assessed Job Satisfaction and Ischaemic Heart Disease Mortality: A 10-Year Follow-Up of Urban Bus Drivers. *International Journal of Epidemiology*, **22**, 51–56.

Nettleton, S. (1995). *The sociology of health and illness*. Cambridge: Polity Press.

Neumayer, E. (2004). Recessions lower (some) mortality rates: evidence from Germany. *Social Science & Medicine*, **58**, 1037–1047.

Neumayer, E. (2005). The economic business cycle and mortality. *International Journal of Epidemiology*, **34**, 1221–1222.

Nichols, T. (1999). Death and injury at work: A sociological approach. In N. Daykin and L. Doyal (eds.) *Health and Work: Critical Perspectives*, London: Macmillan.

Nickell, S. and Quintini, G. (2002). The recent performance of the UK labour market. *Oxford Review of Economic Policy*, **18**, 202–220.

Niedhammer, I., Teck, M.I., Starke, D. and Siegrist, J. (2004). Effort-Reward Imbalance Model and self-reported health: Cross-sectional and prospective results from the GAZEL Cohort. *Social Science & Medicine*, **58**, 1531–1541.

Norman, P. and Bambra, C. (2007). Incapacity or Unemployment? The utility of an administrative data source as an updatable indicator of population health. *Population, Space and Place*, **13**, 333–352.

North, F., Syme, S., Feeney, A., Shipley, M. and Marmot, M. (1996). Psychosocial work environment and sickness absence among British civil servants: the Whitehall II Study. *American Journal of Public Health*, **86**, 332–340.

Novo, M., Hammerstrom, A. and Janlert, U. (2000). Smoking habits—a question of trend and unemployment? A comparison of young men and women between boom and recession. *Public Health*, **114**, 460–463.

Novo, M., Hammerstrom, A. and Janlert, U. (2001). Do high levels of unemployment influence the health of those who are not unemployed? A gendered comparison of young men and women during boom and recession. *Social Science & Medicine*, **53**, 293–303.

O'Connor, J. (1973). *The Fiscal Crisis of the State*. London: St James.

Offe, C. (1984). *Contradictions of the Welfare State*. London: Hutchinson.

Office for National Statistics. (2009). *A profile of Worklessness*. Available at: http://www.statistics.gov.uk/downloads/theme_compendia/Worklessness-Topic-profile.pdf (accessed 6 July 2011).

Ohisson, K., Attewell, R.G., Pålsson, B., Karlsson, B., Balogh, I., Johnsson, B. *et al.* (1995). Repetitive industrial work and neck and upper limb disorders in females. *American Journal of Industrial Medicine*, **27**, 731–747.

Oliver, M. (1990). *The Politics of Disablement*. London: Macmillan.

Oliver, M. and Barnes, C. (1998). *Disabled people and social policy*. London: Longman.

Organisation for Economic Cooperation and Development (OECD). (1996). *Benefits and Wages: OECD Indicators*. Paris: OECD.

Organisation for Economic Cooperation and Development (OECD). (2003). *Transforming disability into ability: policies to promote work and income security for disabled people*. Paris: OECD.

Organisation for Economic Cooperation and Development (OECD). (2006). *Benefits and Wages: OECD Indicators*. Paris: OECD.

Organisation for Economic Cooperation and Development (OECD). (2008). *Indicators of Employment Protection*. Paris: OECD.

Organisation for Economic Cooperation and Development (OECD). (2009). *Sickness, Disability and Work: Background paper*. Paris: OECD.

Orwell, G. (1937 [1981]). *The Road to Wigan Pier*. London: Penguin.

Ostry, A.S., Kelly, S., Demers, P.A., Mustard, C. and Hertzman, C. (2003). A Comparison between the Effort-Reward Imbalance and Demand Control Models. *BioMed Central*, **3**, 10.

Ozmen, C.A., Nazaroglu, H., Yildiz, T. Bayrak, A.H., Senturk, S. Ates, G. *et al*. (2010). MDCT Findings of Denim-Sandblasting-Induced Silicosis: a cross-sectional study. *Environmental Health*, **9**, 17.

Paoliello, M.M.B. and De Capitani, E.M. (2007). Occupational and environmental human lead exposure in Brazil. *Environmental Research*, **103**, 288–297.

Paugam and Zhou. (2007). In D. Gallie (ed.) *Employment regimes and the quality of work*, New York: Oxford University Press.

Parent-Thirion, A., Fernández Macías, E., Hurley, J. and Vermeylen, G. (2007). *European Foundation for the Improvement of Living and Working Conditions. Fourth European Working Conditions Survey*. Dublin: European Foundation.

Parkes, K.R., Carnell, S. and Farmer, E. (2005). *Musculoskeletal disorders, mental health and the work environment. Health and Safety Executive Research Report 316*. Available at: http://www.hse.gov.uk/research/rrpdf/rr316.pdf (accessed 6 July 2011).

Pärnänen, A., Sutela, H. and Mahler, S. (2008). *Combining family and full-time work. Report for the European Foundation for the Improvement of Living and Working Conditions 2007*. Dublin: European Foundation.

Parsons, T. (1951 [1991]). *The Social System*. London, Routledge.

Passchier-Vermeer, W. and Passchier, W.F. (2000). Noise Exposure and Public Health. *Environmental Health Perspectives*, **108**, 123–131.

Paterniti, S., Niedhammer, I., Lang, T. and Consoli, S.M. (2002). Psychosocial factors at work, personality traits and depressive symptoms. Longitudinal results from the GAZEL Study. *British Journal of Psychiatry*, **181**, 111–117.

Pattinson, K. and Peace, D. (2010). *No Redemption*. London: Flambard Press.

Peck. J. (1996). *Work-place: Social regulation of labour markets*. London: Routledge.

Pelucchi, C., Pira, E., Piolatto, G., Coggiola, M., Carta, P. and La Vecchia, C. (2006). Occupational silica exposure and lung cancer risk: a review of epidemiological studies 1996–2005. *Annals of Oncology*, **17**, 1039–1050.

Persson Waye, K., Rylander, R., Benton, S. and Leventhall, H.G. (1997). Effects on performance and work quality due to low frequency ventilation noise. *Journal of Sound and Vibration*, **205**, 467–474.

Persson Waye, K., Bengtsson, J., Rylander, R., Hucklebridge, F., Evans, P. and Clow, A. (2002). Low frequency noise enhances cortisol among noise sensitive subjects during work performance. *Life Sciences*, 70, 745–758.

Peterson, C. (1999). *Stress at Work: A Sociological Perspective*. New York: Baywood.

Pierson, C. (1991). *Beyond the Welfare State*. London: Polity.

Pierson, C. (1994). Continuity and Discontinuity in the Emergence of the Post-Fordist Welfare State. In: R. Burrows and B. Loader (eds.) *Towards a Post-Fordist Welfare State?* pp. 95–116, London: Routledge.

Pierson, C. (1998). Theory in British Social Policy. In: C. Pierson and N. Ellison (eds.) *Developments in British Social Policy*, pp. 17–30, London: Macmillan.

Pierson, P. (1994). *Dismantling the Welfare State: Reagan, Thatcher and the Politics of Retrenchment*. Cambridge: Cambridge University Press.

Piggott, L. and Grover, L. (2009). Retrenching Incapacity Benefit: Employment Support Allowance and Paid Work. *Social Policy and Society*, 8, 159–170.

Pikhart, H., Bobak, M., Pajak, A., Malyutina, S., Kubinova, R., Topor, R. *et al.* (2004). Psychosocial factors at work and depression in three countries of Central and Eastern Europe. *Social Science & Medicine*, 58, 1475–1482.

Pilcher, J., Lambert, B. and Huffcutt, A. (2000). Differential effects of permanent and rotating shifts on self-report sleep length: a meta-analytic review. *Sleep*, 23, 155–63.

Piven, F. and Cloward, R. (1971[1993]). *Regulating the Poor: the Functions of Public Welfare*. New York: Vintage Books.

Plaisier, I., de Bruijn, J.G.M., de Graaf, R., ten Have, M. Beekman, A.T.F. and Penninx, B.W.J.H. (2007). The contribution of working conditions and social support to the onset of depressive and anxiety disorders among male and female employees. *Social Science & Medicine*, 64, 401–410.

Platt, S. (1986). Parasuicide and unemployment. *British Journal of Psychiatry*, 149, 401–405.

Police, R., Zhao, Y., Russell, M. and Foster, T. (2009). A systematic review of the burden, epidemiology, costs and treatment of chronic low back pain. *The Journal of Pain*, 10, S5.

Pope, D. and Bambra, C. (2005). Has the disability discrimination act closed the employment gap? *Disability and Rehabilitation*, 27, 1261–1266.

Pope, M., Magnusson, M., Lundström, R, Hulshof, C, Verbeek, J. (2002). Guidelines for Whole Body Vibration Health Surveillance. *Journal of Sound and Vibration*, 253, 131–167.

Popham, F. and Bambra, C. (2010). Evidence from the 2001 English Census on the contribution of employment status to the social gradient in self-rated health. *Journal of Epidemiology and Community Health*, 64, 277–280.

Poulantzas, N. (1975). *Classes in Contemporary Capitalism*. London: New Left Books.

Poverty site. (2010). *Key facts on poverty*. Available at: http://www.poverty.org.uk/ summary/key%20facts.shtml (accessed 6 July 2011).

Prasad, L.R. and Nazareth, B. (2000). Contamination of allotment soil with lead: managing potential risks to health. *Journal of Public Health Medicine*, 22, 525–530.

Punnett, L. and Wegman, D.H. (2004). Work-related musculoskeletal disorders: the epidemiologic evidence and the debate. *Journal of Electromyography and Kinesiology*, 14, 13–23.

Punnett, L., Prüss-Ustün, A., Nelson, D.I., Fingerhut, M.A., Leigh, J. Tak, S.W. *et al.* (2005). Estimating the global burden of low back pain attributable to combined occupational exposures. *American Journal of Industrial Medicine*, **48**, 459–469.

Putnam, R. (2000). *Bowling Alone: The Collapse and Revival of American Community*. New York: Simon and Schuster.

Quinlan, M., Mayhew, C. and Bohle, P. (2001). The Global Expansion of Precarious Employment, Work Disorganisation, and Consequences for Occupational Health: a Review of Recent Research. *International Journal of Health Services*, **31**, 335–414.

Rajaratnam, S. and Arendt, J. (2001). Health in a 24-h society. *Lancet*, **358**, 999–1005.

Rantakeisu, U., Starrin, B. and Hagquist, C. (1997). Unemployment, shame and ill health—an exploratory study. *Scandinavian Journal of Social Welfare*, **5**, 13–23.

Rees, D. and Murray, J. (2007). Silica, silicosis and tuberculosis. *International Journal of Tuberculosis and Lung Disease*, **11**, 474–484.

Rhodes, M. (1997). The Welfare State: internal challenges, external constraints, in M. Rhodes and A. Vincent (ed.) *Developments in Western European politics*; pp. 57–74, London: Macmillan.

Richmond, R., Wodak, A., Bourne, S. and Heather, N. (1998). Screening for unhealthy lifestyle factors in the workplace. *Australian and New Zealand Journal of Public Health*, **22**, 324–331.

Ritakallio, V.M. and Fritzell, J. (2004). *Societal Shifts and Changed Patterns of Poverty*. Luxembourg Income Study Working Paper Series.

Ritchie, H., Casebourne, J. and Rick, J. (2005). *Understanding workless people and communities: A literature review. Department for Work and Pensions Research Report No 255*. Leeds: Corporate Document Services.

Ritchie, J., Ward, K. and Duldig, W. (1993). *GPs and IVB. A qualitative study of the role of general practitioners in the award of Invalidity benefit*. London: Her Majesty's Stationery Office.

Riva, M., Bambra, C., Easton, S. and Curtis, S.E. (2011). Hard times or Good times? Inequalities in the health effects of economic change. *International Journal of Public Health*, **56**, 3–5.

Rivara, F.P. and Thompson, D.C. (2000). Prevention of falls in the construction industry: evidence for program effectiveness. *American Journal of Preventive Medicine*, **18**, 23–26.

Roberts, S., Heaver, C., Hill, K., Rennison, J., Staffors, B., Howat, N. *et al.* (2004). *Disability in the workplace: Employers' and service providers responses to the Disability Discrimination Act in 2003 and preparations for the 2004 changes*. London: DWP.

Robinson, P. (1998). Beyond Workfare: Active Labour Market Policies. *IDS Bulletin*, **29**, 86–93.

Robinson, P. (2000). Active Labour Market Policies: A Case of Evidence Based Policy Making. *Oxford Review of Economic Policy*, **16**, 1.

Rodriguez, E. (2001). Keeping the unemployed healthy: the effect of means-tested and entitlement benefits in Britain, Germany and the United States. *American Journal of Public Health*, **91**, 1403–1411.

Ronen, S. and Primps, S. (1981). The Compressed Working Week as organisational change: Behavioral and attitudinal outcomes. *Academy of Management Review*, **6**, 61–74.

Rose, G. (1992). *The Strategy of Preventive Medicine*, Oxford, Oxford University Press.

Rosengren, A., Hawken, S., Ôunpuu, S., Sliwa, K., Zubaid, M., Almahmeed, W.A. *et al.*, for the INTERHEART investigators. (2004). Association of psychosocial risk factors with risk of acute myocardial infarction in 11,119 cases and 13,648 controls from 52 countries (the INTERHEART study): case-control study. *Lancet*, 364, 953–962.

Ross, M.H. and Murray, J. (2004). Occupational respiratory disease in mining. *Occupational Medicine*, 54, 304–310.

Rossignol, A.M., Morse, E.P., Summers, V. and Pagnotto, L.D. (1987). Video display terminal use and reported health symptoms among Massachusetts clerical workers. *Journal of Occupational Medicine*, 29, 112–118.

Rosskam, E. (2009). Measuring the protection of workers' health: a national work security index, in P. Schnall, M. Dobson, E. Rosskam (ed.) *Unhealthy Work: Causes, Consequences, Cures*, New York: Baywood.

Roulstone, A. (2000). Disability, Dependency and the New Deal for Disabled People. *Disability & Society*, 15, 427–444.

Roulstone, A. and Barnes, C. (ed.) (2005). *Working Futures: disabled people, policy and social inclusion*. Bristol: Policy Press.

Roulstone, A. and Warren, J. (2006). Applying a barriers approach to monitoring disabled people's employment: implications for the Disability Discrimination. *Disability and Society*, 21, 115–131.

Rudas, N., Tondo, L., Musio, A. and Masia, M. (1991). Unemployment and depression: results of a psychometric evaluation. *Minerva Psichiatr*, 32, 205–209.

Ruhm, C.J. (1995). Economic conditions and alcohol problems. *Journal of Health Economics*, 14, 583–603

Ruhm, C.J. (2000). Are recessions good for your health? *Quarterly Journal of Economics*, 617–650.

Ruhm, C.J. and Black, W.E. (2002). Does drinking really decrease in bad times? *Journal of Health Economics*, 21, 659–678.

Ruhm, C.J. (2003). Good times make you sick. *Journal of Health Economics*, 22, 637–658.

Ruhm, C.J. (2004). Healthy living in hard times. *Journal of Health Economics*, 24, 341–363.

Russell, M. (2002). What disability civil rights cannot do: employment and political economy. *Disability & Society*, 17, 117–135.

Saarela, J. (2006). Replacement rates and labour market behaviour. *Socio-Economic Planning Sciences*, 40, 187–211.

Sainsbury, R. and Davidson, J. (2006). *Routes onto Incapacity Benefits: Findings from Qualitative Research. Department for Work and Pensions Research Report 350.* Leeds: Corporate Document Services.

Salavecz, G., Chandola, T., Pikhart, H., Dragano, N., Siegrist, J., Jöckel, K-H. *et al.* (2010). Work stress and health in Western European and post-Communist countries: an East-West comparison study. *Journal of Epidemiology and Community Health*, 64, 57–62.

Sanders, A., Slade, G., John, M., Steele, J., Suominen-Taipale, A., Lahti, S. *et al.* (2009). A cross-national comparison of income gradients in oral health quality of life in four welfare states: application of the Korpi and Palme typology. *Journal of Epidemiology and Community Health*, **63**, 569–574.

Sandover, J. (1998). The fatigue approach to vibration and health: is it a practical and viable way of predicting the effects on people? *Journal of Sound and Vibration*, **215**, 699–721.

Schins, R.P.F. and Borm, P.J.A. (1999). Mechanisms and Mediators in Coal Dust Induced Toxicity: A Review. *The Annals of Occupational Hygiene*, **43**, 7–33.

Schnall, P., Dobson, M., Rosskam, E. and Landsbergis, P. (2009). Curing unhealthy work. In: P. Schnall, M. Dobson and E. Rosskam (eds.) *Unhealthy Work: Causes, Consequences, Cures*, New York: Baywood.

Schumpeter, A. (1942 [2010]). *Capitalism, Socialism and Democracy*. London, Routledge.

Schuring, M., Burdorf, A., Kunst, A.E., and Mackenbach, J. (2007). The effect of ill health on entering and maintaining paid employment: evidence in European countries. *Journal of Epidemiology and Community Health*, **61**, 597–604.

Schuring, M., Burdorf, A., Voorham, A., der Weduwe, K. and Mackenbach, J. (2009). Effectiveness of a health promotion programme for long-term unemployed subjects with health problems: a randomised controlled trial. *Journal of Epidemiology and Community Health*, **63**, 893–899.

Scott-Samuel, A. (1984). Unemployment and health. *Lancet*, **324**, 1465.

Seedhouse, D. (1986). *Health: the foundations for achievement.* Chichester: Wiley.

Sekine, M., Chandola, T., Martikainen, P., Marmot, M. and Kagamimori, S. (2009). Socioeconomic inequalities in physical and mental functioning of British, Finnish, and Japanese civil servants: Role of job demand, control, and work hours. *Social Science & Medicine*, **69**, 1417–1425.

Seixas, N.S, Goldman, B., Sheppard, L., Neitzel, R., Norton, S. and Kujawa, S.G (2005). Prospective noise induced changes to hearing among construction industry apprentices. *Occupational and Environmental Medicine*, **62**, 309–317.

Serrano Pascual, A. and Magnusson, L. (2007). *Reshaping welfare states and activation regimes in Europe.* Brussels: Peter Lang.

Shakespeare, T. (2006). *Disability, Rights and Wrongs.* London: Routledge.

Shaw, C., Blakely, T., Atkinson, J. and Crampton, P. (2005). Do social and economic reforms change socioeconomic inequalities in child mortality? A case study: New Zealand 1981–1999. *Journal of Epidemiology and Community Health*, **59**, 638–644.

Shiels, C., Gabbay, M.B. and Ford, F.M. (2004). Patient factors associated with duration of certified sickness absence and transition to long-term incapacity. *British Journal of General Practice*, **54**, 86–91.

Showler, B. and Sinfield, A. (ed.) (1981). *The Workless State: a study of unemployment.* Oxford: M Robertson.

Siegrist, J. (1996). Adverse health effects of high effort–low reward conditions at work. *Journal of Occupational Health Psychology*, **1**, 27–43.

Siegrist, J. (2005). Social reciprocity and health: New scientific evidence and policy implications. *Psychoneuroendocrinology*, **30**, 1033–1038.

Siegrist, J. and Marmot, M. (2004). Health inequalities and the psychosocial environment–two scientific challenges. *Social Science & Medicine*, **58**, 1463–1473.

Siegrist, J. and Theorell, T. (2006). Socio-economic position and health: the role of work and employment. In: J. Siegrist and M. Marmot (eds.) *Social Inequalities in Health: New Evidence and Policy Implications*; pp. 73–1007, Oxford: Oxford University Press.

Siegrist, J., Siegrist, K. and Weber, I. (1986). Sociological concepts in the etiology of chronic disease: the case of ischemic heart disease. *Social Science & Medicine*, **22**, 247–53.

Siegrist, J., Starke, D., Chandola, T., Godin, I., Marmot, M., Niedhammer, I. *et al.* (2004). The measurement of effort–reward imbalance at work:European comparisons. *Social Science & Medicine*, **58**, 1483–1499.

Siegrist, J., Benach, J., McKnight, A., Goldblatt, P. and Muntaner, C. (2009). *Employment arrangements, work conditions and health inequalities. Report on new evidence on health inequality reduction, produced by Task Group 2 for the Strategic Review of Health Inequalities post 2010.* Available at: http://www.ucl.ac.uk/gheg/marmotreview/ consultation/Employment_arrangements__work_conditions_report.

Sinfield, A. (1993). *Poverty, inequality and justice. New Waverley Papers*, **6**, Edinburgh.

Skalická, V., Lenthe, F., Bambra, C., Krokstad, S. and Mackenbach J. (2009). Material, psychosocial, behavioural and biomedical factors in the explanation of socio-economic inequalities in mortality: evidence from the HUNT study. *International Journal of Epidemiology*, **38**, 1272–1284.

Smith, B.E. (1983). Black lung: The social production of disease. In: V. Navarro and D. Berman (eds.) *Health and Work under Capitalism: an international perspective*, New York: Baywood.

Smith, K.E., Bambra, C. and Joyce, K. (2010). 'Striking out': Shifting labour markets, welfare to work policy and the renegotiation of gender performances. *Critical Social Policy*, **30**, 74–98.

Smith, R. (1985). 'Bitterness, shame, emptiness, waste': an introduction to unemployment and health, *British Medical Journal*, **291**, 1024–1027.

Smith, R. (1993). Workfare and health: There just might be benefits, *British Medical Journal*, **306**, 474.

Smith, L., Folkard, S., Tucker, P. and MacDonald, I. (1998). Work shift duration: a review comparing eight hour and 12 hour shift systems. *Occupational and Environmental Medicine*, **55**, 217–229.

Solantaus, T., Leinonen, J. and Punamaki, R. (2004). Children's mental health in times of economic recession: Replication and extension of the family economic stress model in Finland. *Developmental Psychology*, **40**, 412–429.

Stafford, M and McCarthy, M. (2006). Neighbourhoods, housing and health. In: M. Marmot and R. Wilkinson (eds.) *The Social Determinants of Health*; pp. 297–317, Oxford: Oxford University Press.

Stanistreet, D., Bambra, C. and Scott-Samuel, A. (2005). Is patriarchy the source of male mortality? *Journal of Epidemiology and Community Health*, **59**, 873–876.

Stansfeld, S.A. (2002). *Work, personality and mental health. British Journal of Psychiatry*, **181**, 96–98.

Stansfeld, S.A., North, F.M., White, I. and Marmot, M.G. (1995). Work characteristics and psychiatric disorder in civil servants in London. *Journal of Epidemiology and Community Health*, **49**, 48–53.

Stansfeld, S.A., Rael, E., Head, J., Head, J. and Marmot, M.G. (1997). Social support and psychiatric sickness absence: a prospective study of British civil servants. *Psychological Medicine*, **27**, 35–48.

Stansfeld, S.A., Fuhrer, R., Shipley, M.J. and Marmot, M.G. (1999).Work characteristics predict psychiatric disorder: prospective results from the Whitehall II study. *Occupational Environmental Medicine*, **56**, 302–307.

Stansfeld, S.A., Head, J., Fuhrer, R., Wardle, J., Cattell, V. (2003). Social inequalities in depressive symptoms and physical functioning in the Whitehall II study: Exploring a common cause explanation. *Journal of Epidemiology and Community Health*, **57**, 361–367.

Starfield, B. (2007). Pathways to influence on equity in health. *Social Science & Medicine*, **64**, 1355–1362.

Stanton, R. (2009). Who will take responsibility for obesity in Australia? *Public Health*, **123**, 280–282.

Stirbu, I. (2008). *Inequalities in health: does health care matter?* Rotterdam: Erasmus MC.

Steenland, K., Loomis, D., Shy, C. and Simonsen, N. (1996). Review of occupational lung carcinogens. *American Journal of Industrial Medicine*, **29**, 474–490.

Stone, D.A. (1978). The deserving sick: income-maintenance policy towards the ill and disabled. *Policy Sciences*, **10**, 133–155.

Stone, D.A. (1986). *The disabled state.* Basingstoke: Macmillan.

Strazdins, L. and Bammer, G. (2004). Women, work and musculoskeletal health. *Social Science & Medicine*, **58**, 997–1005.

Stuckler, D., Basu, S., Suhrcke, M., Coutts, A. and McKee, M. (2009). The public health effect of economic crises and alternative policy responses in Europe: an empirical analysis. *Lancet*, **374**, 315–323.

Swerdlow, A. (2003). *Shift work and breast cancer: a critical review of the epidemiological literature. Health and Safety Executive Research Report 132.* London: HSE.

Szasz, T.S. (1964). *The myth of mental illness: foundations of a theory of personal conflict.* New York: Harper & Row.

Tapia Granados, J.A. (2005a). Increasing mortality during the expansions of the US economy, 1900–1996. *International Journal of Epidemiology*, **34**, 1194–1202.

Tapia Granados, J.A. (2005b). Recessions and Mortality in Spain, 1980–1997. *European Journal of Population*, **21**, 393–422.

Tapia Granados, J.A. and Ionides, E.L. (2008). The reversal of the relation between economic growth and health progress: Sweden in the 19th and 20th centuries. *Journal of Health Economics*, **27**, 544–563.

Taylor, A., Angerer, J., Arnaud, J., Claeys, F., Kristiansen, J., Mazarrasa, O. *et al.* (2007). Differences in national legislation for the implementation of lead regulations included in the European directive for the protection of the health and safety of workers with occupational exposure to chemical agents (98/24/EC). *International Archives of Environmental Health*, **80**, 254–264.

Tausig, M.F.R. (1999). Recession and Wellbeing. *Journal of Health and Social Behavior*, **40**, 1–16.

Theodore, N. (2007). New Labour at work: long-term unemployment and the geography of opportunity. *Cambridge Journal of Economics*, **31**, 927–939.

Thomas, L.T. and Ganster, D.C. (1995). Impact of family-supportive work variables on work-family conflict and strain: A control perspective. *Journal of Applied Psychology*, **80**, 6–15.

Thomson, W.M., Williams, S.M., Dennison, P.J. and Peacock, D.W. (2002). Were NZ's structural changes to the welfare state in the early 1990s associated with a measurable increase in oral health inequalities among children? *The Australian and New Zealand Journal of Public Health*, **26**, 525–530.

Thornton, C., Livermore, G., Stapleton, D., Kregel, J., Silva, T., O'Day, B. *et al.* (2004). *Evaluation of the Ticket to Work program: Initial evaluation report.* Washington: Mathematica Policy Research Inc.

Thornton, I. Rautiu, R. and Brush, S. (2001). *Lead: the facts.* London: Imperial College Consultants Ltd.

Timio, M. and Gentili, S. (1976). Adrenosympathetic overactivity under conditions of work stress. *British Journal of Preventative & Social Medicine*, **30**, 262–265.

Timio, M., Gentili, S. and Pede, S. (1979). Free adrenaliane and noradrenaline excretion related to occupational stress. *British Heart Journal*, **42**, 471–474.

Torfing, J. (1999a). Towards a Schumpeterian Workfare Post-National Regime: Path shaping and Path Dependency in Danish Welfare State Reform. *Economy and Society*, **28**, 369–402.

Torfing, J. (1999b). Workfare with Welfare: Recent Reforms of the Danish Welfare State. *Journal of European Social Policy*, **9**, 5–28.

Tsutsumi, A., Kayaba, K., Theorell, T. and Siegrist, J. (2001). Association between job stress and depression among Japanese employees threatened by job loss in comparison between two complementary job-stress models. *Scandinavian Journal of Work, Environment & Health*, **27**, 146–153.

Tudor-Hart, J. (1971). The inverse care law. *Lancet*, **297**, 405–412.

Turok, I. and Edge, N. (1999). *The Jobs Gap in Britain's Cities: Employment Loss and Labour Market Consequence.* Bristol: Policy Press.

United Nations. (1948). *Universal Declaration of Human Rights.* New York: UN.

Vahtera, J., Pentti, J. and Kivimaki, M. (2004). Sickness absence as a predictor of mortality among male and female employees. *Journal of Epidemiology and Community Health*, **58**, 321–326.

Valkonen, T. (1989). Adult mortality and level of education: a comparison of six countries. In: A.J. Fox (ed.) *Health inequalities in European countries*, pp. 142–160, Aldershot: Gower.

Valkonen, T., Martikainen, P., Jalovaara, M., Koskinen, S., Martelin, T. and Makela, P. (2000). Changes in socioeconomic inequalities in mortality during an economic boom and recession among middle-aged men and women in Finland. *European Journal of Public Health*, **10**, 274–280.

van der Doef, M. and Maes, S. (1999). The Job Demand-Control (-Support) Model and psychological well-being: a review of 20 years of empirical research. *Work and Stress*, **13**, 87–114.

van der Klink, J.J.L., Blonk, R.W.B., Schene, A.H. and van Dijk, F.J.H. (2001). The benefits of interventions for work-related stress. *American Journal of Public Health*, **91**, 270–276.

van der Molen, H.F., Sluiter, J.K., Hulshof, C.T., Vink, P. and Frings-Dresen, M.H. (2005). Effectiveness of measures and implementation strategies in reducing physical work demands due to manual handling at work. *Scandinavian Journal of Work, Environment & Health*, **31**, S75–S87.

van der Wel, K.A. (2011). Long-term effects of poor health on employment: the significance of life stage and educational level. *Sociology of Health and Illness*. Doi: 10.1111/j.1467-9566.2011.01346.x.

van der Wel, K.A., Dahl, E. and Thielens, K. (2010). Health inequalities and employment in European welfare states: A multi-level analysis of EU-SILC. *13th Biennial Congress of the European Society for Health and Medical Sociology*, 26–28 August 2010 Ghent, Belgium.

van der Windt, D., Pope, D., de Winter, A., Macfarlane, G., Bouter, L. and Silman, A. (2000). Occupational risk factors for shoulder pain: a systematic review. *Occupational and Environmental Medicine*, **57**, 433–442.

van Doorslaer, E., Wagstaff, A. and Bleichrodt, H. (1997). Income related inequalities in health: some international comparisons, *Journal of Health Economics*, **16**, 93–112.

van Kempen, E., Kruize, H., Boshuizen, H., Ameling, C., Staatsen, B. and de Hollander, A. (2002). The association between noise exposure and blood pressure and ischemic heart disease: a meta-analysis. *Environmental Health Perspectives*, **110**, 307–317.

van Orschot, W. (2006). Making the difference in social Europe: deservingness perceptions among citizens of European welfare states. *Journal of European Social Policy*, **16**, 23–42.

van Rossum, C.T.M., Shipley, M.J., van de Mheen, H., Grobbee, D.E. and Marmot, M.G. (2000). Employment grade differences in cause specific mortality. A 25 year follow up of civil servants from the first Whitehall study. *Journal of Epidemiology and Community Health*, **54**, 178–184.

van Vegchel, N., de Jonge, J., Bosma, H. and Schaufeli, W. (2005). Reviewing the effort-reward imbalance model: drawing up the balance of 45 empirical studies. *Social Science & Medicine*, **60**, 1117–1131.

Viebrock, E. and Clasen, J. (2009). Flexicurity and welfare reform: a review. *Socio-economic review*, **7**, 305–331.

Vinet, A., Vézina, M., Brison, C. and Bernard, P. (1989). Piecework, repetitive work and medicine use in the clothing industry. *Social Science & Medicine*, **28**, 1283–1288.

Virtanen, P., Vahtera, J., Kivimäki, M., Pentti, J. and Ferrie, J. (2002). Employment security and health. *Journal of Epidemiology and Community Health*, **56**, 569–574.

Waddell, G. and Burton, A. (2006). *Is work good for your health and wellbeing?* London: TSO.

Waddell, G., Burton, A.K. and Kendall, N. (2008). *Vocational Rehabilitation What works, for whom, and when?* London: TSO.

Wagner, G.R. (1996). *Screening and surveillance of workers exposed to mineral dust.* Copenhagen: World Health Organisation.

Wagstaff, A. (1985). Time series analysis of the relationship between unemployment and mortality: A survey of econometric critiques and replications of Brenner's studies. *Social Science & Medicine*, **21**, 985–996.

Walker, A. and Wong, C. (2005). *East Asian welfare regimes in transition: From Confucianism to globalisation.* Bristol: Policy Press.

Wanless, D. (2004). *Securing good health for the whole population: final report [The Wanless Report].* London: HM Treasury.

Warr, P. (1990). Decision latitude, job demands, and employee well-being. *Work & Stress*, **4**, 285–294.

Warr, P. (1994). A conceptual framework for the study of work and mental health. *Work & stress*, **8**, 84–97.

Warren, J. (2005). Disabled people, the state and employment: historical lessons and welfare policy, In: A. Roulstone and C. Barnes (eds.) *Working Futures: Disabled people, policy and social inclusion*, Bristol: Policy Press.

Watkins, S. (1986). Economic adversity and health: Policy implications, in F. Eskin (ed.) *Unemployment: a challenge to public health*, pp. 1–72, University of Manchester: Manchester Centre for Professional Development.

Webster, D. (2000). The geographical concentration of labour market disadvantage. *Oxford Review of Economic Policy*, **16**, 114–28.

Webster, D. (2006). Welfare Reform: Facing up to the Geography of Worklessness. *Local Economy*, **21**, 107–16.

Webster, J. (1996). *Shaping women's work: gender, employment and information technology.* London: Longman.

Wedderburn, Z. and Rankin, D. (2001). *An intervention using a self-help guide to improve the coping behavior of nightshift workers and its evaluation. Health and Safety Executive Report 365.* London: Health and Safety Executive Books.

Welshman, J. (2006). The concept of the unemployable. *The Economic History Review*, **59**, 570–606.

Westerlund, H., Bergström, A. and Theorell, T. (2004). Changes in anabolic and catabolic activity among women taking part in an alternative labour market programme. *Integrative Physiological and Behavioural Science*, **39**, 3–15.

Whitehead, M. (2007). A typology of actions to tackle social inequalities in health. *Journal of Epidemiology and Community Health*, **61**, 473–478.

Whitehead, M., Clayton, S., Holland, P., Drever, F., Barr, B., Gosling, R. *et al.* (2009). *Helping Chronically Ill or Disabled people into work: what can we learn from international comparative analyses?* York, Public Health Research Consortium. Available at: http://www.york.ac.uk/phrc/PHRC%20C2–06_%20RFR.pdf (accessed 6 July 2011).

Wikström, B, Kjellberg, A. and Landström, U. (1994). Health effects of long-term occupational exposure to whole-body vibration: A review. *International Journal of Industrial Ergonomics*, **14**, 273–292.

Wilding, P. (1982). *Professional Power and Social welfare* London: Routledge.

Wilkinson, R. and Pickett, K. (2009). *The Spirit Level: Why more equal societies almost always do better.* London: Penguin.

Williams, G.H. (2010). Understanding Incapacity. In: G. Scambler and S. Scambler (eds.) *New Directions in the Sociology of Chronic and Disabling Conditions: Assaults on the Lifeworld*, London: Palgrave.

Wilson, J. (2002). The impact of shift patterns on healthcare professionals. *Journal of Nursing Management*, **10**, 211–219.

Woods, L.M., Rachet, B., Riga, M., Stone, N., Shah, A. and Coleman, M.P. (2005). Geographical variation in life expectancy at birth in England and Wales is largely explained by deprivation. *Journal of Epidemiology and Community Health*, **59**, 115–120.

World Health Organization. (1983). *Indoor Air Pollutants: Exposure and Health Effects, World Health Organization EURO Reports and Studies 78.* Copenhagen: World Health Organization.

World Health Organization. (1989). *Occupational Exposure Limit for Asbestos. Reports prepared by a WHO Meeting.* United Kingdom: Oxford.

World Health Organization. (2000a). *Asbestos.* Available at: http://www.euro.who.int/document/aiq/6_2_asbestos.pdf (accessed 22 April 2010).

World Health Organization. (2000b). *Silicosis. Fact Sheet No. 238.* Available at: http://www.who.int/mediacentre/factsheets/fs238/en/print.html (accessed 6 July 2011).

World Health Organization. (2000c). *Elimination of Silicosis.* Available at: http://www.who.int/occupational_health/publications/newsletter/gohnet12e.pdf (accessed 6 July 2011).

World Health Organization. (2003). *Preventing musculoskeletal disorders in the workplace.* Available at: http://www.who.int/occupational_health/publications/en/oehmsd3.pdf (accessed 6 July 2011).

World Health Organization. (2006). *Elimination of asbestos related diseases.* Available at: http://www.who.int/mediacentre/factsheets/fs343/en/(accessed 6 July 2011).

World Health Organization. (2008). *Closing the gap in a generation: Health equity through action on the social determinants of health. Report of the WHO Commission on the Social Determinants of Health.* Geneva: World Health Organization.

Wright, E.O. (1985). *Classes.* London: Verso.

Wright Mills, C. (1959). *The Sociological Imagination.* New York: Oxford University Press.

Yamada, Y., Kameda, M., Noborisaka, Y., Suzuki, H., Honda, M. and Yamada, S. (2001). Excessive fatigue and weight gain among cleanroom workers after changing from an 8-hour to a 12-hour shift. *Scandinavian Journal of Work, Environment & Health,* **27**, 318–326.

Yassi, A. 1997. Repetitive strain injuries. *Lancet,* **349**, 943–947.

Yelin, E. and Katx, P. (1994). Making work more central to work disability policy. *Milbank Quarterly,* **72**, 593–619.

Yngwe, M., Fritzell, J., Lundberg, O., Diderichsen, F. and Burstrom, B. (2003). Exploring relative deprivation: Is social comparison a mechanism in the relation between income and health? *Social Science & Medicine,* **57**, 1463–1473.

Zambon, A., Boyce, W., Cois, E., Currie, C., Lemma, P., Dalmasso, P. *et al.* (2006). Do welfare regimes mediate the effect of socioeconomic position on health in adolescence? A cross-national comparison in Europe, North America, and Israel. *International Journal of Health Services,* **36**, 309–329.

Zola, I.K. (1972). Medicine as an Institution of Social Control. *Sociological Review,* **20**, 487–504.

Index